D1369526

Sweet!

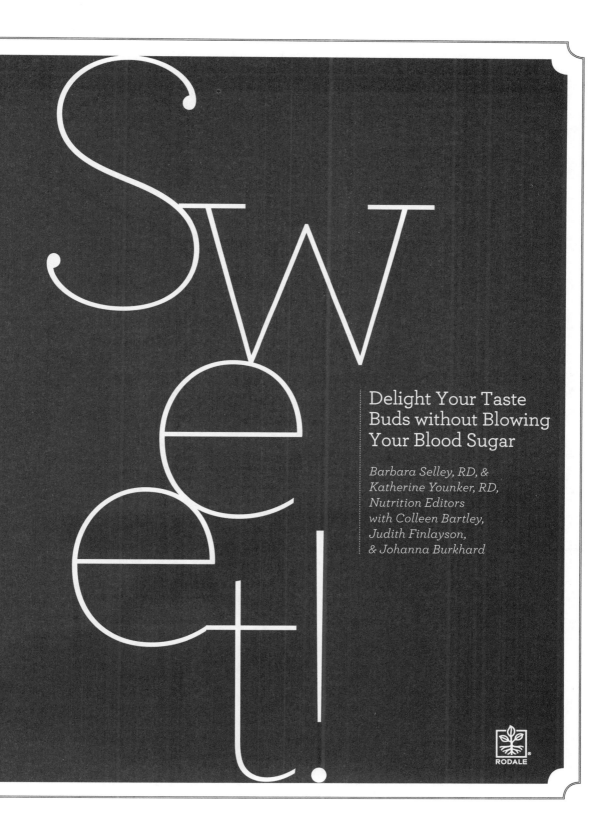

Sweet!

Delight Your Taste Buds without Blowing Your Blood Sugar

Barbara Selley, RD, &
Katherine Younker, RD,
Nutrition Editors
with Colleen Bartley,
Judith Finlayson,
& Johanna Burkhard

RODALE

Printed in the United States of America
Rodale Inc. makes every effort to use acid-free ∞, recycled paper ♲.

Contributing Authors: See page 321.
Cover Photograph: Chocolate Chip Refrigerator Cookies, page 98
Photography: Anna Williams
Food Styling: Stephana Bottom
Prop Styling: Pam Morris
Book Design: Barbara Reyes

Portions of this book were previously published by Robert Rose Inc., as *150 Best Diabetes Desserts* © 2008, *America's Complete Diabetes Cookbook* © 2005, and *America's Best Cookbook for Kids with Diabetes* © 2005. The Rodale Inc. direct mail edition is published in 2009 under license from Robert Rose Inc.

Library of Congress Cataloging-in-Publication Data
Sweet! : delight your taste buds without blowing your blood sugar / Barbara Selley and Katherine Younker, nutrition editors ; with Colleen Bartley, Judith Finlayson, and Johanna Burkhard.
    p. cm.
   Includes index.
   "Portions of this book were previously published by Robert Rose Inc., as *150 Best Diabetes Desserts* , 2008, America's Complete Diabetes Cookbook, 2005, and America's Best Cookbook for Kids with Diabetes, 2005."
   ISBN-13: 978-1-60529-546-6 hardcover
   ISBN-10: 1-60529-546-9 hardcover
   1. Diabetes—Diet therapy—Recipes.   2. Desserts.   I. Selley, Barbara.   II. Younker, Katherine E.
RC662.S94 2008
641.5'6314—dc22   2009029067

  4 6 8 10 9 7 5 3   direct mail hardcover

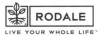

RODALE
LIVE YOUR WHOLE LIFE™

We inspire and enable people to improve their lives and the world around them
For more of our products visit **rodalestore.com** or call 800-848-4735

CONTENTS

	vii	*Preface*
	ix	*Introduction*
1	*xviii*	MUFFINS, LOAVES & SCONES
2	50	BISCOTTI & SHORTBREAD
3	74	COOKIES
4	120	BARS, SQUARES & BROWNIES
5	154	CAKES, COFFEE CAKES & CHEESECAKES
6	208	PIES, TARTS, CRISPS & FRUIT DESSERTS
7	254	FROZEN, CHILLED & OTHER DESSERTS
8	294	BEVERAGES
	307	*Appendix A*
	309	*Appendix B*
	311	*Appendix C*
	313	*Appendix D*
	321	*Contributing Authors*
	324	*Index*

PREFACE

THIS BOOK OF DESSERTS is for people living with diabetes and for their families and friends—just about everyone! By 2010, 10% of the population of the United States will have diabetes, so it's a rare person who does not know someone with this disease.

The recipes selected for this book were not specifically developed for people with diabetes, but we have chosen ones that can be worked into most people's meal plans. Many are special-occasion treats, but some can fit in more often.

To help you include these recipes in your meals, each recipe has a breakdown of calories, carbohydrate, fiber and other nutrients, plus Exchanges.

In the introduction, we look at

- *who has diabetes and why we should be concerned about this disease*

- *food and nutrition recommendations for people with diabetes; and*

- *"budgeting" for desserts: how you can plan to include these treats in your meals*

In addition, in case you don't wind up with the same number of cookies as we did when preparing a recipe, we've included a "cookie calculator" that allows you to recalculate a single serving.

Following the introduction, you will find a table of nutrient values for common dessert ingredients, as well as two worksheets, so you can figure out how to fit your own favorite desserts into your meal plan. Would you like to know the Exchanges for a serving of a favorite recipe? The worksheet on pages 314–315 will help you estimate them.

Throughout the book, you will find "Dietitian's Notes" and other tips that will help you prepare and enjoy these recipes.

Whether you're controlling your diabetes through diet and exercise alone, or with the help of oral medication or insulin, I hope you'll enjoy the recipes in this book and find the tips helpful.

INTRODUCTION

WHO HAS DIABETES?

In North America, 6% to 7% of adults and children have diabetes—about 20.8 million people in the United States alone. These numbers have been rising steadily in recent years and are expected to reach 10% of the population by 2010.

Diabetes is a serious disease. Untreated, it can lead to a wide variety of sometimes life-threatening complications involving the heart, eyes, kidneys, nerves and circulatory system.

Diabetes affects us all. Because about one person in fifteen lives with diabetes, almost every one of us knows someone with the disease.

What Is Diabetes?

There are three main types of diabetes. In each instance, blood glucose (sugar) levels are above normal because glucose isn't being metabolized properly.

In **type 1 diabetes**, the pancreas doesn't produce insulin, the hormone that allows the body to use glucose as fuel. About 10% of people with diabetes have type 1.

Type 2 diabetes is much more prevalent, affecting about 90% of people with diabetes. It occurs when the pancreas doesn't produce enough insulin, or when the body can't use it properly, a condition known as insulin resistance. Until recently, type 2 diabetes was generally considered to be a condition of middle age, but it is now occurring in children and teenagers.

Gestational diabetes occurs in about 4% of pregnant women. While it usually disappears after the baby is born, both mother and child are at higher risk for type 2 diabetes later in life.

In addition to those with known diabetes, millions of North Americans of all ages have **pre-diabetes:** their blood glucose readings are above normal, but the levels are not high enough for a diagnosis of diabetes. Although pre-diabetes can develop into type 2 diabetes, we now know it's possible to prevent this progression.

WHAT CAN I DO TO MANAGE DIABETES?

Whether you have type 1, type 2, gestational diabetes or pre-diabetes, the cornerstones of effective management are:

- *managing food intake to control blood glucose;*

- *increasing physical activity;*

- *achieving or maintaining a healthy weight;*

- *quitting smoking if you smoke;*

- *monitoring blood glucose;*

- *taking medication (insulin or oral medications) if required; and*

- *maintaining blood pressure in a healthy range.*

It is important to become educated about diabetes and to work closely with your physician, dietitian, pharmacist and other members of your health care team.

For more information about diabetes, its prevention and its treatment, contact the American Diabetes Association at www.diabetes.org.

Healthy eating recommendations for people with diabetes are very similar to those for the general population. It is not necessary to prepare separate meals or buy special foods.

WHAT SHOULD PEOPLE WITH DIABETES EAT?

Healthy eating recommendations for people with diabetes are very similar to those for the general population. It is not necessary to prepare separate meals or buy special foods.

The following information is general. Your dietitian's recommendations for you may differ in some ways.

Carbohydrate

Carbohydrate, found mainly in grain products, vegetables, legumes (dried peas and beans), fruits and milk products, should make up about 50% of your calories. You may be surprised to learn that it's okay for people with diabetes to eat sugar (see "What's the Story on Sugar?" on the next page).

FIBER

To achieve the recommended fiber intake of at least 25 grams per day, carbohydrate food choices should consist mainly of whole-grain products, legumes and vegetables.

What's the Story on Sugar?

There are many types of sugar. Milk, vegetables and fruit all contain naturally occurring sugars (such as lactose, glucose or fructose). Added sugars (such as granulated sugar, honey or corn syrup) are those added either when food products are manufactured or when we ourselves prepare our meals and beverages.

People with diabetes used to be advised to avoid added sugars altogether, but we now know this ban was unnecessary. Added sugars, however, do not provide vitamins and minerals, so they should replace only small amounts of carbohydrate from other sources. The key word is "replace." Any food eaten in excess of what you need will lead to weight gain and/or elevated blood glucose levels.

Current guidelines allow for people with diabetes to consume up to 10% of total daily energy (calories) as added sugars from all sources, including processed foods. If you eat 2,000 calories per day, this translates to 50 grams of carbohydrate—a little over 3 Other Carbohydrate Exchanges (equivalent to 10 teaspoons of sugar).

Remember that this 50 grams includes both sugar you can see (added to your coffee, for example) and hidden sugar in sweet foods.

Fat

Fat should make up no more than 30% of your calories. At 2,000 calories per day, this is equivalent to 66 grams. Remember, this includes fat from all sources: meat, fish, poultry, eggs, oils and spreads, nuts and seeds, and combination foods such as cookies and muffins.

- *Saturated and trans fats* together should make up no more than one-third of your total fat intake, or 22 grams if you consume 2,000 calories per day.

- *Polyunsaturated fat* should also not exceed one-third of total fat intake, and should include omega-3 fatty acids from fatty fish and plant sources, such as canola oil, walnuts and flaxseed.

- *Monounsaturated fat,* which is the remaining fat you consume, at least one-third of daily fat intake and preferably more, should come from monounsaturated sources, such as canola oil, olive oil and soybean oil. Often called "healthy fats," monounsaturated fats can help lower your LDL ("bad") cholesterol.

Protein

Protein from all sources (meat, fish, poultry, eggs, dairy products, legumes and other plant sources) should make up about 15% to 20% of

There's a wide range of sugar substitutes and artificial sweeteners in the marketplace. On page 307 you can read about the various types and how they are used.

your calories. At an intake of 2,000 calories per day, this is equivalent to 75 to 100 grams of protein. Higher amounts are not recommended, as they may increase the work that the kidneys need to do.

Sodium

People with diabetes should follow the recommendation for the general population: a maximum of 2,300 mg of sodium per day, about the amount in 1 teaspoon of salt. This does not mean, however, that you can add a teaspoon of salt to your meals. Up to 75% of the sodium we consume comes from processed foods, not from what we use in cooking or add at the table. So, when you're grocery shopping, it's important to check sodium on the Nutrition Facts panels.

WHAT NUTRIENTS ARE FOUND IN DESSERT INGREDIENTS?

Carbohydrate

Carbohydrate in desserts comes mainly from flour, other grain products (such as rolled oats) and sugar. Fresh and dried fruit, chocolate and cocoa supply smaller amounts. Here are some other points to keep in mind:

- *Whole-grain ingredients, such as whole wheat flour, rolled oats, oat bran and wheat bran, help boost fiber intake.*

- *All sources of sugar—whether granulated sugar, brown sugar, fructose, honey, maple syrup, corn syrup, jam or jelly—contain about 5 grams of carbohydrate per teaspoon.*

Fats and Oils

Soft non-hydrogenated margarine and canola oil are the best choices. They are low in saturated fat, contain no trans fats and supply omega-3 fatty acids. However, some recipes do not work well with these preferred fats, calling instead for butter or shortening. Although they contain the same total amount of fat as margarine or oil, butter and shortening are high in saturated fat. Shortening also contains trans fats (the levels are lower than in the past, but still significant).

If you have a choice in a recipe between margarine and butter, for example, always choose to use soft non-hydrogenated margarine. If a recipe specifies butter or shortening, it likely will not work if another fat is substituted. In that case, limit your enjoyment of the recipe to special occasions.

Sodium

Sodium is a nutrient you don't usually need to be concerned about in desserts:

- *While salt, baking powder and baking soda are all high in sodium, only a very small amount is present in a single serving.*

- *Margarine and butter containing salt add sodium, but again the amount is small.*

- *Flour, sugar and fruit contain almost no sodium; milk and eggs have moderate amounts.*

HOW CAN I "BUDGET" TO ALLOW ROOM IN MY MEAL PLAN FOR DESSERTS?

We plan ahead when we budget money. It's just as important to plan ahead when you will be having a dessert or another food item you don't routinely eat. The key is to find a food or foods somewhere else in your meal that contains the same Exchanges as the dessert you intend to eat, and then replace it with your dessert.

Example: You usually have a slice of bread with a teaspoon of margarine at dinner. Tonight, you would like to have a cookie that contains 1 Other Carbohydrate Exchange and 1 Fat Exchange. If you replace the bread and margarine with the cookie, you'll be on budget.

Why Is It Important to Measure Ingredients Accurately?

Careful measuring is important for a couple of reasons. First, the Exchange values accompanying the recipes are based on the ingredient quantities and number of servings stated. If you change ingredient amounts (or the portion size), the stated Exchanges will no longer be correct. Second, baked goods may not rise properly if ingredient amounts are inaccurate.

For information about measuring cups and other measures, see page 173. You will find tips for accurate measuring on page 53.

We plan ahead when we budget money. It's just as important to plan ahead when you will be having a dessert or another food item you don't routinely eat.

WHAT DO I NEED TO KNOW ABOUT SERVING SIZE?

We live in an age of ever-larger dinner plates and food packages, and therefore serving sizes. It's often hard to remember what the more reasonable sizes of 10 or 20 years ago looked like. As a result, some of the portions specified in this book may be smaller than you're accustomed to. Be sure to use the serving sizes in the recipes and don't be led astray by the "portion distortion" that is all around us.

Cookie Calculator to the Rescue

If you're making a batch of cookies and you end up with a different number of cookies than stated in the yield on the recipe, the ingredient quantities in each cookie will be different, as will the number of cookies that correspond to the Exchanges listed with the recipe.

Using Oatmeal Raisin Cookies (page 78) as an example, here's how you can calculate a new portion size:

You can also use the cookie calculator for other baked goods, such as muffins. For example, you might get 16 muffins from a recipe that says it makes 12. Using the calculator, you can work out how many of your muffins match the nutrients and Exchanges on the recipe.

Example: Raisin Oatmeal Cookies

This recipe has a yield of 18 cookies, and the serving size is 2 cookies. But when you prepare the recipe, you make smaller cookies and end up with 24. In the table below, enter

- *in box t1, the stated yield of the recipe (18 cookies);*

- *in box s1, the number of cookies per serving according to the recipe (2); and*

- *in box t2, your yield from the recipe (24 cookies).*

COOKIES	TOTAL	PER SERVING
Recipe	t1	s1
You get	t2	s2

So, once the table is filled in, it will look like this:

COOKIES	TOTAL	PER SERVING
Recipe	18	2
You get	24	?

To calculate the number of cookies in your serving (box s2), you will:

• *Divide the total number of cookies you get (t2) by the total number in the recipe (t1), then*

• *Multiply by the number of cookies per serving stated in the recipe (s1).*

That is, s2 = (t2 ÷ t1) x s1. In this example, s2 = (24 ÷ 18) x 2 = 2.7 cookies per serving (for box s2).

COOKIE CALCULATOR ROUNDING TABLE

IF YOUR RESULT FOR S2 EQUALS	ROUND TO
0.3–0.7	½
0.8–1.2	1
1.3–1.7	1½
1.8–2.2	2
2.3–2.7	2½
2.8–3.2	3
3.3–3.7	3½
3.8–4.2	4

If your result includes a fraction, round it off to the nearest half-cookie, referring to the ranges in the table below. In this example, the result is 2.7, which should be rounded to 2½. So, if you get 24 cookies from the Raisin Oatmeal Cookie recipe, your serving size will be 2½ cookies.

Here's an example for you to work out:

Example: Best-Ever Chocolate Cookies
You've made a batch of Best-Ever Chocolate Cookies (page 96). The recipe says it makes 42 cookies and the serving size is 2 cookies. But you only have 30 cookies (yours are larger). What should your serving size be?

COOKIES	TOTAL	PER SERVING
Recipe	t1	s1
You get	t2	s2

ROUNDED ....

Answer: (30 ÷ 42) × 2 = 1.4, rounded according to the table above = 1½ If your batch makes only 30 cookies, a serving will be 1½ cookies (not 2).

MORE INFORMATION
For additional information about meal planning and all aspects of managing diabetes, contact:

The American Diabetes Association
www.diabetes.org

Sweet!

MUFFINS, LOAVES & SCONES

1 | Streusel Apple Muffins
2 | Orange Cranberry Muffins
3 | Banana Date Muffins
4 | Big-Batch Banana Blueberry Muffins
5 | Banana Applesauce Muffins
6 | Blueberry Banana Muffins
7 | Kiwi Raspberry Muffins
8 | Blueberry Lemon Cornmeal Muffins
9 | Chocolate Chip Oatmeal Muffins
10 | Banana Chocolate Chunk Muffins
11 | Peanut Butter Surprise Muffins
12 | Wheat Muffins
13 | Honey Whole Wheat Muffins
14 | Blueberry Wheat Germ Muffins
15 | Perfect Bran Muffins
16 | Yogurt Bran Muffins
17 | Triple B Health Muffins
18 | Pumpkin Bran Muffins
20 | Oat Berry Muffins
21 | Pineapple Carrot Date Muffins
22 | Sunrise Zucchini Muffins
24 | Sweet Potato Muffins

26 | Pumpkin Molasses Raisin Loaf
27 | Carrot Pineapple Zucchini Loaf
28 | Lemon Poppy Seed Loaf
29 | Banana Nut Raisin Loaf
30 | Carrot, Apple & Coconut Loaf
31 | Rhubarb Orange Bread
32 | Poppy Seed Oat Bread
33 | Blueberry Banana Oat Bread
34 | Blueberry Buckwheat Bread
35 | Peach Blueberry Quick Bread
36 | Low-Fat Applesauce Raisin Bread
37 | Fruited Barm Brack
38 | Oat Bran Banana Bread
40 | Banana Walnut Bread
41 | Irish Whole Wheat Soda Bread
42 | Pumpkin Spice Nut Bread
44 | Pumpkin Raisin Scones
46 | Scottish Oatmeal Scones
47 | Whole Wheat Poppy Biscuits
48 | Lemon Yogurt Biscuits
49 | Pecan Cinnamon Biscuits

STREUSEL APPLE MUFFINS

Preheat oven to 375°F
12-cup muffin tin, sprayed with nonstick vegetable spray

½	cup packed brown sugar
½	cup applesauce
¼	cup vegetable oil
1	egg
1	tsp vanilla
1	cup all-purpose flour
1	tsp baking soda
1	tsp baking powder
½	tsp ground cinnamon
¾	cup diced peeled apple

Topping

2	tbsp packed brown sugar
2	tsp all-purpose flour
½	tsp ground cinnamon
1	tsp margarine

1. In a large bowl, combine brown sugar, applesauce, oil, egg and vanilla until well mixed. Combine flour, baking soda, baking powder and cinnamon; stir into bowl just until incorporated. Stir in apple. Pour into muffin cups, filling two-thirds full.

2. *Topping:* In a small bowl, combine sugar, flour and cinnamon; cut in margarine until crumbly. Sprinkle evenly over muffins. Bake for 20 minutes or until tops are firm to the touch.

Makes 12 muffins (1 muffin per serving)

DIETITIAN'S NOTE *These muffins can also be made without the topping. It contributes about 2 g carbohydrate per muffin.*

TIPS When using margarine, choose a soft (non-hydrogenated) version to limit consumption of trans fats.

Prepare up to a day before. Freeze for up to 6 weeks.

NUTRIENTS PER SERVING

Calories	142
Carbohydrate	22 g
Fiber	1 g
Protein	2 g
Fat, total	5 g
Fat, saturated	1 g
Cholesterol	16 mg
Sodium	141 mg

EXCHANGES PER SERVING

½	Starch
1	Other Carbohydrates
1	Fat

ORANGE CRANBERRY MUFFINS

VARIATION Substitute fresh or frozen blueberries for the cranberries.

NUTRIENTS PER SERVING

Calories	179
Carbohydrate	27 g
Fiber	1 g
Protein	3 g
Fat, total	7 g
Fat, saturated	1 g
Cholesterol	16 mg
Sodium	159 mg

EXCHANGES PER SERVING

1 Starch
1 Other Carbohydrates
1½ Fat

Preheat oven to 375°F
12-cup muffin tin, lightly greased or lined with paper cups

1½	cups all-purpose flour
¾	cup granulated sugar
2	tsp baking powder
1	tsp baking soda
1	whole navel orange
1	egg
½	cup milk
⅓	cup vegetable oil
1	cup fresh cranberries (or frozen, thawed)

1. In a large bowl, combine flour, sugar, baking powder and baking soda.

2. Cut off ends of orange, then cut into quarters, without peeling. Remove seeds.

3. In food processor, process orange (including peel), egg, milk and oil until blended. Stir into flour mixture until just moistened. Gently stir in cranberries.

4. Divide batter evenly among prepared muffin cups.

5. Bake in preheated oven for 20 to 25 minutes or until tops are firm to the touch and a tester inserted in the center of a muffin comes out clean. Let cool in tin for 10 minutes, then remove to a wire rack to cool completely.

Makes 12 muffins (1 muffin per serving)

BANANA DATE MUFFINS

Preheat oven to 375°F
12-cup muffin tin, sprayed with vegetable spray

¼	cup margarine or butter
1	medium banana, mashed
¾	cup granulated sugar
1	egg
1	tsp vanilla
¾	cup all-purpose flour
½	cup bran or corn flakes cereal
1	tsp baking powder
1	tsp baking soda
¾	cup chopped pitted dates
½	cup 2% yogurt

1. In a large bowl, combine margarine, banana, sugar, egg and vanilla; mix well.

2. In a bowl, combine flour, bran flakes cereal, baking powder and baking soda. Add to wet ingredients and stir just until mixed. Stir in dates and yogurt, just until smooth.

3. Spoon batter into prepared muffin cups and bake for 15 to 20 minutes or until tops are firm and tester inserted in center comes out clean.

Makes 12 muffins (1 muffin per serving)

TIPS These muffins will be fairly flat due to the weight of the dates.

When using margarine, choose a soft (non-hydrogenated) version.

Prepare up to a day ahead, or freeze for up to 3 weeks.

NUTRIENTS PER SERVING

Calories	168
Carbohydrate	31 g
Fiber	2 g
Protein	2 g
Fat, total	5 g
Fat, saturated	1 g
Cholesterol	16 mg
Sodium	202 mg

EXCHANGES PER SERVING

½	Starch
½	Fruit
1	Other Carbohydrates
1	Fat

BIG-BATCH BANANA BLUEBERRY MUFFINS

TIP Ripe bananas can be thrown in the freezer, peel and all. To use, just thaw, peel and mash. You can also mash bananas and freeze in amounts appropriate for your recipes.

NUTRIENTS PER SERVING

Calories	185
Carbohydrate	25 g
Fiber	5 g
Protein	4 g
Fat, total	8 g
Fat, saturated	1 g
Cholesterol	16 mg
Sodium	141 mg

EXCHANGES PER SERVING

½ Starch
½ Fruit
½ Other Carbohydrate
1½ Fat

Preheat oven to 350°F
Three 12-cup muffin tins, lightly greased or lined with paper cups

3	cups whole wheat flour
3	cups ground flaxseed
2	cups lightly packed brown sugar
1	tbsp baking powder
1	tbsp baking soda
	Pinch salt
3	eggs
3	ripe bananas, mashed (about 1⅓ cups)
1	jar (4½ oz) baby food prunes or unsweetened applesauce
⅔	cup vegetable oil
2	tsp vanilla
2	cups fresh or frozen blueberries

1. In a large bowl, combine flour, flaxseed, brown sugar, baking powder, baking soda and salt.

2. In a very large bowl, combine eggs, bananas, prunes, oil and vanilla. Fold in flour mixture until just combined. Fold in blueberries.

3. Divide batter evenly among prepared muffin cups.

4. Bake in preheated oven for 20 minutes, rotating pans halfway through, or until tops are firm to the touch and a tester inserted in the center of a muffin comes out clean. Let cool in tin for 10 minutes, then remove to a wire rack to cool completely.

Makes 36 muffins (1 muffin per serving)

BANANA APPLESAUCE MUFFINS

Preheat oven to 400°F
12-cup muffin tin, lightly greased or lined with paper cups

2	cups whole wheat flour
1	tbsp baking powder
1	tsp baking soda
½	tsp salt
3	ripe bananas, mashed (about 1⅓ cups)
1	egg, lightly beaten
1	cup unsweetened applesauce
½	cup granulated sugar
¼	cup vegetable oil

1. In a large bowl, combine flour, baking powder, baking soda and salt.

2. In a medium bowl, combine bananas, egg, applesauce, sugar and oil. Stir into flour mixture until just combined.

3. Divide batter evenly among prepared muffin cups.

4. Bake in preheated oven for 15 to 20 minutes or until tops are firm to the touch and a tester inserted in the center of a muffin comes out clean. Let cool in tin for 10 minutes, then remove to a wire rack to cool completely.

Makes 12 muffins (1 muffin per serving)

NUTRIENTS PER SERVING

Calories	183
Carbohydrate	32 g
Fiber	3 g
Protein	4 g
Fat, total	5 g
Fat, saturated	1 g
Cholesterol	16 mg
Sodium	274 mg

EXCHANGES PER SERVING

1	Starch
½	Fruit
½	Other Carbohydrate
1	Fat

BLUEBERRY BANANA MUFFINS

TIPS A 9- by 5-inch loaf pan can also be used; bake for 30 to 40 minutes, or until tester comes out dry.

Use the ripest bananas possible for the best flavor.

Bake up to a day before or freeze for up to 6 weeks.

NUTRIENTS PER SERVING

Calories	151
Carbohydrate	21 g
Fiber	1 g
Protein	2 g
Fat, total	7 g
Fat, saturated	1 g
Sodium	138 mg
Cholesterol	18 mg

EXCHANGES PER SERVING

½ Starch
⅔ Other Carbohydrate
⅓ Fruit
1½ Fat

Preheat oven to 375°F
12-cup muffin tin, sprayed with vegetable spray

¾	cup pureed bananas (about 1½ bananas)
½	cup granulated sugar
⅓	cup vegetable oil
1	egg
1	tsp vanilla
1	cup all-purpose flour
1	tsp baking powder
1	tsp baking soda
¼	cup 2% yogurt or light sour cream
½	cup blueberries

1. In a large bowl, beat together bananas, sugar, oil, egg and vanilla until well mixed.

2. Combine flour, baking powder and baking soda; stir into bowl. Stir in yogurt; fold in blueberries.

3. Pour batter into prepared cups. Bake for about 20 minutes, or until tops are firm to the touch.

Makes 12 muffins (1 per serving)

KIWI RASPBERRY MUFFINS

Preheat oven to 400°F
12-cup muffin tin, sprayed with vegetable spray or lined with paper liners

1	cup all-purpose flour
1	cup whole wheat flour
1	tbsp baking powder
½	tsp baking soda
2	peeled chopped kiwis
½	cup fresh or frozen raspberries
1	egg, lightly beaten
¼	cup margarine or butter
⅓	cup skim milk
1	tsp vanilla

1. In a large bowl, mix together flour, whole wheat flour, baking powder and baking soda. Add kiwis and raspberries, mixing well. Make a well in the center.

2. In another bowl, combine egg, margarine, milk and vanilla. Add to the flour mixture, stirring only until moistened and blended. Do not overmix.

3. Spoon batter into prepared muffin cups, filling them to the top. Bake in preheated oven for 15 to 20 minutes.

Makes 12 muffins (1 per serving)

NUTRIENTS PER SERVING

Calories	126
Carbohydrate	19 g
Fiber	2 g
Protein	3 g
Fat, total	5 g
Fat, saturated	1 g
Sodium	219 mg
Cholesterol	18 mg

EXCHANGES PER SERVING

1 Starch
1 Fat

BLUEBERRY LEMON CORNMEAL MUFFINS

TIPS Fresh blueberries are always best tasting, especially the small ones available in the summer. If using frozen berries, do not thaw. The flour will help to absorb the excess liquid.

When using margarine, choose a soft (non-hydrogenated) version.

Bake up to 2 days in advance; store in an airtight container.

Freeze for up to 6 weeks.

NUTRIENTS PER SERVING

Calories	156
Carbohydrate	27 g
Fiber	1 g
Protein	2 g
Fat, total	5 g
Fat, saturated	1 g
Cholesterol	16 mg
Sodium	201 mg

EXCHANGES PER SERVING

1 Starch
½ Fruit
½ Other Carbohydrate
1 Fat

Preheat oven to 350°F
12-cup muffin tin, sprayed with vegetable spray

¾	cup granulated sugar
¼	cup margarine or butter
1	egg
3	tbsp freshly squeezed lemon juice
3	tbsp 2% milk
1½	tsp grated lemon zest
1	cup all-purpose flour
¼	cup cornmeal
1½	tsp baking powder
1	tsp baking soda
½	cup 2% plain yogurt
1¼	cups fresh or frozen blueberries
2	tsp all-purpose flour

1. In a large bowl, with an electric mixer, beat sugar, margarine, egg, lemon juice, milk and lemon zest until well blended. (Mixture may appear curdled.)

2. In another bowl, stir together flour, cornmeal, baking powder and baking soda. Add flour mixture and yogurt alternately to creamed mixture. In a small bowl, toss blueberries with flour; fold into batter. Divide batter among prepared muffin cups.

3. Bake for 20 to 25 minutes or until tops are firm to the touch and tester inserted in center comes out clean.

Makes 12 muffins (1 muffin per serving)

CHOCOLATE CHIP OATMEAL MUFFINS

Preheat oven to 400°F
12-cup muffin tin, lightly greased or lined with paper cups

1½	cups whole wheat flour
½	cup quick-cooking rolled oats
¼	cup ground flaxseed
¼	cup granulated sugar
2	tsp baking powder
½	tsp baking soda
½	tsp salt
1	egg
1	cup milk
¼	cup vegetable oil
¼	cup liquid honey
½	cup semisweet chocolate chips or dried fruit
½	cup chopped nuts (optional)

1. In a large bowl, combine flour, oats, flaxseed, sugar, baking powder, baking soda and salt.

2. In a small bowl, whisk together egg, milk, oil and honey. Stir into flour mixture until just combined. Fold in chocolate chips and nuts (if using).

3. Divide batter evenly among prepared muffin cups.

4. Bake in preheated oven for 15 to 20 minutes or until tops are firm to the touch and a tester inserted in the center of a muffin comes out clean. Let cool in tin for 10 minutes, then remove to a wire rack to cool completely.

Makes 12 muffins (1 muffin per serving)

DIETITIAN'S NOTE *Substituting dried fruit, such as raisins, for the chocolate chips will trim ½ Fat Exchange from the total. Adding the optional chopped nuts will add ½ Fat Exchange.*

TIPS If you choose to use dried fruit instead of chocolate chips, you will add nutrition and fiber to your muffins.

For the nuts, try walnuts, pecans or almonds.

NUTRIENTS PER SERVING

Calories	239
Carbohydrate	31 g
Fiber	4 g
Protein	5 g
Fat, total	12 g
Fat, saturated	2 g
Cholesterol	17 mg
Sodium	211 mg

EXCHANGES PER SERVING

1	Starch
1	Other Carbohydrates
2½	Fat

BANANA CHOCOLATE CHUNK MUFFINS

TIP Store tightly wrapped in foil in the freezer for up to 2 weeks.

NUTRIENTS PER SERVING

Calories	163
Carbohydrate	25 g
Fiber	1 g
Protein	3 g
Fat, total	7 g
Fat, saturated	4 g
Cholesterol	26 mg
Sodium	159 mg

EXCHANGES PER SERVING

½ Starch

1 Other Carbohydrates

1½ Fat

Preheat oven to 375°F, with rack in lower middle position
Stand mixer
12-cup muffin tin, lightly greased

2 ¼	cups unbleached all-purpose flour
2	tsp baking powder
1	tsp salt
½	tsp baking soda
1	cup granulated sugar
½	cup unsalted butter, softened
2	eggs
1	cup mashed bananas (about 2)
1	cup lower-fat plain yogurt
1	cup semisweet chocolate chunks or chips

1. In a medium bowl, combine flour, baking powder, salt and baking soda. Set aside.

2. Place sugar and butter in the mixer bowl. Attach the flat beater and mixer bowl to the mixer. Set to Speed 4 and beat until light and fluffy, about 2 minutes. Stop mixer to scrape down bowl. Set to Speed 4 and add eggs, one at a time, beating well after each addition. Add bananas and beat well. Stop mixer to scrape down bowl. Set to Speed 2 and beat in flour mixture alternately with yogurt, making 3 additions of dry and 2 of wet. Stop mixer to scrape down bowl. Set to Stir and mix in chocolate chunks.

3. Divide batter evenly among muffin cups. Bake in middle of pre-heated oven for 25 to 30 minutes or until golden brown. Let cool in tin on a wire rack for 5 minutes. Serve warm or let cool completely.

Makes 12 muffins (½ muffin per serving)

DIETITIAN'S NOTE *Half of this muffin is a serving, so share this one with a friend.*

PEANUT BUTTER SURPRISE MUFFINS

Preheat oven to 400°F
12-cup muffin tin, sprayed with vegetable spray or lined with paper liners

1	cup all-purpose flour
½	tsp salt
1	tbsp baking powder
1	tbsp granulated sugar
½	cup cornmeal
1	cup milk
1	egg, beaten
¼	cup peanut butter
1	tbsp margarine or butter, melted

1. In a large bowl, combine flour, salt, baking powder and sugar. Stir in cornmeal, mixing to blend well.

2. In a small bowl, combine milk, egg, peanut butter and melted margarine. Add to dry ingredients, stirring until moistened and blended.

3. Spoon batter into prepared muffin cups, filling them three-quarters full. Bake in preheated oven for about 20 minutes.

Makes 12 muffins (1 per serving)

NUTRIENTS PER SERVING

Calories	120
Carbohydrate	16 g
Fiber	1 g
Protein	4 g
Fat, total	5 g
Fat, saturated	1 g
Sodium	170 mg
Cholesterol	18 mg

EXCHANGES PER SERVING

1 Starch

1 Fat

WHEAT MUFFINS

TIP To keep muffins at their best, freeze any which won't be used in the first 2 days after baking. Thaw at room temperature or reheat in the microwave.

NUTRIENTS PER SERVING

Calories	138
Carbohydrate	21 g
Fiber	2 g
Protein	4 g
Fat, total	5 g
Fat, saturated	1 g
Sodium	290 mg
Cholesterol	18 mg

EXCHANGES PER SERVING

1	Starch
⅓	Other Carbohydrate
1	Fat

Preheat oven to 400°F
12-cup muffin tin, sprayed with vegetable spray or lined with paper liners

1	cup all-purpose flour
1	cup unsifted whole wheat flour
2	tsp baking powder
1	tsp salt
1	egg, lightly beaten
¼	cup molasses
1	cup milk
¼	cup margarine or butter, melted

1. In a large bowl, combine flour, whole wheat flour, baking powder and salt. Make a well in the center.

2. In another bowl, combine egg, molasses, milk and margarine. Add to flour mixture, stirring just until blended. Do not overmix.

3. Spoon batter into prepared muffin cups, filling them three-quarters full. Bake in preheated oven for 25 minutes, or until golden brown.

Makes 12 muffins (1 per serving)

HONEY WHOLE WHEAT MUFFINS

Preheat oven to 400°F
12-cup muffin tin, sprayed with vegetable spray or lined with paper liners

1	cup	whole wheat flour
1	cup	all-purpose flour
1	tbsp	baking powder
1	tsp	salt
1		egg
1	cup	milk
¼	cup	vegetable oil
¼	cup	honey

1. In a large bowl, combine whole wheat flour, flour, baking powder and salt. Make a well in the center.

2. In another bowl, whisk together egg, milk and oil. Add the honey. Stir into flour mixture until moist and lumpy.

3. Spoon batter into prepared muffin cups, dividing evenly. Bake in preheated oven for 20 to 25 minutes, or until lightly browned.

Makes 12 muffins (1 per serving)

NUTRIENTS PER SERVING

Calories	152
Carbohydrate	23 g
Fiber	2 g
Protein	4 g
Fat, total	5 g
Fat, saturated	1 g
Sodium	260 mg
Cholesterol	18 mg

EXCHANGES PER SERVING

1	Starch
⅓	Other Carbohydrate
1	Fat

BLUEBERRY WHEAT GERM MUFFINS

NUTRIENTS PER SERVING

Calories	161
Carbohydrate	24 g
Fiber	1 g
Protein	4 g
Fat, total	6 g
Fat, saturated	1 g
Sodium	170 mg
Cholesterol	18 mg

EXCHANGES PER SERVING

1 Starch

⅓ Fruit

⅓ Other Carbohydrate

1 Fat

Preheat oven to 400°F
12-cup muffin tin, sprayed with vegetable spray or lined with paper liners

1¾	cups all-purpose flour
⅓	cup wheat germ
⅓	cup granulated sugar
1	tbsp baking powder
1½	tsp grated lemon zest
½	tsp salt
1	egg
1	cup milk
¼	cup vegetable oil
1	cup fresh blueberries or frozen blueberries, drained

1. In a large bowl, combine flour, wheat germ, sugar, baking powder, zest and salt. Make a well in the center.

2. In another bowl, whisk together egg, milk and oil. Add to dry ingredients, stirring just until moist and blended. Fold in berries.

3. Spoon batter into prepared muffin cups, filling them three-quarters full. Bake in preheated oven for 20 to 25 minutes.

Makes 12 muffins (1 per serving)

PERFECT BRAN MUFFINS

Preheat oven to 375°F
12-cup muffin tin, lined with paper liners or sprayed with nonstick spray

1½	cups natural wheat bran
1	cup buttermilk
1	cup all-purpose flour
1	tsp baking soda
1	tsp baking powder
½	tsp salt
1	egg
⅔	cup packed brown sugar
⅓	cup vegetable oil
½	tsp vanilla
½	cup golden raisins

1. In a bowl, soak bran with buttermilk for 5 minutes. In another bowl, whisk together flour, baking soda, baking powder and salt. Set aside.

2. In a large bowl, whisk together egg, brown sugar, oil and vanilla until blended. Add bran mixture and flour mixture and, using a wooden spoon, stir just until moistened. Fold in raisins.

3. Scoop into prepared muffin tin. Bake in preheated oven until firm to the touch and a toothpick inserted into center comes out clean, 15 to 20 minutes. Let cool in tin on a wire rack for 10 minutes. Transfer to rack to cool completely.

Makes 12 muffins (1 muffin per serving)

TIP Make sure you wait the entire 5 minutes for the bran to soak up the buttermilk or the muffins will be very dry.

VARIATION You can add ½ cup of fresh berries such as raspberries, blackberries, etc. with the raisins.

NUTRIENTS PER SERVING

Calories	188
Carbohydrate	31 g
Fiber	4 g
Protein	4 g
Fat, total	7 g
Fat, saturated	1 g
Cholesterol	16 mg
Sodium	257 mg

EXCHANGES PER SERVING

1	Starch
1	Other Carbohydrates
1½	Fat

YOGURT BRAN MUFFINS

NUTRIENTS PER SERVING

Calories	142
Carbohydrate	24 g
Fiber	2 g
Protein	3 g
Fat, total	5 g
Fat, saturated	1 g
Cholesterol	16 mg
Sodium	173 mg

EXCHANGES PER SERVING

½ Starch
1 Other Carbohydrates
1 Fat

Preheat oven to 375°F
12-cup muffin tin, sprayed with nonstick vegetable spray

½	cup brown sugar
¼	cup margarine
1	tbsp molasses
1	egg
1	tsp vanilla
¾	cup wheat bran cereal
½	cup all-purpose flour
⅓	cup whole wheat flour
¾	tsp baking powder
½	tsp baking soda
½	cup 2% yogurt
⅓	cup raisins

1. In a large bowl, combine brown sugar, margarine, molasses, egg and vanilla until well blended.

2. Combine cereal, all-purpose and whole wheat flours, baking powder and baking soda; add to bowl alternately with yogurt. Stir in raisins. Pour into prepared muffin cups; bake for 15 to 18 minutes or until tops are firm to the touch.

Makes 12 muffins (1 muffin per serving)

DIETITIAN'S NOTES *For added fiber, use whole wheat flour whenever you can. In most recipes, you can replace up to half the all-purpose flour with whole wheat without affecting the finished product.*

Because whole wheat flour contains the germ of the wheat, it can become rancid if kept for a long time. Buy it in small quantities and store in a cool place.

TRIPLE B HEALTH MUFFINS

Preheat oven to 400°F
12-cup muffin tin, lightly greased or lined with paper cups

1	cup whole wheat flour
1	cup natural wheat bran or oat bran
1	cup fresh or frozen blueberries
1	tsp baking soda
1	tsp baking powder
2	ripe bananas, mashed (about 1 cup)
1	egg, lightly beaten
½	cup granulated sugar
½	cup milk
¼	cup vegetable oil
1	tsp vanilla

1. In a medium bowl, combine flour, wheat bran, blueberries, baking soda and baking powder.

2. In a large bowl, combine bananas, egg, sugar, milk, oil and vanilla. Fold in flour mixture until just combined.

3. Divide batter evenly among prepared muffin cups, filling each two-thirds full.

4. Bake in preheated oven for 20 to 25 minutes or until tops are firm to the touch and a tester inserted in the center of a muffin comes out clean. Let cool in tin for 10 minutes, then remove to a wire rack to cool completely.

Makes 12 muffins (1 muffin per serving)

NUTRIENTS PER SERVING

Calories	153
Carbohydrate	25 g
Fiber	4 g
Protein	3 g
Fat, total	6 g
Fat, saturated	1 g
Cholesterol	16 mg
Sodium	139 mg

EXCHANGES PER SERVING

½	Starch
½	Fruit
½	Other Carbohydrate
1	Fat

PUMPKIN BRAN MUFFINS

TIPS If you don't have buttermilk for a baking recipe, sour milk is a great substitute. Simply add 1 tbsp lemon juice or vinegar to each cup of regular milk. Let stand for 10 minutes before using.

You can substitute 1 cup natural bran for the bran cereal.

The batter will keep in the refrigerator for up to 1 week, so there's no need to bake the muffins all at once.

If you don't have left-over cooked pumpkin, you can use canned pumpkin purée (not pie filling).

Two 12-cup muffin tins, lightly greased or lined with paper cups

2	cups bran cereal
1¼	cups all-purpose flour
1¼	cups whole wheat flour
1	cup raisins
½	cup sesame seeds
½	cup ground flaxseed
¼	cup wheat germ
2½	tsp baking soda
½	tsp salt
2	eggs, lightly beaten
2	cups buttermilk or sour milk
1½	cups lightly packed brown sugar
1	cup mashed cooked pumpkin
½	cup vegetable oil

1. In a large bowl, combine bran cereal, all-purpose flour, whole wheat flour, raisins, sesame seeds, flaxseed, wheat germ, baking soda and salt.

2. In a very large bowl, combine eggs, buttermilk, brown sugar, pumpkin and oil. Gradually fold in bran mixture until well combined. Bake immediately or cover and refrigerate for up to 1 week. Preheat oven to 400°F.

3. Scoop about ⅓ cup batter per muffin into prepared muffin cups.

4. Bake for 15 to 20 minutes or until tops are firm to the touch and a tester inserted in the center of a muffin comes out clean. Let cool in tins for 10 minutes, then remove to a wire rack to cool completely.

Makes 24 muffins (1 muffin per serving)

DIETITIAN'S NOTES *When purchasing canned pumpkin, read the label carefully and make sure you're not buying pumpkin pie filling by mistake. Canned pumpkin may also contain squash but has nothing else added to it. Pumpkin pie filling contains sugar, salt and other ingredients.*

We've seen a lot of "portion distortion" in muffins in recent years. It's not hard to find coffee-shop muffins that are three to four times the size of the ones in this book. When you make a muffin recipe (or any other recipe) from this book, take the opportunity to remember the size and the nutrients and Exchanges it contains. This will help you make better choices when you're eating away from home.

NUTRIENTS PER SERVING

Calories	216
Carbohydrate	34 g
Fiber	5 g
Protein	5 g
Fat, total	8 g
Fat, saturated	1 g
Cholesterol	16 mg
Sodium	262 mg

EXCHANGES PER SERVING

1 Starch
½ Fruit
1 Other Carbohydrates
1½ Fat

OAT BERRY MUFFINS

TIP If using frozen berries, keep them frozen until you are ready to add them to the batter to prevent the color from tinting the batter.

VARIATION You can use one type of berry, but I enjoy a multi-colored muffin you get by using a mixture of varieties.

NUTRIENTS PER SERVING

Calories	176
Carbohydrate	30 g
Fiber	2 g
Protein	3 g
Fat, total	5 g
Fat, saturated	3 g
Cholesterol	27 mg
Sodium	195 mg

EXCHANGES PER SERVING

1 Starch
1 Other Carbohydrates
1 Fat

Preheat oven to 400°F
12-cup muffin tin, lined with paper liners or sprayed with nonstick spray

1	cup all-purpose flour
1	cup old-fashioned rolled oats
1	tbsp baking powder
½	tsp salt
¼	cup unsalted butter, softened
¾	cup packed brown sugar
1	egg
1	cup buttermilk
1	cup mixed berries, frozen or fresh

1. In a bowl, whisk together flour, oats, baking powder and salt. Set aside.

2. In a mixer bowl fitted with paddle attachment, cream butter and brown sugar until fluffy, for 2 minutes. Beat in egg and buttermilk. Using a wooden spoon, stir in flour mixture just until moistened. Fold in berries.

3. Scoop into prepared muffin tin. Bake in preheated oven until light brown and a toothpick inserted into center comes out clean, 20 to 24 minutes. Let cool in tin on a wire rack for 10 minutes. Transfer to rack to cool completely.

Makes 12 muffins (1 muffin per serving)

PINEAPPLE CARROT DATE MUFFINS

Preheat oven to 375°F
12-cup muffin tin, sprayed with vegetable spray

¾	cup granulated sugar
⅓	cup vegetable oil
1	egg
1	tsp vanilla
½	cup grated carrots
½	cup canned pineapple, drained and crushed
⅓	cup finely chopped dates
⅓	cup light sour cream or 2% yogurt
1	cup all-purpose flour
⅔	cup rolled oats
1	tsp baking powder
1	tsp baking soda
1	tsp ground cinnamon
¼	tsp ground nutmeg

1. In a large bowl, combine sugar, oil, egg and vanilla; mix well.

2. Stir in carrots, pineapple, dates and sour cream.

3. In a bowl, combine flour, oats, baking powder, baking soda, cinnamon and nutmeg. Add to wet ingredients and mix just until combined. Spoon into prepared muffin cups and bake for 15 to 18 minutes or until tops are firm to the touch and tester inserted in center comes out clean.

Makes 12 muffins (1 muffin per serving)

DIETITIAN'S NOTE *For baking, always use plain, unflavored oats. Fifty grams of plain rolled oats of any type contains about 33 grams of total carbohydrate, including 5 grams of fiber. In 50 grams of flavored sweetened instant oats, however, you will find only 2 to 3 grams of fiber. This is because only two-thirds of the sweetened variety is actually oats—the rest is sugar.*

TIP Prepare up to a day ahead. Freeze for up to 6 weeks.

NUTRIENTS PER SERVING

Calories	195
Carbohydrate	30 g
Fiber	1 g
Protein	3 g
Fat, total	7 g
Fat, saturated	1 g
Cholesterol	16 mg
Sodium	143 mg

EXCHANGES PER SERVING

1	Starch
1	Other Carbohydrates
1½	Fat

SUNRISE ZUCCHINI MUFFINS

Preheat oven to 400°F, with rack in lower middle position
Stand mixer
12-cup muffin tin, greased and floured

2	cups unbleached all-purpose flour
1	cup shredded zucchini
½	cup whole wheat flour
½	cup raisins
½	cup granulated sugar
1	tbsp baking powder
1	tbsp grated orange zest
1	tsp baking soda
¾	tsp salt
½	tsp ground cinnamon
¼	tsp ground nutmeg
2	eggs, beaten
½	cup homogenized (whole) milk
⅓	cup vegetable oil
¼	cup freshly squeezed orange juice

1. Place all-purpose flour, zucchini, whole wheat flour, raisins, sugar, baking powder, orange zest, baking soda, salt, cinnamon and nutmeg in the mixer bowl. Attach the flat beater and mixer bowl to the mixer. Set to Stir and mix until combined.

2. In a small bowl, combine eggs, milk, oil and orange juice. Add to the mixer bowl and mix until just combined.

3. Divide batter evenly among muffin cups. Bake in middle of pre-heated oven for 10 minutes, then reduce temperature to 375°F and bake until golden, about 10 minutes. Remove muffins from tins and let cool on a wire rack. Serve warm or let cool completely.

Makes 12 muffins (1 muffin per serving)

DIETITIAN'S NOTES *Bleached and unbleached flour are inter-changeable in recipes. Vitamin E is destroyed by the bleaching process, but other nutrients are unaffected.*

Baking powder, baking soda and salt all contribute sodium to baked goods. If you reduce the salt in this recipe to ½ tsp, the sodium in each muffin will be lowered by 50 mg. It's not a good idea, however, to decrease the amount of baking powder or baking soda because the muffins won't rise properly. When you reduce the salt, you may want to increase the quantities of spices and other flavorings in this recipe, such as the orange zest, cinnamon and nutmeg.

NUTRIENTS PER SERVING

Calories	224
Carbohydrate	35 g
Fiber	2 g
Protein	5 g
Fat, total	8 g
Fat, saturated	1 g
Cholesterol	32 mg
Sodium	333 mg

EXCHANGES PER SERVING

1½ Starch
½ Fruit
½ Other Carbohydrate
1½ Fat

SWEET POTATO MUFFINS

TIP For the mixed dried fruit, try raisins, blueberries, cherries and cranberries.

Preheat oven to 400°F
12-cup muffin tin, lightly greased or lined with paper cups

1	cup	quick-cooking rolled oats
1	cup	buttermilk (approx.)
½	cup	all-purpose flour
½	cup	whole wheat flour
¼	cup	granulated sugar
1	tbsp	wheat germ
1	tbsp	baking powder
1	tsp	salt
½	tsp	baking soda
1	cup	mixed dried fruit
1	egg, beaten	
½	cup	grated sweet potato
¼	cup	lightly packed brown sugar
¼	cup	vegetable oil
1	tsp	grated orange zest

1. Place oatmeal in a large bowl and pour in buttermilk; stir to combine. Cover and let stand for 10 minutes.

2. Meanwhile, in a small bowl, combine all-purpose flour, whole wheat flour, granulated sugar, wheat germ, baking powder, salt and baking soda. Stir in dried fruit.

3. In another small bowl, combine egg, sweet potato, brown sugar, oil and orange zest. Stir into oatmeal mixture. Gradually fold in flour mixture until just moistened. If too stiff, add a little more buttermilk.

4. Divide batter evenly among prepared muffin cups, filling almost to the top (these muffins do not rise much).

5. Bake for 20 minutes or until a tester inserted in the center of a muffin comes out clean. Let cool in tin for 10 minutes, then remove to a wire rack to cool completely.

Makes 12 muffins (1 muffin per serving)

DIETITIAN'S NOTES *This recipe contains ¼ cup oil. In recipes for 12 muffins that call for more than this amount, you can often reduce it. Use ¼ cup oil and add unsweetened applesauce or mashed banana to make up the difference in volume.*

Cut dried fruit into small pieces to spread its flavor through a batter or dough.

These muffins contain more salt than most homemade muffins, so they are higher in sodium. To lower sodium by 100 mg per muffin, reduce the salt to ½ teaspoon. At the same time, you may want to increase the quantity of orange zest.

When you look for new recipes, keep your eye out for ones with nutritious ingredients. This one contains rolled oats, whole wheat flour and wheat germ, all of which boost fiber. Wheat germ is also rich in B vitamins and vitamin E. The dried fruit and sweet potato add vitamins and bursts of flavor and sweetness, but they don't contain much sugar—there's only 1 tsp per muffin.

NUTRIENTS PER SERVING

Calories	185
Carbohydrate	31 g
Fiber	3 g
Protein	4 g
Fat, total	6 g
Fat, saturated	1 g
Cholesterol	16 mg
Sodium	342 mg

EXCHANGES PER SERVING

1 Starch
½ Fruit
½ Other Carbohydrate
1 Fat

PUMPKIN MOLASSES RAISIN LOAF

TIPS When using margarine, choose a soft (non-hydrogenated) version to limit consumption of trans fats.

Can be prepared up to 2 days ahead.

NUTRIENTS PER SERVING

Calories	170
Carbohydrate	32 g
Fiber	1 g
Protein	3 g
Fat, total	4 g
Fat, saturated	1 g
Cholesterol	19 mg
Sodium	110 mg

EXCHANGES PER SERVING

½ Starch

½ Fruit

1 Other Carbohydrates

1 Fat

Preheat oven to 350°F
9- by 5-inch loaf pan, sprayed with vegetable spray

1¼	cups brown sugar
⅓	cup margarine or butter
2	eggs
2	tbsp molasses
1	tsp vanilla
1	cup canned pumpkin purée (not pie filling)
1	cup raisins
1⅓	cups all-purpose flour
⅔	cup whole wheat flour
2¼	tsp ground cinnamon
1½	tsp baking powder
½	tsp baking soda
¼	tsp ground ginger
½	cup 2% yogurt

1. In a large bowl, beat sugar and margarine together until crumbly. Add eggs and mix until smooth. Beat in molasses, vanilla and pumpkin. (Mixture may appear curdled.) Stir in raisins.

2. In a bowl, combine flour, whole wheat flour, cinnamon, baking powder, baking soda and ginger. Add to wet ingredients alternately with the yogurt; stir just until combined. Pour into pan and bake for 55 to 60 minutes or until a cake tester inserted in center comes out clean.

Makes 20 half-slices (1 half-slice per serving)

DIETITIAN'S NOTE *Serving the correct portion size is important. This recipe makes 20 servings, but it's often difficult to cut a loaf of this size into 20 slices. Instead, cut it into 10 slices and then cut each slice in half to make 20 servings.*

CARROT PINEAPPLE ZUCCHINI LOAF

Preheat oven to 350°F
9- by 5-inch loaf pan, sprayed with nonstick vegetable spray

¼	cup margarine
1	cup granulated sugar
1	egg
1	egg white
2	tsp ground cinnamon
1½	tsp vanilla
¼	tsp ground nutmeg
¾	cup grated carrot
¾	cup grated zucchini
½	cup drained crushed pineapple
⅓	cup raisins
1¼	cups all-purpose flour
½	cup whole wheat flour
1	tsp baking powder
1	tsp baking soda

1. In a large bowl or food processor, cream margarine with sugar. Add egg, egg white, cinnamon, vanilla and nutmeg; beat well. Stir in carrot, zucchini, pineapple and raisins, blending until well combined.

2. Combine all-purpose and whole wheat flours, baking powder and soda; add to bowl and mix just until combined. Pour into loaf pan and bake for 35 to 45 minutes or until a tester inserted into center comes out dry.

Makes 20 half-slices (1 half-slice per serving)

TIPS If you like muffins, fill 12 muffin cups and bake for 20 minutes or until tops are firm to the touch.

Make up to 2 days in advance or freeze for up to 2 months.

NUTRIENTS PER SERVING

Calories	118
Carbohydrate	22 g
Fiber	1 g
Protein	2 g
Fat, total	3 g
Fat, saturated	0 g
Cholesterol	9 mg
Sodium	116 mg

EXCHANGES PER SERVING

½	Starch
½	Fruit
½	Other Carbohydrate
½	Fat

LEMON POPPY SEED LOAF

TIP When using margarine, choose a soft (non-hydrogenated) version to limit consumption of trans fats.

Bake a day before or freeze for up to 6 weeks.

NUTRIENTS PER SERVING

Calories	102
Carbohydrate	16 g
Fiber	0 g
Protein	2 g
Fat, total	4 g
Fat, saturated	1 g
Cholesterol	10 mg
Sodium	94 mg

EXCHANGES PER SERVING

½ Starch
½ Other Carbohydrate
1 Fat

Preheat oven to 350°F
9- by 5-inch loaf pan, sprayed with nonstick vegetable spray

¾	cup granulated sugar
⅓	cup soft margarine
1	egg
2	tsp grated lemon zest
3	tbsp freshly squeezed lemon juice
⅓	cup 2% milk
1¼	cups all-purpose flour
1	tbsp poppy seeds
1	tsp baking powder
½	tsp baking soda
⅓	cup 2% yogurt or light sour cream

Glaze

¼	cup confectioner's sugar
2	tbsp freshly squeezed lemon juice

1. In a large bowl or food processor, beat together sugar, margarine, egg, lemon zest and juice, mixing well. Add milk, mixing well.

2. Combine flour, poppy seeds, baking powder and baking soda; add to bowl alternately with yogurt, mixing just until incorporated. Do not overmix. Pour into pan and bake for 35 to 40 minutes or until a tester inserted into center comes out dry.

3. *Glaze:* Prick holes in top of loaf with fork. Combine confectioner's sugar with lemon juice; pour over loaf.

Makes 20 half-slices (1 half-slice per serving)

DIETITIAN'S NOTE *The lemon glaze on this loaf adds a lot of flavor but only a small amount of carbohydrate. The small quantity of icing sugar contributes about 2 grams of carbohydrate per serving.*

BANANA NUT RAISIN LOAF

Preheat oven to 375°F
9- by 5-inch loaf pan, sprayed with nonstick vegetable spray

2	large ripe bananas
⅓	cup soft margarine
½	cup granulated sugar
1	egg
1	egg white
¼	cup hot water
1⅓	cups whole wheat flour
¾	tsp baking soda
¼	cup raisins
⅓	cup chopped pecans or walnuts

1. In a bowl or food processor, beat bananas and margarine; beat in sugar, egg, egg white and water until smooth.

2. Combine flour and baking soda; stir into batter along with raisins and all but a few of the pecans, mixing just until blended. Do not over-mix. Pour into pan; arrange reserved nuts down middle of mixture. Bake for 35 to 45 minutes or until a tester inserted into center comes out dry.

Makes 20 half-slices (1 half-slice per serving)

TIPS When using margarine, choose a soft (non-hydrogenated) version to limit consumption of trans fats.

Bake up to 2 days in advance or freeze for up to 6 weeks.

NUTRIENTS PER SERVING

Calories	110
Carbohydrate	16 g
Fiber	1 g
Protein	2 g
Fat, total	5 g
Fat, saturated	1 g
Cholesterol	9 mg
Sodium	95 mg

EXCHANGES PER SERVING

½	Starch
½	Other Carbohydrate
1	Fat

DIETITIAN'S NOTE *Serving the correct portion size is important. This recipe makes 20 servings, but it's often difficult to cut a loaf of this size into 20 slices. Instead, cut it into 10 slices and then cut each slice in half to make 20 servings.*

CARROT, APPLE & COCONUT LOAF

TIPS Grate carrots or chop and process them in food processor just until finely diced.

Prepare up to a day ahead, or freeze up to 4 weeks.

VARIATION Chopped, pitted dates can replace the raisins.

NUTRIENTS PER SERVING

Calories	111
Carbohydrate	17 g
Fiber	1 g
Protein	2 g
Fat, total	4 g
Fat, saturated	2 g
Sodium	121 mg
Cholesterol	22 mg

EXCHANGES PER SERVING

½ Fruit
⅔ Other Carbohydrate
1 Fat

Preheat oven to 350°F
9- by 5-inch loaf pan, sprayed with vegetable spray

⅔	cup granulated sugar
¼	cup margarine or butter
2	eggs
1½	tsp ground cinnamon
¼	tsp ground nutmeg
1	tsp vanilla
1¼	cup grated carrots
⅔	cup finely chopped peeled apple
⅓	cup unsweetened shredded coconut
⅓	cup raisins
⅔	cup all-purpose flour
½	cup whole wheat flour
1	tsp baking powder
1	tsp baking soda
⅓	cup 2% yogurt

1. In large bowl or food processor, cream together sugar and margarine. Add eggs, cinnamon, nutmeg and vanilla; beat well. Stir in carrots, apple, coconut and raisins.

2. In bowl, combine flour, whole wheat flour, baking powder and baking soda; add to batter alternately with yogurt, mixing until just combined.

3. Pour batter into prepared loaf pan. Bake in preheated oven for 40 to 45 minutes, or until tester inserted in center comes out clean.

Makes 1 loaf or 10 slices (½ slice per serving)

DIETITIAN'S NOTE *Orange fruits and vegetables—such as carrots, squash and mangoes—are good sources of beta-carotene and vitamin A.*

RHUBARB ORANGE BREAD

Preheat oven to 350°F
9- by 5-inch loaf pan, lightly greased

1¾	cups finely chopped rhubarb
⅓	cup granulated sugar
2	cups all-purpose flour
2	tsp baking powder
¾	tsp baking soda
½	tsp salt
2	tbsp grated orange zest
½	cup chopped walnuts
3	tbsp vegetable oil
1	egg
⅔	cup orange juice
1	tsp vanilla

1. In a bowl combine rhubarb and sugar; set aside for 10 to 15 minutes.

2. In a large bowl, stir together flour, baking powder, baking soda, salt and zest. Stir in walnuts.

3. In a separate bowl, using an electric mixer, beat oil, egg, juice and vanilla until combined. Stir in reserved rhubarb mixture. Pour over dry ingredients and stir just until combined. Spoon into prepared pan.

4. Bake in preheated oven for 70 to 80 minutes, or until a cake tester inserted in the center comes out clean. Let cool in pan on rack for 10 minutes. Remove from pan and let cool completely on rack.

Makes 1 loaf or 12 slices (1 slice per serving)

TIP The rhubarb must be finely chopped; otherwise, the finished loaf tends to crumble when sliced.

VARIATION Substitute pecans or pistachios for the walnuts and lemon zest for the orange.

NUTRIENTS PER SERVING

Calories	178
Carbohydrate	25 g
Fiber	1 g
Protein	4 g
Fat, total	7 g
Fat, saturated	1 g
Sodium	214 mg
Cholesterol	18 mg

EXCHANGES PER SERVING

1½	Starch
1½	Fat

POPPY SEED OAT BREAD

VARIATION Substitute sesame seeds or flaxseeds for the poppy seeds.

NUTRIENTS PER SERVING

Calories	174
Carbohydrate	32 g
Fiber	2 g
Protein	6 g
Fat, total	3 g
Fat, saturated	1 g
Sodium	254 mg
Cholesterol	19 mg

EXCHANGES PER SERVING

½ Starch
⅔ Other Carbohydrate
½ Fat

Preheat oven to 350°F
9- by 5-inch loaf pan, lightly greased

1	cup	whole wheat flour
1	cup	all-purpose flour
1	cup	quick-cooking oats
1	tsp	baking powder
1	tsp	baking soda
½	tsp	salt
¼	cup	poppy seeds
1		egg
1¾	cups	buttermilk
⅓	cup	honey

1. In a large bowl, stir together whole wheat flour, flour, oats, baking powder, baking soda, salt and poppy seeds.

2. In a separate bowl, using an electric mixer, beat egg and buttermilk until combined. Add honey while mixing. Pour mixture over dry ingredients and stir just until combined. Spoon into prepared pan.

3. Bake in preheated oven for 70 to 80 minutes, or until a cake tester inserted in the center comes out clean. Let cool in pan on rack for 10 minutes. Remove from pan and let cool completely on rack.

Makes 1 loaf or 12 slices (1 slice per serving)

BLUEBERRY BANANA OAT BREAD

Preheat oven to 350°F
9- by 5-inch loaf pan, lightly greased

1¾	cups all-purpose flour
¼	cup quick-cooking oats
2	tbsp oat bran
½	cup granulated sugar
2	tsp baking powder
½	tsp salt
2	tbsp vegetable oil
1	egg
1½	cups mashed bananas
¾	cup frozen blueberries (see Tip)

1. In a large bowl, stir together flour, oats, oat bran, sugar, baking powder and salt.

2. In a separate bowl, using an electric mixer, beat oil, egg and bananas until combined. Pour mixture over dry ingredients and stir just until combined. Gently fold in frozen blueberries. Spoon into prepared pan.

3. Bake in preheated oven for 70 to 80 minutes, or until a cake tester inserted in the center comes out clean. Let cool in pan on rack for 10 minutes. Remove from pan and serve warm.

Makes 1 loaf or 12 slices (1 slice per serving)

TIPS Leave blueberries in the freezer until just before using. This will help to prevent them from "bleeding" into the bread.

Use ripe bananas for the best flavor.

VARIATION Try natural wheat bran instead of the oat bran.

NUTRIENTS PER SERVING

Calories	169
Carbohydrate	32 g
Fiber	2 g
Protein	3 g
Fat, total	3 g
Fat, saturated	0 g
Sodium	138 mg
Cholesterol	18 mg

EXCHANGES PER SERVING

1	Starch
⅓	Fruit
⅔	Other Carbohydrate
½	Fat

BLUEBERRY BUCKWHEAT BREAD

TIP Leave blueberries in the freezer until just before using. This will help to prevent them from "bleeding" into the bread.

VARIATION Try substituting frozen sour cherries or cranberries for half or all of the blueberries.

NUTRIENTS PER SERVING

Calories	158
Carbohydrate	28 g
Fiber	1 g
Protein	4 g
Fat, total	4 g
Fat, saturated	0 g
Sodium	181 mg
Cholesterol	0 mg

EXCHANGES PER SERVING

1 Starch
⅔ Other Carbohydrate
1 Fat

Preheat oven to 350°F
9- by 5-inch loaf pan, lightly greased

1⅔	cups all-purpose flour
⅓	cup buckwheat flour
1	tbsp baking powder
½	tsp salt
1	tsp grated lemon zest
3	tbsp vegetable oil
2	egg whites
1¼	cups plain yogurt
⅓	cup honey
½	cup frozen blueberries (see Tip)

1. In a large bowl, stir together flour, buckwheat flour, baking powder, salt and zest.

2. In a separate bowl, using an electric mixer, beat oil, egg whites, yogurt and honey until combined. Pour mixture over dry ingredients and stir just until combined. Gently fold in frozen blueberries. Spoon into prepared pan.

3. Bake in preheated oven for 70 to 80 minutes, or until a cake tester inserted in the center comes out clean. Let cool in pan on rack for 10 minutes. Remove from pan and let cool completely on rack.

Makes 1 loaf or 12 slices (1 slice per serving)

PEACH BLUEBERRY QUICK BREAD

Preheat oven to 350°F
9- by 5-inch loaf pan, lightly greased

1¾	cups all-purpose flour
2½	tsp baking powder
¾	tsp salt
½	tsp ground cardamom
⅓	cup margarine
⅔	cup granulated sugar
2	eggs
⅓	cup milk
1	cup chopped fresh peaches
½	cup fresh or frozen blueberries

1. In a large bowl, stir together flour, baking powder, salt and cardamom.

2. In a separate large bowl, using an electric mixer, cream margarine, sugar and eggs until light and fluffy. Stir in dry ingredients alternately with milk, making 3 additions of dry ingredients and 2 of milk; stir just until combined. Gently fold in peaches and blueberries. Spoon into prepared pan.

3. Bake in preheated oven for 70 to 80 minutes, or until a cake tester inserted in the center comes out clean. Let cool in pan on rack for 10 minutes. Remove from pan and let cool completely on rack.

Makes 1 loaf or 12 slices (1 slice per serving)

VARIATION For a milder spice flavor, use mace or nutmeg instead of the cardamom.

NUTRIENTS PER SERVING

Calories	180
Carbohydrate	28 g
Fiber	1 g
Protein	3 g
Fat, total	6 g
Fat, saturated	1 g
Sodium	266 mg
Cholesterol	36 mg

EXCHANGES PER SERVING

1	Starch
⅔	Other Carbohydrate
1	Fat

DIETITIAN'S NOTE *Blueberries are becoming very popular as a source of antioxidants with disease-fighting properties.*

LOW-FAT APPLESAUCE RAISIN BREAD

TIP Instead of using egg whites, try using 1 whole egg. This will increase the fat content slightly, but it yields a softer-textured loaf.

VARIATION Substitute dates for the raisins and ground ginger or nutmeg for the cinnamon.

NUTRIENTS PER SERVING

Calories	123
Carbohydrate	29 g
Fiber	1 g
Protein	2 g
Fat, total	0 g
Fat, saturated	0 g
Sodium	95 mg
Cholesterol	0 mg

EXCHANGES PER SERVING

1 Starch
1 Fruit

Preheat oven to 350°F
9- by 5-inch loaf pan, lightly greased

2	cups all-purpose flour
½	cup granulated sugar
1	tsp baking powder
½	tsp baking soda
¼	tsp salt
½	tsp ground cinnamon
1	cup raisins
2	egg whites
1¼	cups unsweetened applesauce

1. In a large bowl, stir together flour, sugar, baking powder, baking soda, salt and cinnamon. Stir in raisins.

2. In a separate bowl, using an electric mixer, beat egg whites and applesauce until combined. Pour mixture over dry ingredients and stir just until combined. Spoon into prepared pan.

3. Bake in preheated oven for 70 to 80 minutes, or until a cake tester inserted in the center comes out clean. Let cool in pan on rack for 10 minutes. Remove from pan and let cool completely on rack.

Makes 1 loaf or 16 slices (1 slice per serving)

FRUITED BARM BRACK

Preheat oven to 350°F
9- by 5-inch loaf pan, lightly greased

2	cups all-purpose flour
½	cup packed brown sugar
2	tsp baking powder
½	tsp baking soda
½	tsp salt
1	tsp ground cinnamon
1	tsp ground nutmeg
½	cup snipped dried apricots
½	cup currants
½	cup dried cranberries
2	tbsp vegetable oil
1	egg
1	cup tea, at room temperature

1. In a large bowl, stir together flour, brown sugar, baking powder, baking soda, salt, cinnamon and nutmeg. Stir in dried apricots, currants and dried cranberries.

2. In a separate bowl, using an electric mixer, beat oil, egg and tea until combined. Pour mixture over dry ingredients and stir just until combined. Spoon into prepared pan.

3. Bake in preheated oven for 70 to 80 minutes, or until a cake tester inserted in the center comes out clean. Let cool in pan on rack for 10 minutes. Remove from pan and let cool completely on rack.

Makes 1 loaf or 12 slices (1 slice per serving)

TIPS *Barm brack*, meaning "yeast bread" in Gaelic, is an Irish bread with raisins or currants and candied fruit peel—although it is not always made with yeast.

Snip dried apricots into ¼-inch pieces with sharp scissors.

VARIATION Try replacing one or more of the fruits with an equal quantity of dried cherries, dried apples or fresh dates.

NUTRIENTS PER SERVING

Calories	186
Carbohydrate	37 g
Fiber	2 g
Protein	3 g
Fat, total	3 g
Fat, saturated	0 g
Sodium	192 mg
Cholesterol	18 mg

EXCHANGES PER SERVING

1	Starch
⅔	Fruit
⅔	Other Carbohydrate
½	Fat

OAT BRAN BANANA BREAD

TIP When using margarine, choose a non-hydrogenated version to limit consumption of trans fats.

Preheat oven to 325°F
9- by 5-inch loaf pan, lightly greased

1½	cups whole wheat flour
½	cup oat bran
⅓	cup ground flaxseed
1	tsp baking powder
1	tsp baking soda
2	egg whites
1	egg
½	cup granulated sugar
¼	cup vegetable oil or margarine
1	tsp vanilla
¾	cup low-fat plain yogurt
3	ripe bananas, mashed (about 1⅓ cups)
2	tbsp whole flaxseed (optional)

1. In a medium bowl, combine flour, oat bran, ground flaxseed, baking powder and baking soda.

2. In a large bowl, beat egg whites, whole egg, sugar, oil and vanilla for 3 to 4 minutes or until creamy. Stir in yogurt until well combined. Stir in bananas. Gradually fold in flour mixture.

3. Spoon batter into prepared loaf pan and smooth top. Sprinkle with whole flaxseed (if using).

4. Bake in preheated oven for 50 to 60 minutes or until top is firm to the touch and a tester inserted in the center comes out clean. Let cool in pan for 10 minutes, then remove to a wire rack to cool completely.

Makes 12 slices (1 slice per serving)

DIETITIAN'S NOTES *This recipe contains ground flaxseed, a source of omega-3 fatty acids. There is also an optional quantity of whole flax-seed, but the tough coat on it prevents absorption of its nutrients.*

Ground flaxseed goes rancid quickly. Prepare it only as needed or purchase in small quantities and store in the freezer.

NUTRIENTS PER SERVING

Calories	197
Carbohydrate	31 g
Fiber	4 g
Protein	6 g
Fat, total	7 g
Fat, saturated	1 g
Cholesterol	16 mg
Sodium	154 mg

EXCHANGES PER SERVING

1	Starch
½	Fruit
½	Other Carbohydrate
1½	Fat

BANANA WALNUT BREAD

NUTRIENTS PER SERVING

Calories	115
Carbohydrate	14 g
Fiber	1 g
Protein	2 g
Fat, total	6 g
Fat, saturated	3 g
Cholesterol	22 mg
Sodium	146 mg

EXCHANGES PER SERVING

½ Starch
½ Other Carbohydrate
1 Fat

Preheat oven to 375°F
9- by 5-inch loaf pan, sprayed with baking spray

2	ripe bananas, mashed
½	cup butter, softened
½	cup granulated sugar
1	egg
1	egg white
1⅓	cups whole wheat flour
⅓	cup chopped walnuts
1	tsp baking soda
¼	tsp salt
¼	cup hot water
	Sesame seeds or extra chopped walnuts (optional)

1. In a bowl, beat bananas with butter until well mixed. Beat in sugar, whole egg and egg white until fluffy.

2. In another bowl, stir together flour, walnuts, baking soda and salt. Stir into banana mixture along with hot water just until blended. Pour into prepared loaf pan. If desired, sprinkle with sesame seeds or extra chopped walnuts.

3. Bake for 35 to 45 minutes or until a cake tester inserted in center comes out clean. Cool in pan for 5 minutes. Remove from pan and cool on wire rack.

Makes 20 half-slices (1 half-slice per serving)

DIETITIAN'S NOTE *Sesame seeds and additional walnuts are optional in this recipe. One-third cup chopped walnuts or sesame seeds will increase the fat per serving by less than 2 grams.*

IRISH WHOLE WHEAT SODA BREAD

Preheat oven to 400°F
Baking sheet, lightly greased

2	cups whole wheat flour
1	cup all-purpose flour
1	tbsp granulated sugar
1	tsp baking powder
1	tsp baking soda
1	tsp salt
1½	cups buttermilk
	Rice flour for dusting

1. In a large bowl, stir together whole wheat flour, flour, sugar, baking powder, baking soda and salt. Add buttermilk all at once, stirring with a fork to make a soft, but slightly sticky dough.

2. With lightly floured hands, form dough into a ball. On a lightly floured surface, knead the dough gently 8 to 10 times. Pat the dough into a thick, 6-inch round, with a slightly flattened top.

3. Place dough on prepared baking sheet. With a sharp knife or pizza cutter, score the top in the shape of a cross or large X. Bake in pre-heated oven for 35 to 45 minutes. Remove from baking sheet onto a cooling rack immediately. Dust top with rice flour and cut each wedge into 3 slices. Serve warm from the oven.

Makes 1 round loaf or 12 slices (1 slice per serving)

TIP Score the top of the round at least ½ inch deep. This will ensure it breaks easily into wedges.

NUTRIENTS PER SERVING

Calories	123
Carbohydrate	25 g
Fiber	3 g
Protein	5 g
Fat, total	1 g
Fat, saturated	0 g
Sodium	335 mg
Cholesterol	1 mg

EXCHANGES PER SERVING

1½ Starch

PUMPKIN SPICE NUT BREAD

VARIATION Use mini loaf pans to make 12 mini loaves. Bake at the same temperature for 25 minutes, or until a tester comes out clean.

Preheat oven to 350°F
9- by 5-inch loaf pan, lightly greased

1	cup all-purpose flour
¾	cup whole wheat flour
2	tsp ground allspice
1½	tsp baking powder
1	tsp baking soda
½	tsp salt
1	tsp ground cinnamon
½	tsp ground nutmeg
½	tsp ground ginger
1	cup canned pumpkin purée (not pie filling)
¾	cup packed brown sugar
½	cup vegetable oil
2	eggs, lightly beaten
1	tsp vanilla
⅓	cup water (approx.), divided
½	cup chopped pecans or walnuts

1. In a small bowl, combine all-purpose flour, whole wheat flour, allspice, baking powder, baking soda, salt, cinnamon, nutmeg and ginger.

2. In a large bowl, whisk together pumpkin, brown sugar and oil. Whisk in eggs, vanilla and half of the water. Fold in flour mixture (do not overmix). If batter is too thick, stir in the remaining water, a little at a time. Fold in pecans.

3. Spoon batter into prepared loaf pan and smooth top.

4. Bake in preheated oven for 50 to 60 minutes or until top is firm to the touch and a tester inserted in the center comes out clean. Let cool in pan for 10 minutes, then remove to a wire rack to cool completely.

Makes 12 slices (1 slice per serving)

DIETITIAN'S NOTES *Nuts are high in calories because they are high in fat. This fat, however, is primarily the desirable monounsaturated type. The ½ cup of pecans in this recipe contributes about 3 grams of fat per serving, or about ½ Fat Exchange. To reduce the amount of fat, you can decrease the amount of nuts in this recipe. To get the most flavor from nuts, toast them on a rimmed baking sheet at 350°F for about 5 minutes.*

For help in planning your meals, ask your doctor to refer you to a diabetes education center or a dietitian. Local hospitals may also have referral services. On the Internet, look for the "Find a Nutrition Professional" feature at www.eatright.org.

NUTRIENTS PER SERVING

Calories	251
Carbohydrate	30 g
Fiber	2 g
Protein	4 g
Fat, total	14 g
Fat, saturated	1 g
Cholesterol	31 mg
Sodium	252 mg

EXCHANGES PER SERVING

1 Starch
1 Other Carbohydrates
3 Fat

PUMPKIN RAISIN SCONES

Preheat oven to 425°F
Baking sheet, lined with parchment paper or Silpat
Pizza cutter

1½	cups	all-purpose flour
1¼	cups	cake flour
3	tbsp	granulated sugar
1	tbsp	baking powder
1	tsp	salt
1	tsp	ground cinnamon
½	tsp	ground nutmeg
¼	tsp	ground allspice
¼	tsp	ground cloves
6	tbsp	cold vegetable shortening or unsalted butter, cut into chunks
2		eggs, beaten, divided
¼	cup	pumpkin purée (not pie filling)
½	cup	milk, preferably whole
1	tbsp	freshly squeezed lemon juice
½	cup	golden raisins

Mixer Method

1. In a mixer bowl fitted with paddle attachment, beat all-purpose flour, cake flour, sugar, baking powder, salt, cinnamon, nutmeg, allspice and cloves on low speed until blended, for 2 minutes. With mixer running, drop in chunks of shortening or butter, mixing until it resembles coarse crumbs. Set 1 tbsp of the beaten egg aside. Whisk together remaining egg, pumpkin, milk and lemon juice. Pour over the dry ingredients and, using a fork, stir just until dough starts to bind together.

2. Turn dough out onto a lightly floured work surface and knead in raisins. Continue to knead dough just until it holds together, about 6 times. Shape into a ball and pat into a 10-inch circle. Place on prepared baking sheet.

3. Using a pizza cutter or sharp knife, cut into 12 wedges. Do not separate wedges. Brush with reserved egg. Bake in preheated oven until light brown, 18 to 22 minutes. Serve warm.

Food Processor Method
1. In work bowl fitted with metal blade, process all-purpose flour, cake flour, sugar, baking powder, salt, cinnamon, nutmeg, allspice and cloves until combined, about 10 seconds. Add shortening or butter chunks around work bowl; pulse until mixture resembles coarse crumbs, about 10 times. Set 1 tbsp of the beaten egg aside. With motor running, add remaining egg, pumpkin, milk and lemon juice through feed tube and process just until mixture starts to gather. If dough is tacky, refrigerate for 5 minutes. Proceed with Step 2, above.

Makes 12 scones (1 scone per serving)

DIETITIAN'S NOTES *Baking parchment is specially treated paper that does not stick to most foods and can withstand oven temperatures up to 425°F. Waxed paper cannot be used in the same way; it will smoke.*

In this recipe, salt contributes about 200 mg of sodium per scone. Reducing the salt to ½ teaspoon will lower the sodium in each scone by about 100 mg. Doing so, however, may cause the scones to rise less.

Vegetable shortening used to be a common baking ingredient. Because of concern about its trans fat content, we now see it much less often. In most recipes, you can substitute vegetable oil or soft non-hydrogenated margarine. Some people, however, still prefer shortening for biscuits, scones and pastry; the dough is easier to handle and the results are lighter. (See more about ingredient substitutions on page 313.)

NUTRIENTS PER SERVING

Calories	214
Carbohydrate	31 g
Fiber	1 g
Protein	4 g
Fat, total	8 g
Fat, saturated	2 g
Cholesterol	32 mg
Sodium	275 mg

EXCHANGES PER SERVING

1½	Starch
½	Fruit
1½	Fat

SCOTTISH OATMEAL SCONES

TIP To enjoy the next day, split scones in half and reheat in a toaster oven.

VARIATION For a heavier, more traditional oatmeal biscuit, omit the margarine. This will eliminate the Fat Exchange.

NUTRIENTS PER SERVING

Calories	133
Carbohydrate	18 g
Fiber	2 g
Protein	4 g
Fat, total	5 g
Fat, saturated	1 g
Sodium	225 mg
Cholesterol	16 mg

EXCHANGES PER SERVING

1 Starch

1 Fat

Preheat oven to 425°F
Baking sheet, lightly greased

1	cup whole wheat flour
1¼	cups all-purpose flour
½	cup quick-cooking oats
2	tsp baking powder
¾	tsp salt
⅓	cup margarine
1	egg
¾	cup buttermilk

1. In a large bowl, stir together whole wheat flour, flour, oats, baking powder and salt. Using a pastry blender, cut in margarine until mixture resembles coarse crumbs.

2. In a small bowl, whisk together egg and buttermilk. Pour over dry ingredients all at once, stirring with a fork to make a soft, but slightly sticky dough.

3. With lightly floured hands, form dough into a ball. On a lightly floured surface, knead the dough gently 8 to 10 times. Pat or roll out the dough into a 1-inch-thick round.

4. Using a 2-inch floured biscuit cutter, cut out as many rounds as possible. Place on prepared baking sheet. Gently form scraps into a ball, flatten and cut out rounds.

5. Bake in preheated oven for 12 to 15 minutes. Remove from baking sheet onto a cooling rack immediately. Serve warm.

Makes 14 2-inch scones (1 per serving)

WHOLE WHEAT POPPY BISCUITS

Preheat oven to 425°F
Baking sheet, lightly greased
2½-inch round biscuit cutter

1½	cups whole wheat flour
1	cup all-purpose flour
¼	cup granulated sugar
¼	cup poppy seeds
1	tbsp baking powder
½	tsp baking soda
½	tsp salt
⅓	cup margarine
1	cup buttermilk

1. In a large bowl, stir together whole wheat flour, flour, sugar, poppy seeds, baking powder, baking soda and salt. Using a pastry blender, cut in margarine until mixture resembles coarse crumbs. Add buttermilk all at once, stirring with a fork to make a soft, but slightly sticky dough.

2. With lightly floured hands, form dough into a ball. On a lightly floured surface, knead the dough gently 8 to 10 times. Pat or roll out the dough into a ½-inch-thick round.

3. Using a 2-inch floured biscuit cutter, cut out as many rounds as possible. Place on prepared baking sheet. Gently form scraps into a ball, flatten and cut out rounds.

4. Bake in preheated oven for 12 to 15 minutes. Remove from baking sheet onto a cooling rack immediately. Serve warm.

Makes 18 2-inch biscuits (1 per serving)

TIP Adjust the quantity of poppy seeds to your taste. For browner, crisper tops, bake biscuits in the upper third of the oven.

VARIATION Poppy seeds can be replaced with any other small seed—such as sesame, caraway, fennel, anise or mini sunflower seeds. For stronger-flavored seeds, you may wish to reduce the quantity used.

NUTRIENTS PER SERVING

Calories	117
Carbohydrate	17 g
Fiber	2 g
Protein	3 g
Fat, total	5 g
Fat, saturated	1 g
Sodium	193 mg
Cholesterol	0 mg

EXCHANGES PER SERVING

1	Starch
1	Fat

LEMON YOGURT BISCUITS

NUTRIENTS PER SERVING

Calories	141
Carbohydrate	20 g
Fiber	1 g
Protein	3 g
Fat, total	5 g
Fat, saturated	1 g
Sodium	281 mg
Cholesterol	0 mg

EXCHANGES PER SERVING

1 Starch
⅓ Other Carbohydrate
1 Fat

Preheat oven to 425°F
Baking sheet, ungreased
2½-inch round biscuit cutter

2	cups all-purpose flour
2	tbsp granulated sugar
1	tbsp baking powder
½	tsp baking soda
½	tsp salt
2	tsp grated lemon zest
⅓	cup cold margarine or butter
1	cup plain yogurt

1. In a large bowl, stir together flour, sugar, baking powder, baking soda, salt and zest. Using a pastry blender, cut in margarine until mixture resembles coarse crumbs. Add yogurt all at once, stirring with a fork to make a soft, but slightly sticky dough.

2. With lightly floured hands, form dough into a ball. On a lightly floured surface, knead the dough gently 8 to 10 times. Pat or roll out the dough into a 1-inch-thick round. Using a 2-inch floured cutter, cut out as many rounds as possible. Place on baking sheet. Gently form scraps into a ball, flatten and cut out rounds.

3. Bake in preheated oven for 12 to 15 minutes. Remove from baking sheet onto a cooling rack immediately.

Makes 12 2-inch biscuits (1 per serving)

PECAN CINNAMON BISCUITS

Preheat oven to 425°F
Baking sheet, lined with parchment paper or Silpat
2½-inch round biscuit cutter
Blending fork

2	cups all-purpose flour
2	tbsp granulated sugar
4	tsp baking powder
1	tsp ground cinnamon
½	tsp salt
½	cup cold vegetable shortening
¾	cup milk, preferably whole
¼	cup pecans, chopped

1. In a large bowl, using a blending fork, combine flour, sugar, baking powder, cinnamon and salt. Add shortening by spoonfuls, blending with fork until it is well mixed into dry ingredients and resembles coarse meal. Add milk all at once and stir just until dry ingredients are moistened.

2. Turn dough out onto a floured surface and add pecans, kneading a few times just until dough gathers. Pat down. Using a rolling pin, roll dough to about ½-inch thickness. Cut with biscuit cutter, rerolling scraps. Place biscuits close to each other on prepared baking sheet. Bake in preheated oven until biscuits have risen and are light brown, 15 to 22 minutes. Serve warm.

Makes 18 biscuits (1 biscuit per serving)

TIP Silpat is the brand name of a silicone mat used in baking. Its non-stick surface does not require greasing.

NUTRIENTS PER SERVING

Calories	128
Carbohydrate	13 g
Fiber	1 g
Protein	2 g
Fat, total	8 g
Fat, saturated	2 g
Cholesterol	1 mg
Sodium	128 mg

EXCHANGES PER SERVING

1 Starch
1½ Fat

BISCOTTI & SHORTBREAD

51 | Apricot Date Biscotti
52 | Fiber-Power Biscotti
54 | Lemon & Lime Poppy Seed Biscotti
55 | Lemon Almond Biscotti
56 | Mini Hazelnut Biscotti
57 | Pecan Biscotti
58 | Maple Walnut Biscotti
60 | Chocolate Cherry Biscotti
61 | Chocolate Chip Orange Biscotti
62 | Two-Tone Chocolate Orange Biscotti
63 | Gingerbread Biscotti
64 | Chocolate-Wrapped Ginger Biscotti
66 | Holiday Biscotti
68 | Oatmeal Shortbread
69 | Almond Spice Shortbread
70 | Oatmeal Pecan Shortbread
71 | Rice Flour Shortbread
72 | Cornmeal Shortbread
73 | Chunky Chocolate Shortbread

APRICOT DATE BISCOTTI

Preheat oven to 350°F
Baking sheet, sprayed with vegetable spray

⅓	cup margarine or butter
¾	cup granulated sugar
2	eggs
2	tbsp orange juice concentrate, thawed
2	tbsp water
2	tsp grated orange zest
1	tsp vanilla
2⅔	cups all-purpose flour
2¼	tsp baking powder
1	tsp ground cinnamon
⅔	cup chopped pitted dates
⅔	cup chopped dried apricots

1. In a large bowl, cream together margarine and sugar; add eggs, orange juice concentrate, water, orange zest and vanilla and mix well.

2. In a bowl, combine flour, baking powder, cinnamon, dates and apricots; add to wet ingredients and stir just until mixed. Divide dough into 3 portions; shape each portion into a 12-inch-long log, 2 inches wide, and put on prepared baking sheet. Bake for 20 minutes. Let cool for 10 minutes.

3. Cut logs on an angle into ½-inch-thick slices. Put slices flat on baking sheet and bake for another 20 minutes or until lightly browned.

Makes 48 biscotti (1 biscotti per serving)

TIPS Use a serrated knife to cut the logs into slices.

Dried prunes or raisins can replace, or be used in combination with, the apricots and dates.

Orange juice concentrate gives a more intense flavor than just orange juice. Use frozen concentrate, then refreeze the remainder.

Bake cookies up to 2 days ahead for best flavor, keeping tightly covered in cookie tin.

NUTRIENTS PER SERVING

Calories	67
Carbohydrate	12 g
Fiber	1 g
Protein	1 g
Fat, total	2 g
Fat, saturated	0 g
Cholesterol	8 g
Sodium	32 mg

EXCHANGES PER SERVING

½ Starch
½ Fruit
½ Fat

FIBER-POWER BISCOTTI

Preheat oven to 350°F
Baking sheets, lightly greased or lined with parchment paper

2	cups bran cereal, crushed
1½	cups all-purpose flour
1	cup granulated sugar
¾	cup quick-cooking rolled oats
½	cup sliced almonds
½	cup finely chopped dried apricots
2	tsp baking powder
3	eggs, lightly beaten
1	tbsp vegetable oil
2	tsp almond extract
1	tsp vanilla

1. In a large bowl, combine bran cereal, flour, sugar, oats, almonds, apricots and baking powder.

2. In a small bowl, beat eggs, oil, almond extract and vanilla. Stir into bran cereal mixture until well blended (dough will be dry and crumbly).

3. Turn dough out onto a lightly floured surface and knead 10 to 15 times, until dough holds together. Divide dough in half and shape each half into a log about 8 inches long and 3 inches wide. Place on prepared baking sheets.

4. Bake in preheated oven for 30 minutes. Remove from oven and reduce oven temperature to 325°F. Remove logs from baking sheets and let cool on a wire rack for 10 minutes.

5. Using a serrated knife, cut each log into ½-inch-thick slices. Return slices, cut side down, to baking sheets.

6. Bake for 15 minutes. Turn biscotti over and bake for 15 to 20 minutes or until light brown and crisp. Let cool on baking sheets on a wire rack for 5 minutes, then remove to rack to cool completely.

Makes 30 biscotti (1 biscotti per serving)

DIETITIAN'S NOTES *Increase fiber by substituting whole wheat flour for all-purpose flour. Start with one-quarter of the amount; you can usually replace up to half the all-purpose flour in a recipe with whole wheat.*

Use dry ingredient measuring cups for flour and sugar and other dry ingredients. Lightly spoon them in, without packing down, shaking or tapping. Then pass the edge (not the flat side) of a knife or spatula across the rim to remove excess and level off cup contents. Brown sugar is measured a little differently. Pack it down gently before leveling it off; it should hold its shape when turned out.

Although they are not dry, it's easiest to measure margarine, cottage cheese, ricotta cheese, yogurt and sour cream with dry measuring cups.

Use liquid measuring cups on a flat, level surface. Pour in liquid until the required level is reached. It's important to line up the liquid level with the marking, so you'll likely have to bend down to check—or put the measuring cup on a shelf at eye level while you pour.

See page 173 for information about the types of measuring cups and measuring spoons.

NUTRIENTS PER SERVING

Calories	94
Carbohydrate	17 g
Fiber	1 g
Protein	2 g
Fat, total	2 g
Fat, saturated	0 g
Cholesterol	19 mg
Sodium	41 mg

EXCHANGES PER SERVING

½ Starch
½ Other Carbohydrate
½ Fat

LEMON & LIME POPPY SEED BISCOTTI

TIPS If desired, omit lime and use double the quantity of lemon juice and zest.

If dough is sticky when forming into logs, try wetting your fingers.

Store cookies in airtight containers for up to 1 week.

Freeze in airtight containers up to 6 weeks.

NUTRIENTS PER SERVING

Calories	63
Carbohydrate	11 g
Fiber	0 g
Protein	1 g
Fat, total	2 g
Fat, saturated	0 g
Cholesterol	9 mg
Sodium	33 mg

EXCHANGES PER SERVING

½ Starch

½ Other Carbohydrate

½ Fat

Preheat oven to 350°F
Baking sheet, sprayed with vegetable spray

1	cup granulated sugar
¼	cup margarine or butter
2	eggs
1½	tsp grated lime zest
1½	tsp grated lemon zest
2	tbsp freshly squeezed lime juice
2	tbsp freshly squeezed lemon juice
1	tsp vanilla
2½	cups all-purpose flour
2¼	tsp baking powder
2	tsp poppy seeds

1. In a food processor or in a bowl with an electric mixer, beat sugar, margarine and eggs until smooth. Beat in lime zest, lemon zest, lime juice, lemon juice and vanilla.

2. In a separate bowl, stir together flour, baking powder and poppy seeds. Add wet ingredients to dry ingredients, mixing just until combined. Dough will be stiff.

3. Divide dough in half. Form each half into a log 12 inches long and 1½ inches around; transfer to prepared baking sheet. Bake 20 minutes. Cool 10 minutes.

4. Cut logs on an angle into ½-inch slices. Bake 20 minutes.

Makes 40 biscotti (1 biscotti per serving)

LEMON ALMOND BISCOTTI

Preheat oven to 325°F
Greased cookie sheet

1¾	cups all-purpose flour
¾	cup granulated sugar
1	tbsp baking powder
2	tbsp finely grated lemon zest
¾	cup coarsely chopped almonds
2	eggs
⅓	cup olive oil
1	tsp vanilla
½	tsp almond extract

1. In a bowl, mix together flour, sugar, baking powder, lemon zest and almonds. Make a well in the center.

2. In another bowl, whisk eggs, oil, vanilla and almond extract. Pour into well and mix until a soft, sticky dough forms.

3. Divide dough in half. Shape into two rolls about 10 inches long. Place about 2 inches apart on prepared cookie sheet. Bake in preheated oven for 20 minutes.

4. Cool on sheet for 5 minutes, then cut into slices ½ inch thick. Return to sheet and bake for 10 minutes. Turn slices over and bake for 10 minutes more. Immediately transfer to wire racks.

Makes about 3 dozen biscotti (1 per serving)

NUTRIENTS PER SERVING

Calories	78
Carbohydrate	10 g
Fiber	1 g
Protein	2 g
Fat, total	4 g
Fat, saturated	1 g
Sodium	24 mg
Cholesterol	12 mg

EXCHANGES PER SERVING

½ Starch
½ Fat

MINI HAZELNUT BISCOTTI

TIPS Be prepared—this dough is very stiff, so you will need to work it with your hands to get it smooth. Use a sharp serrated knife to cut biscotti.

Although recipes usually call for an electric mixer to blend ingredients, you can almost always use a wooden spoon when making biscotti. It just takes more physical effort.

VARIATION Substitute almonds or Brazil nuts for the hazelnuts.

NUTRIENTS PER SERVING

Calories	45
Carbohydrate	8 g
Fiber	0 g
Protein	1 g
Fat, total	1 g
Fat, saturated	0 g
Cholesterol	0 mg
Sodium	23 mg

EXCHANGES PER SERVING
½ Other Carbohydrate

Preheat oven to 350°F
Baking sheet, greased or lined with parchment paper

2	cups unbleached all-purpose flour
⅔	cup granulated sugar
½	cup ground hazelnuts
½	tsp baking powder
½	tsp baking soda
¼	tsp salt
1	tsp ground cinnamon
¾	cup whole hazelnuts
⅓	cup liquid honey
2	tsp grated orange zest
⅓	cup orange juice

1. In a large bowl, combine flour, sugar, ground hazelnuts, baking powder, baking soda, salt, cinnamon and whole hazelnuts. Mix to blend.

2. Add honey and orange zest and juice. With a wooden spoon, stir until blended, then, using your hands, knead to form a smooth, stiff dough.

3. Divide dough into halves. Shape each into a roll 15 inches long. Place about 2 inches apart on prepared baking sheet. Bake in preheated oven for 25 to 30 minutes or until set and golden. Cool for 15 minutes on sheet, then transfer to a cutting board. Cut diagonally into ½-inch slices. Place upright about 1 inch apart on baking sheet. Bake for 15 minutes until crisp and golden. Cool for 5 minutes on sheet, then transfer to a rack and cool completely.

Makes 60 biscotti (1 biscotti per serving)

PECAN BISCOTTI

Preheat oven to 350°F
Baking sheet, sprayed with nonstick vegetable spray

2	eggs
¾	cup granulated sugar
⅓	cup margarine
¼	cup water
2	tsp vanilla
1	tsp almond extract
2¾	cups all-purpose flour
½	cup chopped pecans
2¼	tsp baking powder

1. In a large bowl, blend eggs with sugar; beat in margarine, water, vanilla and almond extract until smooth.

2. Add flour, pecans and baking powder; mix until dough forms ball. Divide dough in half; shape each portion into 12-inch-long log and place on baking sheet. Bake for 20 minutes. Let cool for 5 minutes.

3. Cut logs on angle into ½-inch-thick slices. Place slices on sides on baking sheet; bake for 20 minutes or until lightly browned.

Makes 45 biscotti (1 biscotti per serving)

TIPS Instead of pecans, you can use almonds, hazelnuts, pine nuts or a combination.

When using margarine, choose a soft (non-hydrogenated) version to limit consumption of trans fats.

NUTRIENTS PER SERVING

Calories	79
Carbohydrate	13 g
Fiber	0 g
Protein	1 g
Fat, total	3 g
Fat, saturated	0 g
Cholesterol	8 mg
Sodium	644 mg

EXCHANGES PER SERVING

½ Starch
½ Other Carbohydrate
½ Fat

DIETITIAN'S NOTE *Sometimes you will get more or fewer biscotti than stated in the recipe. When this happens, see the cookie calculator on page xvi for help in determining how many cookies make up a serving.*

MAPLE WALNUT BISCOTTI

TIPS When grinding nuts in a food processor, add a little flour or sugar from your recipe to keep them from clumping.

Be sure biscotti are thoroughly dry and cool before packing or they will soften during storage.

VARIATIONS Replace walnuts with pecans.

Omit maple extract. Add 1 tbsp instant espresso coffee powder along with the flour mixture.

Preheat oven to 350°F
Baking sheet, greased or lined with parchment paper

2	cups all-purpose flour
⅓	cup ground walnuts
1¼	tsp baking powder
¼	tsp salt
2	eggs
½	cup packed brown sugar
¼	cup granulated sugar
½	cup vegetable oil
1	tsp maple extract
1	cup coarsely chopped walnuts

1. On a sheet of waxed paper or in a bowl, combine flour, ground walnuts, baking powder and salt. Set aside.

2. In a large bowl, using a wooden spoon, beat eggs, brown and granulated sugars, oil and maple extract until smoothly blended. Add flour mixture, stirring until smooth. Add walnuts. Using your hands, knead to form a smooth dough.

3. Divide dough into halves. Shape each into a roll 8 inches long. Place about 4 inches apart on prepared baking sheet. Flatten rolls to 3 inches wide, leaving top slightly rounded. Bake in preheated oven for 25 to 30 minutes or until light golden. Cool for 15 minutes on sheet, then transfer to a cutting board. Cut into ½-inch slices. Place cut side down on baking sheet. Bake for 10 minutes. Turn slices over and bake for 5 to 10 minutes or until crisp and golden. Cool for 5 minutes on sheet, then transfer to a rack and cool completely.

Makes 30 biscotti (1 biscotti per serving)

DIETITIAN'S NOTES *Did you get a different number of biscotti than the recipe states? Use the cookie calculator on page xvi to help you determine how many of your cookies match the nutrients and Exchanges displayed in the recipe.*

Parchment paper is a great invention. When you line a baking sheet with it, the cookies do not stick—and the baking sheet stays clean. You can use the same sheet of parchment paper several times when you're baking a large batch. If it starts to curl up, sprinkle or spray water on the baking sheet, then smooth the parchment over it.

NUTRIENTS PER SERVING

Calories	120
Carbohydrate	13 g
Fiber	1 g
Protein	2 g
Fat, total	7 g
Fat, saturated	1 g
Cholesterol	12 mg
Sodium	37 mg

EXCHANGES PER SERVING

½ Starch
½ Other Carbohydrate
1½ Fat

CHOCOLATE CHERRY BISCOTTI

BISCOTTI & SHORTBREAD

VARIATION If you don't have dried cherries, dried cranberries work really well.

NUTRIENTS PER SERVING

Calories	93
Carbohydrate	17 g
Fiber	1 g
Protein	2 g
Fat, total	2 g
Fat, saturated	1 g
Cholesterol	14 mg
Sodium	33 mg

EXCHANGES PER SERVING

½ Starch
½ Other Carbohydrate
½ Fat

Preheat oven to 350°F
Baking sheets, lined with parchment paper

3	cups all-purpose flour
2	tsp baking powder
¼	tsp salt
1	cup granulated sugar
3	eggs
2	tbsp vegetable oil
2	tsp vanilla
1½	tsp almond extract
1	cup semisweet chocolate chips
⅔	cup dried sour cherries

1. In a medium bowl, combine flour, baking powder and salt.

2. In a large bowl, using an electric mixer, beat sugar and eggs until thickened and pale, about 4 minutes. Add oil, vanilla and almond extract, beating just until blended. Add flour mixture, beating on low speed just until blended. Stir in chocolate chips and cherries.

3. Divide dough in half. Turn out dough onto prepared baking sheets. Shape each half into a 10-inch-long log and flatten to 1-inch thickness. Bake in preheated oven for 25 to 30 minutes or until lightly browned. Transfer logs to a rack. Let cool for 10 minutes. Reduce oven temperature to 325°F.

4. Transfer logs to a cutting board. Cut each log diagonally into ½-inch slices. Place slices, cut side down, on baking sheet. Bake for 15 to 20 minutes longer or until golden and toasted. The biscotti will be slightly soft in center but will harden as they cool. Transfer to racks and let cool completely.

Makes 40 biscotti (1 biscotti per serving)

CHOCOLATE CHIP ORANGE BISCOTTI

Preheat oven to 350°F
Baking sheets, lined with parchment paper

2¾	cups all-purpose flour
1	cup granulated sugar
2	tsp baking powder
1	tbsp vegetable oil
1	tbsp orange extract
2	tsp grated orange zest
1	tsp vanilla
3	eggs
1	cup semisweet chocolate chips

1. In a medium bowl, combine flour, sugar and baking powder.

2. In a large bowl, using an electric mixer, beat oil, orange extract, orange zest, vanilla and eggs until blended. Add flour mixture, beating until well blended. Stir in chocolate chips.

3. Divide dough in half. Turn out dough onto prepared baking sheets. Shape each half into a 10-inch-long log and flatten to 1-inch thickness. Bake in preheated oven for 25 to 30 minutes or until lightly browned. Transfer logs to a rack. Let cool for 10 minutes. Reduce oven temperature to 325°F.

4. Transfer logs to cutting board. Cut each log diagonally into ½-inch slices. Place slices, cut side down, on baking sheet. Bake for 15 to 20 minutes longer or until golden and toasted. The biscotti will be soft in center but will harden as they cool. Transfer to racks and let cool completely.

Makes 30 biscotti (1 biscotti per serving)

DIETITIAN'S NOTE *Unless otherwise stated, recipes are tested with large eggs. You may not get the same results if you use another size, especially in recipes, such as these biscotti, that contain a very small amount of liquid.*

NUTRIENTS PER SERVING

Calories	108
Carbohydrate	19 g
Fiber	1 g
Protein	2 g
Fat, total	3 g
Fat, saturated	1 g
Cholesterol	19 mg
Sodium	24 mg

EXCHANGES PER SERVING

½ Starch
½ Other Carbohydrate
½ Fat

TWO-TONE CHOCOLATE ORANGE BISCOTTI

TIPS If dough is sticky when forming into logs, try wetting your fingers.

Two colors of dough make these cookies very attractive.

When using margarine, choose a soft (non-hydrogenated) version to limit consumption of trans fats.

Freeze in containers for up to 6 weeks.

NUTRIENTS PER SERVING

Calories	74
Carbohydrate	13 g
Fiber	0 g
Protein	1 g
Fat, total	2 g
Fat, saturated	0 g
Cholesterol	9 mg
Sodium	40 mg

EXCHANGES PER SERVING

½ Starch

½ Other Carbohydrate

½ Fat

Preheat oven to 350°F
Baking sheet, sprayed with vegetable spray

1¼	cups granulated sugar
⅓	cup margarine or butter
2	eggs
2	tbsp orange juice concentrate
1	tbsp grated orange zest
2⅔	cups all-purpose flour
2½	tsp baking powder
3	tbsp unsweetened cocoa powder

1. In a food processor or in a bowl with an electric mixer, beat together sugar, margarine, eggs, orange juice concentrate and orange zest until smooth. Add flour and baking powder; mix just until combined.

2. Divide dough in half; to one half, add cocoa and mix well. Divide chocolate and plain doughs in half to produce 4 doughs. Roll each piece into a long, thin rope approximately 12 inches long and 1 inch wide. Use extra flour if too sticky. Place 1 cocoa dough on top of (or beside) each plain dough. (Ensure the plain and cocoa doughs touch one another.)

3. Bake for 20 minutes. Cool 10 minutes. Cut logs on an angle into ½-inch slices. Bake another 20 minutes.

Makes 40 biscotti (1 biscotti per serving)

GINGERBREAD BISCOTTI

Preheat oven to 350°F
Baking sheet, sprayed with vegetable spray

¾	cup packed brown sugar
¼	cup margarine or butter
¼	cup molasses
2	eggs
1	tsp vanilla
2⅓	cups all-purpose flour
2¼	tsp baking powder
1	tsp ground cinnamon
1	tsp ground ginger
½	tsp ground allspice
¼	tsp ground nutmeg

1. In a food processor or in a bowl with an electric mixer, beat together brown sugar, margarine, molasses, eggs and vanilla until smooth. In a separate bowl, stir together flour, baking powder, cinnamon, ginger, allspice and nutmeg. Add wet ingredients to dry ingredients, mixing just until combined.

2. Divide dough in half. Form each half into a log 12 inches long and 2 inches around; transfer to prepared baking sheet. Bake 20 minutes. Cool 10 minutes.

3. Cut logs on an angle into ½-inch slices. Bake for 20 minutes or until lightly browned.

Makes 40 biscotti (2 biscotti per serving)

DIETITIAN'S NOTE *If you choose to dip these biscotti in chocolate, each cookie will pick up about 1 gram of chocolate, which you don't need to count.*

TIPS To add fiber, use ⅔ cup whole wheat flour and 1⅔ cups all-purpose flour.

For a decadent treat, melt 2 oz semisweet chocolate and dip ends of cookies. Let harden.

NUTRIENTS PER SERVING

Calories	63
Carbohydrate	11 g
Fiber	0 g
Protein	1 g
Fat, total	1 g
Fat, saturated	0 g
Cholesterol	9 mg
Sodium	36 mg

EXCHANGES PER SERVING

½ Starch
½ Other Carbohydrate

CHOCOLATE-WRAPPED GINGER BISCOTTI

TIPS To distribute cocoa evenly and avoid streaks in a dough, knead the dough with your hands on a lightly floured surface.

Cocoa tends to lump during storage. Before mixing, even the smallest amount should be sifted to remove the lumps, as they won't disappear during baking.

A sharp serrated knife works best for cutting biscotti.

Preheat oven to 375°F
Baking sheet, greased or lined with parchment paper

2	cups all-purpose flour
2	tsp baking powder
¼	tsp salt
⅓	cup butter, softened
⅔	cup granulated sugar
2	eggs
2	tbsp unsweetened cocoa powder, sifted
¼	cup finely chopped crystallized ginger
½	cup miniature semisweet chocolate chips
¼	tsp ground ginger

1. On a sheet of waxed paper or in a bowl, combine flour, baking powder and salt. Set aside.

2. In a large bowl, using an electric mixer on medium speed, beat butter and sugar until light and creamy, about 3 minutes. Add eggs, one at a time, beating well after each addition. On low speed, gradually add flour mixture, beating until blended. Divide dough into halves. With a wooden spoon, stir cocoa powder and crystallized ginger into 1 portion and, using your hands, knead until thoroughly integrated. Add mini chocolate chips and ground ginger to the other portion and, using your hands, knead until thoroughly integrated.

3. Divide each portion into halves to make 4 portions. Between two sheets of waxed paper, roll 1 portion of chocolate dough into an 8- by 6-inch rectangle. Remove top sheet of waxed paper. Shape 1 portion of light dough into a roll 8 inches long. Place roll in the center of chocolate dough and wrap chocolate dough around it. Repeat with remaining dough and place the 2 rolls about 4 inches apart on prepared baking sheet. Flatten slightly, leaving top slightly rounded.

4. Bake in preheated oven for 35 to 40 minutes or until set. Cool for 15 minutes on sheet, then transfer to a cutting board. Reduce oven temperature to 325°F. Cut rolls into ½-inch slices. Place upright on baking sheet. Bake for 10 to 15 minutes or until crisp and center is light golden. Cool for 5 minutes on sheet, then transfer to a rack and cool completely.

Makes 30 biscotti (1 biscotti per serving)

DIETITIAN'S NOTES *Did you get a different number of biscotti than the recipe states? Use the cookie calculator on page xvi to help you determine how many of your cookies match the nutrients and Exchanges displayed in the recipe.*

The name of a food can tell us a lot, sometimes in a single word. "Biscotti" is an Italian word meaning "twice cooked" (bis cotti*). To make these hard, dry cookies, the dough is first baked in a loaf, then it is sliced and baked again.*

NUTRIENTS PER SERVING

Calories	98
Carbohydrate	15 g
Fiber	0 g
Protein	2 g
Fat, total	4 g
Fat, saturated	2 g
Cholesterol	18 mg
Sodium	63 mg

EXCHANGES PER SERVING

½ Starch
½ Other Carbohydrate
1 Fat

HOLIDAY BISCOTTI

TIP When using margarine, choose a non-hydrogenated version to limit consumption of trans fats.

VARIATION You can replace the orange zest with 1½ tbsp ground cardamom or 2 tbsp roasted fennel seeds. To roast seeds, place on a baking sheet and bake in preheated 350°F oven until they become aromatic but not brown, about 3 minutes.

Preheat oven to 325°F
Baking sheets, lined with parchment paper

2½	cups all-purpose flour
1	cup slivered almonds or pistachios
1	tbsp grated orange zest
1	tsp baking powder
½	tsp salt
2	eggs
¾	cup granulated sugar
½	cup margarine
2	tsp vanilla or almond extract

1. In a medium bowl, combine flour, almonds, orange zest, baking powder and salt.

2. In a large bowl, beat eggs, sugar, margarine and vanilla until slightly foamy. Fold in flour mixture.

3. Divide dough in half and shape each half into a log about 14 inches long and 2 inches wide. Place on prepared baking sheets. Smooth top and sides with clean hands.

4. Bake in preheated oven for 30 minutes. Remove from oven and reduce oven temperature to 275°F. Remove logs from baking sheets and let cool on a wire rack for 10 minutes.

5. Using a serrated knife, cut each log into ½-inch-thick slices. Place slices upright on baking sheets.

6. Bake for 20 to 25 minutes or until golden and crisp. Let cool on baking sheets on a wire rack for 5 minutes, then remove to rack to cool completely.

Makes 40 biscotti (1 biscotti per serving)

NUTRIENTS PER SERVING

Calories	82
Carbohydrate	10 g
Fiber	1 g
Protein	2 g
Fat, total	4 g
Fat, saturated	1 g
Cholesterol	9 mg
Sodium	70 mg

EXCHANGES PER SERVING

½	Starch
1	Fat

OATMEAL SHORTBREAD

TIP Most bars and squares should be cut after they've cooled, but shortbread and crisp bars should be cut while they're still warm to avoid shattering them. They may not, however, stay completely separated, which is why this recipe includes the instruction to "recut."

NUTRIENTS PER SERVING

Calories	61
Carbohydrate	7 g
Fiber	0 g
Protein	1 g
Fat, total	4 g
Fat, saturated	2 g
Cholesterol	9 mg
Sodium	36 mg

EXCHANGES PER SERVING

½ Starch

1 Fat

Preheat oven to 350°F
13- by 9-inch cake pan, ungreased

1	cup butter, softened
⅔	cup packed brown sugar
1½	cups all-purpose flour
1	tsp ground cinnamon
1¼	cups old-fashioned (large-flake) rolled oats

1. In a bowl, using an electric mixer on medium speed, beat butter and brown sugar until light and creamy, about 3 minutes. Stir in flour, cinnamon and oats, mixing well. Using your hands, knead to form a smooth dough. Press evenly into pan. Prick surface all over with a fork.

2. Bake in preheated oven until light golden, 25 to 30 minutes. Cut into bars or squares just as the pan comes out of the oven, then let cool completely in pan on rack. Recut.

Makes 54 bars (1 bar per serving)

DIETITIAN'S NOTE *In the past, one of the meanings of the word "short" was "crumbly," hence what we know as "shortbread." Its crumbly texture is a result of the high amount of fat (usually butter) in the recipe—two parts butter to one part sugar and three parts flour. Shortbread originated in Scotland, where it was first made with oat flour.*

ALMOND SPICE SHORTBREAD

Preheat oven to 300°F
13- by 9-inch cake pan, ungreased

1	cup butter, softened
¾	cup granulated sugar
1	egg, separated
½	tsp almond extract
2	cups all-purpose flour
1	tsp ground cinnamon
¼	tsp ground nutmeg
¾	cup sliced almonds

1. In a bowl, using an electric mixer on medium speed, beat butter, sugar, egg yolk and almond extract until smooth and creamy. Stir in flour, cinnamon and nutmeg, mixing well. Using your hands, knead to form a smooth dough. Press evenly into pan.

2. In a bowl, whisk egg white lightly (you don't want it to be frothy). Brush lightly over dough. Sprinkle almonds evenly over top.

3. Bake in preheated oven until light golden all over, 30 to 35 minutes. Cut into bars or squares just as the pan comes out of the oven, then let cool completely in pan on rack. Recut.

Makes 54 bars (1 bar per serving)

TIPS When creaming butter and sugar, it's important to have the butter at the right temperature. It should be a spreadable consistency. If it's too hard, it won't mix to a creamy, light texture, and if it's too soft, the dough will be too soft.

Due to the addition of an egg yolk, this dough is a little softer than regular shortbread dough. That's the advantage of bars—the pan holds the shape.

NUTRIENTS PER SERVING

Calories	67
Carbohydrate	7 g
Fiber	0 g
Protein	1 g
Fat, total	4 g
Fat, saturated	2 g
Cholesterol	13 mg
Sodium	36 mg

EXCHANGES PER SERVING

½	Starch
1	Fat

OATMEAL PECAN SHORTBREAD

TIPS Use quick-cooking oats, not instant or old-fashioned large-flake oats, in this recipe.

Use an offset spatula to transfer cookies that are more fragile, such as these, to and from baking sheets.

NUTRIENTS PER SERVING

Calories	115
Carbohydrate	12 g
Fiber	1 g
Protein	1 g
Fat, total	7 g
Fat, saturated	4 g
Cholesterol	16 mg
Sodium	61 mg

EXCHANGES PER SERVING

½ Starch
½ Other Carbohydrate
1½ Fat

Preheat oven to 300°F
2-inch cookie cutters
Baking sheet, ungreased

1½	cups	all-purpose flour
⅔	cup	quick-cooking rolled oats
½	cup	packed brown sugar
¼	cup	finely chopped pecans
½	tsp	ground cinnamon
¾	cup	butter, softened

1. In a large bowl, combine flour, oats, brown sugar, pecans and cinnamon. Mix well. With a wooden spoon, blend in butter until mixture is crumbly. Using your hands, knead to form a soft, smooth dough. If necessary, cover and chill for 30 minutes for easy rolling.

2. Divide dough into halves. On floured surface, roll out one portion at a time to ¼-inch thickness. Dip cutters in flour and cut into desired shapes. Place on baking sheet about 1 inch apart. Bake in preheated oven for 15 to 20 minutes or until light golden. Cool for 5 minutes on sheet, then transfer to a rack and cool completely.

Makes 24 pieces (2 pieces per serving)

DIETITIAN'S NOTE *The bend in the blade near the handle of an offset spatula helps you slide it more easily under what you are lifting.*

RICE FLOUR SHORTBREAD

Preheat oven to 300°F
8-inch square cake pan, ungreased

1½	cups all-purpose flour
⅓	cup superfine granulated sugar
⅓	cup rice flour
¼	tsp salt
¾	cup cold butter, cubed

1. In a bowl, combine all-purpose flour, sugar, rice flour and salt. Using a pastry blender, 2 knives or your fingers, work in butter until mixture resembles coarse crumbs. Knead dough on a lightly floured surface until very smooth, about 5 minutes. Press evenly into pan. Prick surface all over with a fork.

2. Bake in preheated oven until lightly browned around edges, 30 to 35 minutes. Cut into bars or squares just as the pan comes out of the oven, then let cool completely in pan on rack. Recut.

Makes 36 squares (1 square per serving)

NUTRIENTS PER SERVING

Calories	65
Carbohydrate	7 g
Fiber	0 g
Protein	1 g
Fat, total	4 g
Fat, saturated	2 g
Cholesterol	10 mg
Sodium	55 mg

EXCHANGES PER SERVING

½ Other Carbohydrate
1 Fat

CORNMEAL SHORTBREAD

NUTRIENTS PER SERVING

Calories	82
Carbohydrate	8 g
Fiber	0 g
Protein	1 g
Fat, total	5 g
Fat, saturated	3 g
Cholesterol	10 mg
Sodium	40 mg

EXCHANGES PER SERVING

½ Starch

1 Fat

Preheat oven to 350°F
9-inch square cake pan, ungreased

¾	cup whole unblanched almonds
½	cup yellow cornmeal
1¾	cups all-purpose flour
¾	cup granulated sugar
1	cup cold butter, cubed

1. In a food processor, pulse almonds until coarsely chopped. Add cornmeal, flour, sugar and butter. Pulse until mixture resembles coarse crumbs. Press three-quarters of the dough evenly into pan. Using your fingers, scatter remainder on top.

2. Bake in preheated oven until light golden, 25 to 30 minutes. Cut into bars or squares just as the pan comes out of the oven, then let cool completely in pan on rack. Recut.

Makes 48 bars (1 bar per serving)

CHUNKY CHOCOLATE SHORTBREAD

Preheat oven to 350°F
13- by 9-inch cake pan, ungreased

1	cup butter, softened
½	cup superfine granulated sugar
1¾	cups all-purpose flour
¼	cup cornstarch
4	squares (1 oz each) bittersweet chocolate, coarsely chopped
⅔	cup coarsely chopped pecans, toasted

1. In a bowl, beat butter and sugar until light and creamy. Combine flour and cornstarch. Stir into butter mixture, mixing well. Stir in chocolate and pecans. Press evenly into pan.

2. Bake in preheated oven until lightly browned around edges, 30 to 35 minutes. Let cool completely in pan on rack. Cut into bars or squares.

Makes 54 bars (1 bar per serving)

NUTRIENTS PER SERVING

Calories	76
Carbohydrate	7 g
Fiber	0 g
Protein	1 g
Fat, total	5 g
Fat, saturated	3 g
Cholesterol	9 mg
Sodium	35 mg

EXCHANGES PER SERVING

½	Other Carbohydrate
1	Fat

DIETITIAN'S NOTE *This recipe calls for superfine sugar, but it's not necessary to buy it. You can make it by processing granulated sugar in a blender or food processor until fine.*

COOKIES

75 Crispy Oatmeal Cookies
76 Oatmeal Orange Coconut Cookies
77 Cranberry Pecan Oatmeal Cookies
78 Oatmeal Raisin Cookies
79 Oatmeal Raisin Pecan Cookies
80 Oat Bran Raisin Cookies
81 Fruity Oatmeal Cookies
82 Oatmeal Lace Pennies
83 Oatmeal Date Cookies
84 Cranberry Orange Oatmeal Cookies
85 Crunchy Apricot Oat Drops
86 Date Roll-Up Cookies
88 Soft Apple Cinnamon Cookies
89 Lemon Lime Cookies
90 Lemon Poppy Seed Balls
91 Lemon Cranberry Pistachio Wafers
92 Orange Coffee Pecan Slices
93 Crisp Nut Cookies
94 Maple Walnut Slice 'n' Bake Cookies
96 Best-Ever Chocolate Cookies
97 Double Chocolate Raisin Cookies
98 Chocolate Chip Refrigerator Cookies

100 Rugelach (Cinnamon Chocolate Twist Cookies)
102 Cocoa Kisses
103 White Chocolate Cranberry Drops
104 Peanut Butter Cookies
105 Peanut Butter Flaxseed Cookies
106 Peanut Butter Fudge Cookies
107 Peanut Butter Chocolate Chip Cookies
108 Peanut Butter Chip Cookies
109 Applesauce Spice Cookies
110 Whole Wheat Spice Cookies
111 Ginger Cookies
112 Spicy Gingersnaps
114 Vanilla Almond Snaps
115 Sesame Seed Cookies
116 Sesame Snap Wafers
117 Diced Rhubarb Cookies
118 Charlie & Emma's Favorite Carrot Cookies
119 Meringue Candy Canes

CRISPY OATMEAL COOKIES

Preheat oven to 350°F
Stand mixer
Baking sheets, lined with parchment paper

1¼	cups unbleached all-purpose flour
1	tsp salt
1	tsp baking soda
1	tsp ground cinnamon
1½	cups unsalted butter, softened
1	cup lightly packed light brown sugar
½	cup granulated sugar
1	egg
1	tsp vanilla
3	cups old-fashioned rolled oats
2	cups walnut halves, chopped
1	cup dried cranberries

1. In a small bowl, whisk together flour, salt, baking soda and cinnamon.

2. Place butter in the mixer bowl. Attach the flat beater and mixer bowl to the mixer. Set to Speed 4 and beat until soft and creamy. Beat in brown sugar and granulated sugar until light and fluffy. Beat in egg and vanilla. Reduce speed to Stir and mix in flour mixture, in 3 additions. Mix in oats, walnuts and cranberries until evenly incorporated.

3. Drop by rounded teaspoonfuls, 2 inches apart, onto prepared baking sheets. Bake in middle of preheated oven for 8 to 10 minutes, or until lightly browned. Let cool on sheets for 5 minutes, then transfer to wire racks to cool completely.

Makes 72 cookies (1 cookie per serving)

DIETITIAN'S NOTE *You can use salted butter in this recipe, but you should then omit the salt. One-quarter cup salted butter contains about ¼ tsp salt.*

TIP Store in an airtight container in the freezer for up to 4 weeks.

VARIATION Substitute pecans or slivered almonds for the walnuts.

NUTRIENTS PER SERVING

Calories	96
Carbohydrate	10 g
Fiber	1 g
Protein	1 g
Fat, total	6 g
Fat, saturated	3 g
Cholesterol	13 mg
Sodium	53 mg

EXCHANGES PER SERVING

½ Other Carbohydrate
1 Fat

OATMEAL ORANGE COCONUT COOKIES

TIPS When using margarine, choose a soft (non-hydrogenated) version to limit consumption of trans fats.

Bake cookies up to a day ahead, keeping tightly covered in a cookie tin. Freeze cookie dough for up to 2 weeks.

NUTRIENTS PER SERVING

Calories	109
Carbohydrate	19 g
Fiber	1 g
Protein	1 g
Fat, total	3 g
Fat, saturated	1 g
Cholesterol	9 mg
Sodium	86 mg

EXCHANGES PER SERVING

½ Starch
½ Other Carbohydrate
½ Fat

Preheat oven to 350°F
Baking sheets, sprayed with vegetable spray

¼	cup margarine or butter
¼	cup brown sugar
½	cup granulated sugar
1	egg
1	tsp vanilla
2	tbsp orange juice concentrate, thawed
½	tsp grated orange zest
⅔	cup all-purpose flour
½	tsp baking powder
½	tsp baking soda
½	tsp ground cinnamon
1	cup corn flakes or bran flakes cereal
⅔	cup raisins
½	cup rolled oats
¼	cup coconut

1. In a large bowl, cream together margarine, brown sugar and granulated sugar. Add egg, vanilla, orange juice concentrate and orange zest and mix well.

2. In another bowl, combine flour, baking powder, baking soda, cinnamon, corn flakes, raisins, rolled oats and coconut just until combined. Add to sugar mixture and mix until just combined

3. Drop by heaping teaspoons onto prepared baking sheets, 2 inches apart, and press down with back of fork; bake for approximately 10 minutes or until browned.

Makes 40 cookies (2 cookies per serving)

DIETITIAN'S NOTE *The cookies will have more fiber if you use bran flakes. Flaked cereals can generally be substituted for one another, but bran flakes are not interchangeable with raw bran or the very high-fiber bran cereals.*

CRANBERRY PECAN OATMEAL COOKIES

Preheat oven to 350°F
Baking sheet, greased or lined with parchment paper

¾	cup all-purpose flour
¾	tsp baking soda
¼	tsp salt
1	tsp ground cinnamon
¾	cup butter, softened
¾	cup packed brown sugar
½	cup granulated sugar
1	egg
2	tbsp milk
3	cups quick-cooking rolled oats
1	cup dried cranberries
¾	cup chopped pecans
⅓	cup sunflower seeds

1. On a sheet of waxed paper or in a bowl, combine flour, baking soda, salt and cinnamon. Set aside.

2. In a large bowl, using an electric mixer on medium speed, beat butter, brown and granulated sugars, egg and milk until light and creamy, about 3 minutes. On low speed, gradually add flour mixture, beating until blended. With a wooden spoon, stir in oats, cranberries, pecans and sunflower seeds.

3. Drop dough by tablespoonfuls, about 2 inches apart, on prepared baking sheet. Press flat with a fork dipped in flour. Bake in preheated oven for 11 to 15 minutes (see Tip). Cool for 5 minutes on sheet, then transfer to a rack and cool completely.

Makes 48 cookies (1 cookie per serving)

TIP Bake the minimum time for chewy cookies. They will look like they are not quite done when you take them out of the oven, but they will continue to cook on the sheet. Bake longer, until golden, if you prefer crisp cookies.

VARIATION Omit cinnamon. Replace milk with orange juice and 1 tbsp grated orange zest.

NUTRIENTS PER SERVING

Calories	104
Carbohydrate	14 g
Fiber	1 g
Protein	2 g
Fat, total	5 g
Fat, saturated	2 g
Cholesterol	12 mg
Sodium	65 mg

EXCHANGES PER SERVING

1 Other Carbohydrates
1 Fat

OATMEAL RAISIN COOKIES

NUTRIENTS PER SERVING

Calories	160
Carbohydrate	24 g
Fiber	2 g
Protein	3 g
Fat, total	6 g
Fat, saturated	4 g
Cholesterol	34 mg
Sodium	79 mg

EXCHANGES PER SERVING

½ Fruit
1 Other Carbohydrates
1 Fat

Preheat oven to 375°F
Baking sheet, sprayed with baking spray

6	tbsp packed brown sugar
¼	cup butter, softened
1	egg
1	tsp vanilla
½	cup rolled oats
½	cup raisins
¼	cup whole wheat flour
¼	cup wheat germ
½	tsp baking powder

1. In a bowl, cream brown sugar with butter. Beat in egg and vanilla. In another bowl, stir together oats, raisins, whole wheat flour, wheat germ and baking powder. Stir into creamed mixture just until blended.

2. Drop batter by teaspoonfuls onto prepared baking sheet, leaving 2 inches between cookies. Bake for 10 to 12 minutes or until golden. Cool on wire racks.

Makes 18 cookies (2 cookies per serving)

DIETITIAN'S NOTE *Wheat germ is the nutritious heart of a wheat kernel. Together with fiber-containing bran, it is removed when white flour is manufactured. To avoid rancidity, buy wheat germ in small quantities and keep it in the refrigerator.*

OATMEAL RAISIN PECAN COOKIES

Preheat oven to 350°F
Baking sheets, sprayed with nonstick vegetable spray

½	cup brown sugar
¼	cup soft margarine
1	egg
1	tsp vanilla
½	cup rolled oats
¼	cup whole wheat flour
¼	cup wheat germ
¼	cup pecan pieces
¼	cup raisins
½	tsp baking powder

1. In a large bowl or food processor, beat together brown sugar, margarine, egg and vanilla until well blended.

2. Add rolled oats, flour, wheat germ, pecans, raisins and baking powder; mix just until incorporated.

3. Drop by heaping teaspoonfuls, 2 inches apart, onto prepared baking sheets. Bake for 12 to 15 minutes or until browned.

Makes 30 cookies (2 cookies per serving)

TIPS These cookies are soft and chewy if baked for a shorter time; crisp if baked longer.

If wheat germ is not available, substitute another ¼ cup rolled oats.

When using margarine, choose a soft (non-hydrogenated) version.

Dough can be frozen for up to 2 weeks.

NUTRIENTS PER SERVING

Calories	106
Carbohydrate	14 g
Fiber	1 g
Protein	2 g
Fat, total	5 g
Fat, saturated	1 g
Cholesterol	12 mg
Sodium	57 mg

EXCHANGES PER SERVING

1 Other Carbohydrates

1 Fat

OAT BRAN RAISIN COOKIES

TIP This recipe makes a smaller batch of cookies than usual, but it can be doubled, if desired.

NUTRIENTS PER SERVING

Calories	86
Carbohydrate	12 g
Fiber	1 g
Protein	2 g
Fat, total	4 g
Fat, saturated	1 g
Sodium	53 mg
Cholesterol	0 mg

EXCHANGES PER SERVING

⅔ Other Carbohydrate

½ Fat

Preheat oven to 350°F
Greased cookie sheet

⅔	cup uncooked oat bran cereal
¼	cup old-fashioned rolled oats
3	tbsp all-purpose flour
½	tsp baking powder
3	tbsp softened margarine
¼	cup firmly packed brown sugar
1	egg white, lightly beaten
2	tsp water
¼	tsp vanilla
2	tbsp raisins

1. In a bowl, mix together oat bran, rolled oats, flour and baking powder.

2. In another bowl, beat together margarine and brown sugar until smooth and creamy. Stir in egg white, water and vanilla, mixing until thoroughly incorporated. Add flour mixture and mix well. Fold in raisins.

3. Drop by level tablespoonfuls, about 2 inches apart, onto prepared cookie sheet. Using a fork or the bottom of a glass, flatten slightly. Bake in preheated oven for 12 to 15 minutes or until bottoms are slightly browned. Cool on sheet for 3 minutes, then transfer to wire racks to cool completely.

Makes about 1 dozen cookies (1 per serving)

FRUITY OATMEAL COOKIES

Preheat oven to 350°F
Baking sheets, lightly greased or lined with parchment paper

2	cups old-fashioned rolled oats
1¼	cups whole wheat flour
1	cup semisweet chocolate chips
1	cup dried fruit
¾	cup ground flaxseed
1	tsp baking soda
½	tsp salt
2	large bananas, mashed
¾	cup liquid honey
½	cup margarine

1. In a large bowl, combine oats, flour, chocolate chips, dried fruit, flaxseed, baking soda and salt.

2. In another large bowl, combine bananas, honey and margarine. Fold in oats mixture.

3. Drop dough by tablespoonfuls, about 2 inches apart, onto prepared baking sheets. Flatten with a fork.

4. Bake in preheated oven for about 10 minutes or until lightly browned. Let cool on baking sheets on a wire rack for 5 minutes, then remove to rack to cool completely.

Makes 36 cookies (1 cookie per serving)

TIP When using margarine, choose a non-hydrogenated version to limit consumption of trans fats.

VARIATIONS Replace the semisweet chocolate chips with white chocolate or butterscotch chips, or leave them out entirely for a fruitier cookie.

Try rice syrup or fancy molasses instead of honey.

NUTRIENTS PER SERVING

Calories	130
Carbohydrate	20 g
Fiber	2 g
Protein	2 g
Fat, total	5 g
Fat, saturated	1 g
Cholesterol	0 mg
Sodium	104 mg

EXCHANGES PER SERVING

½	Starch
1	Other Carbohydrates
1	Fat

OATMEAL LACE PENNIES

**NUTRIENTS
PER SERVING**

Calories	32
Carbohydrate	4 g
Fiber	0 g
Protein	0 g
Fat, total	2 g
Fat, saturated	1 g
Sodium	32 mg
Cholesterol	7 mg

**EXCHANGES
PER SERVING**

½ Other Carbohydrate
½ Fat

Preheat oven to 350°F
Cookie sheet lined with foil, bright side up

1	cup old-fashioned rolled oats
1	cup granulated sugar
3	tbsp all-purpose flour
¼	tsp baking powder
½	tsp salt
1	egg, beaten
½	cup margarine or butter, melted
½	tsp vanilla

1. In a bowl, mix together oats, sugar, flour, baking powder and salt.

2. In another bowl, beat egg, margarine and vanilla. Add flour mixture and mix well. (If dough seems too soft, chill for 15 to 20 minutes to firm.)

3. Drop by rounded teaspoonfuls, about 2 inches apart, onto prepared cookie sheet. Bake in preheated oven for 8 to 10 minutes. Cool for 2 minutes on foil, then transfer to wire racks to cool completely.

Makes about 5 ½ dozen cookies (1 per serving)

OATMEAL DATE COOKIES

Preheat oven to 350°F
Baking sheets, sprayed with vegetable spray

⅓	cup margarine or butter
⅓	cup granulated sugar
1	egg
1	tsp vanilla
⅔	cup all-purpose flour
1	tsp baking powder
¾	tsp ground cinnamon
¾	cup rolled oats
¾	cup bran flakes or corn flakes cereal
⅔	cup chopped pitted dates

1. In a large bowl, cream together margarine and sugar. Add egg and vanilla and mix well.

2. In another bowl, combine flour, baking powder, cinnamon, rolled oats, cereal and dates. Add to sugar mixture and mix until just combined.

3. Drop by heaping teaspoonfuls onto prepared baking sheets, 2 inches apart, and press down with back of fork; bake for approximately 10 minutes or until browned.

Makes 32 cookies (2 cookies per serving)

NUTRIENTS PER SERVING

Calories	117
Carbohydrate	18 g
Fiber	1 g
Protein	2 g
Fat, total	5 g
Fat, saturated	1 g
Cholesterol	12 mg
Sodium	84 mg

EXCHANGES PER SERVING

½ Starch
½ Fruit
1 Fat

DIETITIAN'S NOTES *For baking, use one of the soft, non-hydrogenated margarines. They contain 55% to 80% less saturated fat than butter and no trans fat. Do not use margarines that come in a stick or block; they are high in saturated and trans fat.*

Flaked cereals can generally be substituted for one another, but bran flakes are not interchangeable with raw bran or the very high-fiber bran cereals. For maximum fiber, use bran flakes in this recipe.

CRANBERRY ORANGE OATMEAL COOKIES

TIP Freeze cranberries before chopping or grinding them to ease cleanup.

NUTRIENTS PER SERVING

Calories	86
Carbohydrate	13 g
Fiber	1 g
Protein	1 g
Fat, total	4 g
Fat, saturated	1 g
Sodium	69 mg
Cholesterol	7 mg

EXCHANGES PER SERVING

½	Starch
⅓	Other Carbohydrate
½	Fat

Preheat oven to 375°F
Greased cookie sheet

2	cups all-purpose flour
1	tsp baking powder
¼	tsp baking soda
½	tsp salt
2	cups quick-cooking oats
1	cup softened margarine or butter
1½	cups granulated sugar
2	eggs
1	tsp vanilla
1	cup raisins
1	cup coarsely chopped cranberries, fresh or frozen
1	tbsp grated orange zest

1. In a bowl, mix together flour, baking powder, baking soda, salt and oats.

2. In another bowl, beat margarine and sugar until smooth and creamy. Beat in eggs, one at a time, until well incorporated. Mix in vanilla. Add flour mixture and mix well. Fold in raisins, cranberries and orange zest.

3. Drop by rounded teaspoonfuls, about 2 inches apart, onto prepared cookie sheet. Bake in preheated oven for 10 to 12 minutes or until edges are lightly browned. Immediately transfer to wire racks to cool.

Makes about 5 dozen cookies (1 per serving)

CRUNCHY APRICOT OAT DROPS

Preheat oven to 350°F
Baking sheet, greased or lined with parchment paper

¾	cup unbleached all-purpose flour
½	tsp baking soda
¼	tsp salt
½	tsp ground cinnamon
½	cup butter, softened
¾	cup packed brown sugar
1	egg
¾	cup quick-cooking rolled oats
⅓	cup wheat germ
1	cup crisp rice cereal
¾	cup chopped dried apricots
⅓	cup unsweetened flaked coconut
¼	cup sunflower seeds

1. On a sheet of waxed paper or in a bowl, combine flour, baking soda, salt and cinnamon. Set aside.

2. In a large bowl, using an electric mixer on medium speed, beat butter, brown sugar and egg until light and creamy, about 3 minutes. On low speed, gradually add flour mixture, beating until blended. With a wooden spoon, stir in oats and wheat germ. Add cereal, apricots, coconut and sunflower seeds. Mix well.

3. Drop dough by tablespoonfuls, about 2 inches apart, onto prepared baking sheet. Bake in preheated oven for 8 to 12 minutes or until golden. Cool for 5 minutes on sheet, then transfer to a rack and cool completely.

Makes 36 cookies (2 cookies per serving)

TIPS Do not use light or whipped margarine when baking. These products are lower in fat and often contain water, which may result in baked goods that aren't acceptable.

When baking, always place cookie dough on a cool sheet. Cookies will spread too much if the sheet is warm.

VARIATION Replace apricots with dried cranberries, raisins or chopped dates.

NUTRIENTS PER SERVING

Calories	171
Carbohydrate	24 g
Fiber	2 g
Protein	3 g
Fat, total	8 g
Fat, saturated	4 g
Cholesterol	24 mg
Sodium	145 mg

EXCHANGES PER SERVING

½	Starch
1	Other Carbohydrates
1½	Fat

DATE ROLL-UP COOKIES

TIPS For maximum freshness, store cookies in airtight containers in the freezer; remove as needed.

Try this recipe with dried figs or apricots.

When using margarine, choose a soft (non-hydrogenated) version to limit consumption of trans fats.

Prepare date mixture and freeze until needed.

Preheat oven to 350°F
Large baking sheet, sprayed with vegetable spray

Filling

8 oz	pitted dates
1	cup orange juice
¼	tsp ground cinnamon

Dough

2 ¼	cups all-purpose flour
⅔	cup granulated sugar
¼	cup margarine or butter
¼	cup vegetable oil
¼	cup 2% plain yogurt
3	tbsp water
1	tsp vanilla
1	tsp grated orange zest

1. *Filling:* In a saucepan, bring dates, orange juice and cinnamon to a boil; reduce heat to medium-low and cook 10 minutes or until soft. Mash with a fork until liquid is absorbed. Refrigerate.

2. *Dough:* In a food processor, combine flour, sugar, margarine, oil, yogurt, water, vanilla and orange zest; process until dough forms. Add up to 1 tbsp more water, if necessary. Divide dough in half; form each half into a ball, wrap and refrigerate for 15 minutes or until chilled.

3. Between 2 sheets of waxed paper sprinkled with flour, roll one of the dough balls into a rectangle, approximately 12 by 10 inches and ⅛ inch thick. Remove top sheet of waxed paper. Spread half of date mixture over rolled dough. Starting at short end and using the waxed paper as an aid, roll up tightly. Cut into ½-inch slices and place on prepared baking sheet. Repeat with remaining dough and filling.

4. Bake 25 minutes or until lightly browned.

Makes 32 cookies (1 cookie per serving)

DIETITIAN'S NOTE *We are all familiar with peanut butter, but "butter" can also be made from other nuts, including cashews and almonds. Regardless of the type of nut, or whether it's smooth or chunky, all nut butters contain 8 to 10 grams of fat per tablespoon. The unsalted varieties contain almost no sodium, but salted varieties have around 80 milligrams of sodium per tablespoon.*

NUTRIENTS PER SERVING

Calories	101
Carbohydrate	17 g
Fiber	1 g
Protein	1 g
Fat, total	3 g
Fat, saturated	0 g
Cholesterol	0 mg
Sodium	21 mg

EXCHANGES PER SERVING

½ Fruit
½ Other Carbohydrate
½ Fat

SOFT APPLE CINNAMON COOKIES

**NUTRIENTS
PER SERVING**

Calories	86
Carbohydrate	13 g
Fiber	1 g
Protein	1 g
Fat, total	3 g
Fat, saturated	2 g
Cholesterol	15 mg
Sodium	76 mg

**EXCHANGES
PER SERVING**

1 Other Carbohydrates
½ Fat

Preheat oven to 400°F
Baking sheets, lightly greased or lined with parchment paper

2	cups all-purpose flour
1	tbsp ground cinnamon
1	tsp baking powder
½	tsp baking soda
½	tsp salt
3	large apples (unpeeled), grated
1	cup packed brown sugar
⅔	cup butter
2	eggs
½	cup sour milk or buttermilk
2	cups quick-cooking rolled oats

1. In a small bowl, sift together flour, cinnamon, baking powder, baking soda and salt.

2. Sprinkle grated apples with ½ cup of the flour mixture.

3. In a large bowl, cream brown sugar and butter. Add eggs, one at a time, beating well after each addition. Add milk, then oats, and blend well. Fold in remaining flour mixture. Stir in apples.

4. Drop dough by tablespoonfuls, about 2 inches apart, onto prepared baking sheets.

5. Bake in preheated oven for 8 to 10 minutes or until lightly browned. Let cool on baking sheets on a wire rack for 5 minutes, then remove to rack to cool completely.

Makes 48 cookies (1 cookie per serving)

DIETITIAN'S NOTE *To make ½ cup sour milk, place 1½ tsp vinegar or lemon juice in a measuring cup and add milk to make up the full amount. Let stand for 5 minutes before using.*

LEMON LIME COOKIES

Preheat oven to 350°F
2-inch round cookie cutter
Baking sheet, ungreased

3½	cups all-purpose flour
2	tsp baking powder
½	tsp salt
1	cup butter, softened
1¼	cups granulated sugar
2	eggs
2	tbsp grated lemon zest
2	tbsp grated lime zest
½	tsp lemon extract

1. On a sheet of waxed paper or in a bowl, combine flour, baking powder and salt. Set aside.

2. In a large bowl, using an electric mixer on medium speed, beat butter and sugar until light and creamy, about 3 minutes. Add eggs, one at a time, beating well after each addition. Add lemon zest, lime zest and lemon extract. On low speed, gradually add flour mixture, beating until dough becomes too stiff for the mixer, then finish mixing with a wooden spoon. Using your hands, knead to form a smooth dough.

3. On a floured surface, roll out dough to ⅛-inch thickness. Using cutter dipped in flour, cut into rounds. Place about 1 inch apart on baking sheet. Bake in preheated oven for 7 to 11 minutes or until lightly browned around edges. Cool for 5 minutes on sheet, then transfer to a rack and cool completely.

Makes 72 cookies (2 cookies per serving)

TIPS I prefer combining the dry ingredients on a piece of waxed paper instead of dirtying a bowl. Then I use the paper as a funnel when adding them to the butter mixture.

Try not to use too much flour when rolling. It will toughen any dough. You need just enough on the surface of the dough, your hands and the rolling pin to prevent sticking. If you use a pastry cloth and rolling pin cover, you'll have no problems with the dough sticking.

NUTRIENTS PER SERVING

Calories	121
Carbohydrate	16 g
Fiber	0 g
Protein	2 g
Fat, total	6 g
Fat, saturated	3 g
Cholesterol	24 mg
Sodium	103 mg

EXCHANGES PER SERVING

½	Starch
½	Other Carbohydrate
1	Fat

LEMON POPPY SEED BALLS

COOKIES

VARIATION For a plain cookie, omit the poppy seeds and lemon zest. Add 1 tsp vanilla or ½ tsp almond extract.

NUTRIENTS PER SERVING

Calories	144
Carbohydrate	16 g
Fiber	1 g
Protein	2 g
Fat, total	8 g
Fat, saturated	5 g
Cholesterol	28 mg
Sodium	105 mg

EXCHANGES PER SERVING

½ Starch
½ Other Carbohydrate
1½ Fat

Preheat oven to 325°F
Baking sheet, ungreased

2½	cups all-purpose flour
2	tbsp poppy seeds
¼	tsp salt
1	cup butter, softened
⅔	cup granulated sugar
1	egg
1	tbsp grated lemon zest

1. On a sheet of waxed paper or in a bowl, combine flour, poppy seeds and salt. Set aside.

2. In a large bowl, using an electric mixer on medium speed, beat butter, sugar, egg and lemon zest until light and creamy, about 3 minutes. On low speed, gradually add flour mixture, beating until dough becomes too stiff for the mixer, then finish mixing with a wooden spoon until smooth. Using your hands, knead to form a smooth dough.

3. Shape dough into 1-inch balls. Place about 1 inch apart on baking sheet. Bake in preheated oven for 15 to 19 minutes or until golden around edges. Cool for 5 minutes on sheet, then transfer to a rack and cool completely.

Makes 48 cookies (2 cookies per serving)

LEMON CRANBERRY PISTACHIO WAFERS

Baking sheet, ungreased

1¾	cups all-purpose flour
¼	tsp baking powder
¼	tsp salt
¾	cup butter, softened
½	cup confectioner's sugar, sifted
1	egg
1	tbsp grated lemon zest
⅓	cup finely chopped pistachios
¼	cup chopped dried cranberries

1. On a sheet of waxed paper or in a bowl, combine flour, baking powder and salt. Set aside.

2. In a large bowl, using an electric mixer on medium speed, beat butter, confectioner's sugar, egg and lemon zest until light and creamy, about 3 minutes. On low speed, gradually add flour mixture, beating until blended. With a wooden spoon, stir in pistachios and cranberries. Shape into a roll 12 inches long. Wrap and chill until firm, at least 3 hours.

3. Fifteen minutes before you're ready to bake, preheat oven to 375°F. Cut roll into ¼-inch slices. Place about 1 inch apart on baking sheet. Bake in preheated oven for 8 to 12 minutes or until golden. Cool for 5 minutes on sheet, then transfer to a rack and cool completely.

Makes 48 cookies (3 cookies per serving)

TIPS In refrigerator rolls, ingredients like nuts and fruit are much easier to slice if they are chopped fairly fine.

When cutting dough, always ensure that your knife is sharp. I prefer to use a serrated knife for this dough as it contains nuts.

VARIATIONS Replace lemon zest with orange zest.

Replace dried cranberries with dried cherries.

NUTRIENTS PER SERVING

Calories	166
Carbohydrate	17 g
Fiber	1 g
Protein	2 g
Fat, total	10 g
Fat, saturated	6 g
Cholesterol	35 mg
Sodium	133 mg

EXCHANGES PER SERVING

1 Other Carbohydrates
2 Fat

ORANGE COFFEE PECAN SLICES

TIPS Be sure to remove the zest from oranges and lemons before you cut them to squeeze out the juice. Oranges with a thick, rough skin will give you more zest, but less juice.

One orange should give you about ⅓ cup juice and 4 tsp grated zest.

A thin knife is usually the best choice for cutting dough, but if it contains chunky ingredients, you may find a serrated knife works better. Just make sure your knife is sharp.

NUTRIENTS PER SERVING

Calories	129
Carbohydrate	16 g
Fiber	1 g
Protein	1 g
Fat, total	7 g
Fat, saturated	3 g
Cholesterol	12 mg
Sodium	81 mg

EXCHANGES PER SERVING

1 Other Carbohydrates
1½ Fat

Baking sheet, greased or lined with parchment paper

2¾	cups all-purpose flour
1	tbsp instant espresso coffee powder
2	tsp baking powder
¼	tsp salt
¾	cup butter, softened
1	cup packed brown sugar
1	tbsp grated orange zest
¼	cup orange juice
1	cup chopped pecans

1. On a sheet of waxed paper or in a bowl, combine flour, coffee powder, baking powder and salt. Set aside.

2. In a large bowl, using an electric mixer on medium speed, beat butter, brown sugar and orange zest and juice until smooth. On low speed, gradually add flour mixture, beating until blended. With a wooden spoon, stir in pecans. Divide dough into halves. Shape each into a roll 12 inches long. Wrap and chill until firm, at least 2 hours.

3. Fifteen minutes before you're ready to bake, preheat oven to 375°F. Cut rolls into ¼-inch slices. Place about 1 inch apart on prepared baking sheet. Bake in preheated oven for 7 to 11 minutes or until golden around edges. Cool for 5 minutes on sheet, then transfer to a rack and cool completely.

Makes 96 cookies (3 cookies per serving)

CRISP NUT COOKIES

Preheat oven to 350°F
Baking sheet, sprayed with baking spray

2	eggs
¾	cup granulated sugar
6	tbsp melted butter
¼	cup water
2	tsp vanilla
1	tsp almond extract
2½	cups all-purpose flour
½	cup chopped nuts
2¼	tsp baking powder

1. In a bowl, beat eggs with sugar until well mixed. Beat in butter, water, vanilla and almond extract.

2. In another bowl, stir together flour, nuts and baking powder. Stir into egg-sugar mixture until dough forms a ball. Divide dough in half. Form each half into a log 12 inches long. Put on prepared baking sheet.

3. Bake for 20 minutes. Cool for 5 minutes. Cut on the diagonal into ½-inch-thick slices. Bake for 20 minutes or until golden.

Makes 45 cookies (3 cookies per serving)

TIP Use almonds, pecans, pine nuts or a combination.

NUTRIENTS PER SERVING

Calories	129
Carbohydrate	18 g
Fiber	1 g
Protein	2 g
Fat, total	5 g
Fat, saturated	2 g
Cholesterol	25 mg
Sodium	63 mg

EXCHANGES PER SERVING

1	Other Carbohydrates
1	Fat

MAPLE WALNUT SLICE 'N' BAKE COOKIES

TIPS Although it's not as common as some other extracts, maple extract is an excellent product with a true maple flavor. It's sold in grocery stores where you find vanilla.

To get perfectly round cookies, pack the dough into an appropriate-size used roll from waxed paper, plastic wrap or aluminum foil. Once chilled, simply cut the tube open. When using frozen rolls of dough, let them thaw in the refrigerator overnight or for about 1 hour at room temperature, until they can be sliced easily.

VARIATION Replace maple extract with vanilla and walnuts with pecans.

Baking sheet, ungreased

2⅔	cups all-purpose flour
1	tsp baking powder
½	tsp baking soda
¼	tsp salt
1	cup butter, softened
½	cup granulated sugar
½	cup packed brown sugar
2	eggs
1½	tsp maple extract
1½	cups chopped walnuts

1. On a sheet of waxed paper or in a bowl, combine flour, baking powder, baking soda and salt. Set aside.

2. In a large bowl, using an electric mixer on medium speed, beat butter, granulated and brown sugars, eggs and maple extract until light and creamy, about 3 minutes. On low speed, gradually add flour mixture, beating until blended. With a wooden spoon, stir in walnuts. Divide dough into halves. Shape each into a roll 12 inches long. Wrap and chill until firm, at least 4 hours.

3. Fifteen minutes before you're ready to bake, preheat oven to 375°F. Cut rolls into ¼-inch slices. Place about 1 inch apart on baking sheet. Bake in preheated oven for 8 to 12 minutes or until lightly browned. Cool for 5 minutes on sheet, then transfer to a rack and cool completely.

Makes 96 cookies (3 cookies per serving)

NUTRIENTS PER SERVING

Calories	155
Carbohydrate	16 g
Fiber	1 g
Protein	2 g
Fat, total	10 g
Fat, saturated	4 g
Cholesterol	27 mg
Sodium	111 mg

EXCHANGES PER SERVING

½	Starch
½	Other Carbohydrate
2	Fat

BEST-EVER CHOCOLATE COOKIES

TIP When using margarine, choose a non-hydrogenated version to limit consumption of trans fats.

NUTRIENTS PER SERVING

Calories	207
Carbohydrate	24 g
Fiber	2 g
Protein	3 g
Fat, total	12 g
Fat, saturated	3 g
Cholesterol	18 g
Sodium	247 mg

EXCHANGES PER SERVING

½ Starch
1 Other Carbohydrates
2½ Fat

Preheat oven to 350°F
Baking sheets, ungreased

1	cup all-purpose flour
½	cup unsweetened cocoa powder
1	tsp baking soda
¼	tsp salt
2	eggs
1	cup margarine or butter, softened
¾	cup packed brown sugar
1½	cups quick-cooking rolled oats
1	cup bran cereal (not flakes)
¾	cup white chocolate chips

1. In a small bowl, sift flour, cocoa powder, baking soda and salt.

2. In a large bowl, beat eggs, margarine and brown sugar. Fold in flour mixture. Stir in oats, bran cereal and white chocolate chips.

3. Drop dough by heaping tablespoonfuls, about 2 inches apart, onto baking sheets.

4. Bake in preheated oven for 7 to 9 minutes or until just crisp. Let cool on baking sheets on a wire rack for 5 minutes, then remove to rack to cool completely.

Makes 42 cookies (2 cookies per serving)

DOUBLE CHOCOLATE RAISIN COOKIES

Preheat oven to 350°F
Baking sheets, sprayed with nonstick vegetable spray

¼	cup soft margarine
¾	cup granulated sugar
1	egg
1	tsp vanilla
3	tbsp unsweetened cocoa powder
½	tsp baking soda
½	tsp baking powder
½	cup whole wheat flour
¾	cup all-purpose flour
¼	cup chocolate chips
¼	cup raisins

1. In a large bowl or food processor, beat together margarine, sugar, egg and vanilla until well blended.

2. Combine cocoa, baking soda, baking powder, whole wheat and all-purpose flours; add to bowl and mix until just combined. Stir in chocolate chips and raisins.

3. Drop by heaping teaspoonfuls, 2 inches apart, onto prepared baking sheets. Bake for 12 to 15 minutes or until browned.

Makes 40 cookies (2 cookies per serving)

TIPS Try white chocolate or peanut butter chips for a change.

When using margarine, choose a soft (non-hydrogenated) version to limit consumption of trans fats.

Dough can be frozen for up to 2 weeks.

NUTRIENTS PER SERVING

Calories	99
Carbohydrate	17 g
Fiber	1 g
Protein	2 g
Fat, total	3 g
Fat, saturated	1 g
Cholesterol	9 mg
Sodium	73 mg

EXCHANGES PER SERVING

1 Other Carbohydrates
½ Fat

CHOCOLATE CHIP REFRIGERATOR COOKIES

TIPS When chilling, wrap dough in waxed paper or plastic wrap.

The chocolate chips make cutting a bit difficult, but not to worry. If the rounds aren't even, reshape them on the baking sheet with your fingers. The cookies will look great when baked and taste even better.

Rolls of cookie dough can also be frozen. Thaw for about an hour at room temperature or in the refrigerator overnight, until the dough can be sliced easily.

VARIATIONS Use milk chocolate chips or miniature semisweet chocolate chips.

Omit nuts or replace pecans with your favorite nut.

Baking sheet, ungreased

2¾	cups all-purpose flour
1	tsp baking soda
¼	tsp baking powder
¼	tsp salt
1	cup butter, softened
1	cup packed brown sugar
½	cup granulated sugar
2	eggs
1	tsp vanilla
1	cup semisweet chocolate chips
½	cup finely chopped pecans

1. On a sheet of waxed paper or in a bowl, combine flour, baking soda, baking powder, and salt. Set aside.

2. In a large bowl, using an electric mixer on medium speed, beat butter and brown and granulated sugars until light and creamy, about 3 minutes. Add eggs, one at a time, beating well after each addition. Add vanilla. On low speed, gradually add flour mixture, beating until blended. With a wooden spoon, stir in chocolate chips and pecans. Divide dough into halves. Shape each into a roll 12 inches long. Wrap and chill until firm, at least 4 hours.

3. Fifteen minutes before you're ready to bake, preheat oven to 350°F. Cut rolls into ¼-inch slices. Place about 2 inches apart on baking sheet. Bake in preheated oven for 8 to 12 minutes or until light golden. Cool for 5 minutes on sheet, then transfer to a rack and cool completely.

Makes 96 cookies (2 cookies per serving)

DIETITIAN'S NOTE *Finely chopping the pecans will make it easier to slice the cookies. It also spreads them more evenly through the batter, giving you more of their delicious flavor with every bite. The same rule holds true for chocolate chips, so use mini chips when you can. One cup of mini chocolate chips has the same weight and nutrients as 1 cup of regular chocolate chips.*

NUTRIENTS PER SERVING

Calories	114
Carbohydrate	14 g
Fiber	1 g
Protein	1 g
Fat, total	6 g
Fat, saturated	3 g
Cholesterol	18 mg
Sodium	84 mg

EXCHANGES PER SERVING

1 Other Carbohydrates

1 Fat

RUGELACH (CINNAMON CHOCOLATE TWIST COOKIES)

TIPS These traditionally high-fat cookies are lower in fat and calories because we've used yogurt instead of cream cheese, and cocoa instead of chocolate.

These are best eaten the day they are made; any leftover cookies are best eaten biscotti fashion, dipped in coffee.

When using margarine, choose a soft (non-hydrogenated) version to limit consumption of trans fats.

Prepare dough and freeze for up to 2 weeks. Bake cookies up to a day ahead, keeping tightly covered.

Preheat oven to 350°F
Baking sheets, sprayed with vegetable spray

2 ¼	cups all-purpose flour
⅔	cup granulated sugar
½	cup cold margarine or butter
⅓	cup 2% yogurt
3–4	tbsp water
½	cup brown sugar
⅓	cup raisins
2	tbsp semisweet chocolate chips
1	tbsp unsweetened cocoa powder
½	tsp ground cinnamon

1. In a bowl, combine flour and sugar. Cut in margarine until crumbly. Add yogurt and water, and mix until combined. Roll into a smooth ball, wrap and place in refrigerator for 30 minutes.

2. Put brown sugar, raisins, chocolate chips, cocoa and cinnamon in food processor; process until crumbly, approximately 20 seconds.

3. Divide dough in half. Roll one portion into a rectangle of ¼-inch thickness on a well-floured surface. Sprinkle half of the filling on top of the dough rectangle. Roll up tightly, long end to long end, jelly-roll fashion; pinch ends together. Cut into 1-inch-thick pieces; some filling will fall out. Place on baking sheets, cut side up. Repeat with remaining dough and filling.

4. With the back of a spoon or your fingers, gently flatten each cookie. Bake for 25 minutes, turning the cookies over at the halfway mark (12½ minutes).

Makes 26 cookies (1 cookie per serving)

DIETITIAN'S NOTE *When you will be eating away from home, plan ahead—and bring your meal planning skills with you. How you deal with eating out will depend partly on how you are controlling your diabetes: whether it's through diet and exercise alone or with oral medication and/or insulin. A dietitian or diabetes educator can help you learn to plan for these occasions, whether they are daily occurrences, such as eating at work, or special events.*

In a self-serve situation, such as a buffet dinner, survey the buffet first to identify what you would really like to eat and then decide how to "spend" the food Exchanges you have. If you choose something that turns out not to be as good as expected, don't feel obliged to finish it. Set it aside and search out something you will like better.

Likewise, if you are being served, you don't need to eat everything on your plate. Eat what you know is a healthy portion for you. Most restaurants are happy to provide "doggy bags," so if you really like what you're eating, ask them to pack up the leftovers.

NUTRIENTS PER SERVING

Calories	119
Carbohydrate	20 g
Fiber	1 g
Protein	1 g
Fat, total	4 g
Fat, saturated	1 g
Cholesterol	0 mg
Sodium	52 mg

EXCHANGES PER SERVING

1 Other Carbohydrates

1 Fat

1 Free Food

COCOA KISSES

COOKIES

TIP It's easier to separate eggs when they're cold, but egg whites beat to a greater volume when at room temperature.

NUTRIENTS PER SERVING

Calories	95
Carbohydrate	17 g
Fiber	1 g
Protein	1 g
Fat, total	3 g
Fat, saturated	0 g
Cholesterol	0 mg
Sodium	34 mg

EXCHANGES PER SERVING

1 Other Carbohydrates
½ Fat

Preheat oven to 250°F
Baking sheet, sprayed with baking spray

3	egg whites, at room temperature
1	cup granulated sugar
⅛	tsp salt
1	tsp vanilla
3	tbsp unsweetened cocoa powder
½	cup chopped pecans

1. In a large bowl, beat egg whites until soft peaks form; gradually add sugar and salt, beating until mixture is glossy and stiff peaks form. Beat in vanilla. Sift cocoa into bowl; fold into meringue along with pecans.

2. Put mixture in a pastry bag fitted with star tip; pipe small kisses onto prepared baking sheet (alternatively, drop mixture by teaspoonfuls onto baking sheet). Bake for 1 hour or until firm and dry.

Makes 40 cookies (3 cookies per serving)

DIETITIAN'S NOTES *The leavening ("lightening") agent in these cookies is the air trapped in the meringue (egg whites beaten with sugar).*

Sometimes you will get more or fewer cookies than stated in the recipe. When this happens, see the cookie calculator on page xvi for help in determining how many cookies make up a serving.

WHITE CHOCOLATE CRANBERRY DROPS

Preheat oven to 350°F
Baking sheet, lined with parchment paper

2	cups all-purpose flour
¼	cup cornstarch
1	cup butter, softened
½	cup superfine granulated sugar (see Tip)
1	tsp vanilla
1	cup chopped dried cranberries
¾	cup white chocolate chips

1. On a sheet of waxed paper or in a bowl, combine flour and cornstarch. Set aside.

2. In a large bowl, using an electric mixer on medium speed, beat butter, sugar and vanilla until light and creamy, about 3 minutes. On low speed, gradually add flour mixture, beating until blended. Using your hands, knead to form a smooth dough. Add cranberries and white chocolate chips. Knead well.

3. Drop dough by tablespoonfuls, about 2 inches apart, on prepared baking sheet. Bake in preheated oven for 13 to 18 minutes or until lightly browned around edges. Cool for 5 minutes on sheet, then transfer to a rack and cool completely.

Makes 48 cookies (1 cookie per serving)

TIPS If you don't have superfine sugar, whirl regular granulated sugar in a food processor or blender until fine.

I recommend using parchment paper when baking these cookies, as the white chocolate is likely to stick.

VARIATIONS Replace white chocolate chips with semisweet chocolate chips.

Replace cranberries with dried cherries or dried blueberries.

COOKIES

NUTRIENTS PER SERVING

Calories	86
Carbohydrate	10 g
Fiber	0 g
Protein	1 g
Fat, total	5 g
Fat, saturated	3 g
Cholesterol	10 mg
Sodium	42 mg

EXCHANGES PER SERVING

½ Other Carbohydrate

1 Fat

PEANUT BUTTER COOKIES

TIPS Use a natural, all-peanut type of peanut butter.

When using margarine, choose a soft (non-hydrogenated) version to limit consumption of trans fats.

NUTRIENTS PER SERVING

Calories	107
Carbohydrate	9 g
Fiber	1 g
Protein	2 g
Fat, total	7 g
Fat, saturated	1 g
Cholesterol	9 mg
Sodium	124 mg

EXCHANGES PER SERVING

½ Other Carbohydrate
1½ Fat

Preheat oven to 350°F
Baking sheet, sprayed with baking spray

½	cup peanut butter
½	cup packed brown sugar
⅓	cup margarine
1	egg
1	tsp vanilla
½	cup all-purpose flour
2	tbsp sesame seeds
¾	tsp baking soda
½	tsp ground nutmeg

Coating (optional)

1	egg white, beaten
½	cup wheat germ

1. In a bowl, beat peanut butter, brown sugar, margarine, egg and vanilla until light and fluffy. In another bowl, stir together flour, sesame seeds, baking soda and nutmeg. Stir flour mixture into peanut butter mixture just until combined. Form into 1-inch balls. If desired, dip balls in egg white, then roll in wheat germ. Put on prepared baking sheet.

2. Bake for 10 to 12 minutes or until golden.

Makes 40 cookies (2 cookies per serving)

PEANUT BUTTER FLAXSEED COOKIES

Preheat oven to 350°F
Baking sheets, lightly greased or lined with parchment paper

1¼	cups all-purpose flour
½	cup ground flaxseed
1	tsp baking soda
	Pinch salt
½	cup granulated sugar
½	cup packed brown sugar
½	cup butter, softened
1	egg
1	tsp vanilla
½	cup creamy peanut butter

1. In a small bowl, combine flour, flaxseed, baking soda and salt.

2. In a large bowl, cream granulated sugar, brown sugar and butter. Beat in egg and vanilla. Beat in peanut butter until smooth. Fold in flour mixture.

3. Shape dough into balls, using about 1 tbsp dough per cookie, and place 2 inches apart on prepared baking sheets. Using a fork, flatten cookies in a crisscross pattern.

4. Bake in preheated oven for 8 to 10 minutes or until lightly browned. Let cool on baking sheets on a wire rack for 5 minutes, then remove to rack to cool completely.

Makes 28 cookies (1 cookie per serving)

DIETITIAN'S NOTE *Sometimes you will get more or fewer cookies than stated in the recipe. When this happens, see the cookie calculator on page xvi for help in determining how many cookies make up a serving.*

NUTRIENTS PER SERVING

Calories	120
Carbohydrate	13 g
Fiber	1 g
Protein	2 g
Fat, total	7 g
Fat, saturated	3 g
Cholesterol	16 mg
Sodium	105 mg

EXCHANGES PER SERVING

1	Other Carbohydrates
1½	Fat

PEANUT BUTTER FUDGE COOKIES

TIPS Chopped dates can replace raisins.

Use a natural peanut butter, smooth or chunky.

When using margarine, choose a soft (non-hydrogenated) version to limit consumption of trans fats.

Cookies never last long, but these can be made up to a day ahead, kept tightly covered in a cookie jar or tin.

Prepare cookie dough and freeze for up to 2 weeks, then bake.

NUTRIENTS PER SERVING

Calories	143
Carbohydrate	23 g
Fiber	1 g
Protein	3 g
Fat, total	5 g
Fat, saturated	1 g
Cholesterol	10 mg
Sodium	71 mg

EXCHANGES PER SERVING

1½ Other Carbohydrates
1 Fat

Preheat oven to 350°F
Baking sheets, sprayed with vegetable spray

¼	cup softened margarine or butter
⅓	cup peanut butter
¾	cup granulated sugar
¼	cup brown sugar
1	egg
1	tsp vanilla
1	cup all-purpose flour
¼	cup unsweetened cocoa powder
1	tsp baking powder
¼	cup 2% yogurt
¾	cup raisins
3	tbsp chocolate chips

1. In a large bowl, cream together margarine, peanut butter, sugar and brown sugar. Add egg and vanilla and beat well.

2. In another bowl, combine flour, cocoa and baking powder; add to peanut butter mixture and stir just until combined. Stir in yogurt, raisins and chocolate chips. Drop by heaping teaspoonfuls onto prepared sheets, 2 inches apart, and press down slightly with back of fork. Bake approximately 12 minutes or until firm to the touch and slightly browned.

Makes 40 cookies (2 cookies per serving)

PEANUT BUTTER CHOCOLATE CHIP COOKIES

Preheat oven to 350°F
Baking sheets sprayed with nonstick vegetable spray

½	cup brown sugar
⅓	cup granulated sugar
⅓	cup peanut butter
⅓	cup 2% milk
¼	cup soft margarine
1	egg
1	tsp vanilla
½	cup all-purpose flour
⅓	cup whole wheat flour
1	tsp baking soda
⅓	cup chocolate chips
¼	cup raisins

1. In large bowl or food processor, beat together brown and granulated sugars, peanut butter, milk, margarine, egg and vanilla until well blended.

2. Combine all-purpose and whole wheat flours and baking soda; add to bowl and mix just until incorporated. Do not overmix. Stir in chocolate chips and raisins.

3. Drop by heaping teaspoonfuls 2 inches apart onto baking sheets. Bake for 12 to 15 minutes or until browned.

Makes 40 cookies (1 per serving)

TIPS The longer they bake, the crispier the cookies.

Use natural peanut butter made from peanuts only.

Dough can be frozen up to 2 weeks. Bake just before eating for best flavor.

NUTRIENTS PER SERVING

Calories	70
Carbohydrate	10 g
Fiber	1 g
Protein	1 g
Fat, total	3 g
Fat, saturated	1 g
Sodium	51 mg
Cholesterol	6 mg

EXCHANGES PER SERVING

⅔ Other Carbohydrate
½ Fat

PEANUT BUTTER CHIP COOKIES

TIP For best results, keep your baking ingredients at room temperature. If your margarine is cold, quickly soften it by placing it in a microwaveable bowl and microwaving it, uncovered, for about 15 seconds on Medium-High (70%), just until it is softened but not melted.

NUTRIENTS PER SERVING

Calories	150
Carbohydrate	21 g
Fiber	1 g
Protein	4 g
Fat, total	6 g
Fat, saturated	2 g
Cholesterol	11 mg
Sodium	153 mg

EXCHANGES PER SERVING

½	Starch
1	Other Carbohydrates
1½	Fat

Preheat oven to 350°F
Baking sheets, ungreased

1½	cups all-purpose flour
½	cup quick-cooking rolled oats
½	tsp salt
½	tsp baking soda
½	cup granulated sugar
¼	cup lightly packed brown sugar
¼	cup soft margarine
1	large egg
1	large egg white
½	cup lower-fat peanut butter
½	tsp vanilla
½	cup peanut butter chips

1. In a medium bowl, stir together flour, oats, salt and baking soda.

2. In a large bowl, using an electric mixer or wooden spoon, beat granulated sugar, brown sugar and margarine until light and fluffy. Beat in egg, egg white, peanut butter and vanilla. Stir in flour mixture and mix well. Stir in peanut butter chips.

3. Roll into 40 small balls and place about 2 inches apart on baking sheets. Press flat with a floured fork. Bake in preheated oven for 8 to 10 minutes, or until lightly browned. Cool on baking sheets for 5 minutes, then remove to rack to cool completely.

Makes 40 cookies (2 per serving)

APPLESAUCE SPICE COOKIES

Preheat oven to 350°F
Baking sheets, ungreased

1¼	cups all-purpose flour
1	tsp baking powder
1	tsp pumpkin pie spice
½	tsp baking soda
¼	tsp salt
¾	cup soft margarine
½	cup granulated sugar
¼	cup lightly packed brown sugar
1	large egg
½	tsp vanilla
1	cup unsweetened applesauce
1⅓	cups quick-cooking rolled oats
½	cup currants or raisins

1. In a medium bowl, stir together flour, baking powder, pumpkin pie spice, baking soda and salt.

2. In a large bowl, beat margarine, granulated sugar and brown sugar until light and fluffy. Add egg and vanilla and beat well.

3. Gradually stir in flour mixture alternately with applesauce, making 3 or 4 additions of each, and mix well. Stir in rolled oats and currants.

4. Drop by heaping tablespoonfuls, about 2 inches apart, onto baking sheets. Bake in preheated oven for 12 to 15 minutes, or until lightly browned. Cool on baking sheets for 5 minutes, then remove to rack to cool completely.

Makes 40 cookies (2 per serving)

DIETITIAN'S NOTE *The currants or raisins help to naturally sweeten these flavorful cookies. Paired with yogurt, they make a tasty after-school snack.*

TIPS Out of pumpkin pie spice? Substitute ¾ tsp ground cinnamon and ¼ tsp ground nutmeg or ginger.

These cookies have a muffin-like texture and get softer after storing at room temperature. If you plan to store them for more than 2 days, place them in an airtight container and freeze.

NUTRIENTS PER SERVING

Calories	156
Carbohydrate	20 g
Fiber	1 g
Protein	2 g
Fat, total	8 g
Fat, saturated	1 g
Cholesterol	11 mg
Sodium	162 mg

EXCHANGES PER SERVING

½ Starch
½ Other Carbohydrate
1½ Fat

WHOLE WHEAT SPICE COOKIES

COOKIES

NUTRIENTS PER SERVING

Calories	65
Carbohydrate	11 g
Fiber	0 g
Protein	1 g
Fat, total	2 g
Fat, saturated	0 g
Sodium	87 mg
Cholesterol	12 mg

EXCHANGES PER SERVING (1 COOKIE)

⅔ Other Carbohydrate
½ Fat

Preheat oven to 350°F
Lightly greased cookie sheet

¼	cup vegetable oil
¼	cup molasses
½	cup granulated sugar
¼	cup packed brown sugar
2	eggs
½	cup whole wheat flour
1½	cups all-purpose flour
2	tsp baking soda
¼	tsp salt
1	tsp ground ginger
1	tsp ground cinnamon
1	tsp ground cloves

1. In a bowl, whisk oil, molasses, sugars and eggs until blended.

2. In a large bowl, mix together flours, baking soda, salt, ginger, cinnamon and cloves. Make a well in the center and add the molasses mixture, mixing until thoroughly blended.

3. Drop by teaspoonfuls, about 2 inches apart, onto prepared cookie sheets. Bake in preheated oven for 8 to 10 minutes or until cookies are firm to the touch. Cool on sheets for 5 minutes, then transfer to wire racks to cool completely.

Makes about 3 dozen cookies (1 per serving)

GINGER COOKIES

Preheat oven to 350°F
Baking sheets, lightly greased or lined with parchment paper

1¾	cups	all-purpose flour
1½	tsp	baking powder
1	tsp	ground ginger
1	tsp	ground cinnamon
½	tsp	baking soda
½	tsp	salt
¼	tsp	ground cloves
1		egg
½	cup	granulated sugar
½	cup	vegetable oil
½	cup	fancy molasses

1. In a small bowl, combine flour, baking powder, ginger, cinnamon, baking soda, salt and cloves.

2. In a medium bowl, whisk egg, sugar, oil and molasses until blended. Fold in flour mixture until a moist dough forms.

3. Shape dough into balls, using about 1 tbsp dough per cookie, and place 2 inches apart on prepared baking sheets.

4. Bake in preheated oven for 10 to 12 minutes or until lightly browned and crisp. Let cool on baking sheet on a wire rack for 5 minutes, then remove to rack to cool completely.

Makes 30 cookies (1 cookie per serving)

DIETITIAN'S NOTE *This recipe contains both baking soda and baking powder. These leavening agents cause baked goods to rise by releasing carbon dioxide. Baking soda must be combined with an acidic ingredient (molasses, in this recipe). Baking powder, on the other hand, contains both baking soda and an acid component.*

NUTRIENTS PER SERVING

Calories	91
Carbohydrate	13 g
Fiber	0 g
Protein	1 g
Fat, total	4 g
Fat, saturated	0 g
Cholesterol	6 mg
Sodium	77 mg

EXCHANGES PER SERVING

1 Other Carbohydrates
1 Fat

SPICY GINGERSNAPS

TIP If ground white pepper isn't available, use ¼ tsp freshly ground black pepper. You will notice black specks in the dough.

Preheat oven to 350°F
Baking sheet, ungreased

3¾	cups all-purpose flour
1¼	tsp baking powder
¼	tsp salt
2	tbsp ground ginger
1	tbsp ground cinnamon
½	tsp ground white pepper
¼	tsp ground cloves
1½	cups butter, softened
1¾	cups packed brown sugar
1	egg
1	tbsp grated gingerroot
2	tsp grated lemon zest
¼	cup turbinado sugar

1. On a sheet of waxed paper or in a bowl, combine flour, baking powder, salt, ground ginger, cinnamon, pepper and cloves. Set aside.

2. In a large bowl, using an electric mixer on medium speed, beat butter, brown sugar, egg, gingerroot and lemon zest until smooth and creamy. On low speed, gradually add flour mixture, beating until dough becomes too stiff for the mixer, then finish mixing with a wooden spoon until smooth. Cover and chill dough for 2 hours for easy handling.

3. Shape teaspoonfuls of dough into balls. Place about 1 inch apart on baking sheet. With the bottom of a glass dipped in flour, press down firmly on each to form thin rounds. Sprinkle turbinado sugar evenly over tops. Bake in preheated oven for 10 to 14 minutes or until crisp and golden. Cool for 5 minutes on sheet, then transfer to a rack and cool completely.

Makes 78 cookies (3 cookies per serving)

DIETITIAN'S NOTES *Turbinado sugar is blond-colored coarse crystals of cleaned, partially refined raw sugar. If you don't have it, just omit it.*

If your cookies are larger or smaller than the recipe intends, you won't get the amount indicated, which means the number of your cookies that equal the nutrient Exchanges for a serving will not be the same as stated in the recipe. See the cookie calculator on page xvi for help in figuring out how many of your cookies it takes to match the information in the recipe.

NUTRIENTS PER SERVING

Calories	225
Carbohydrate	30 g
Fiber	1 g
Protein	2 g
Fat, total	11 g
Fat, saturated	7 g
Cholesterol	36 mg
Sodium	152 mg

EXCHANGES PER SERVING

1 Starch

1 Other Carbohydrates

2 Fat

VANILLA ALMOND SNAPS

NUTRIENTS PER SERVING

Calories	97
Carbohydrate	10 g
Fiber	1 g
Protein	3 g
Fat, total	6 g
Fat, saturated	1 g
Cholesterol	0 mg
Sodium	70 mg

EXCHANGES PER SERVING

½ Other Carbohydrate
1 Fat

Preheat oven to 275°F
Baking sheet, lined with parchment paper and sprayed with baking spray

¾	cup whole blanched almonds
¼	cup granulated sugar
¼	tsp salt
2	egg whites
2	tbsp granulated sugar
½	tsp vanilla
	Sliced almonds (optional)

1. In a food processor, grind almonds with ¼ cup sugar and salt until as fine as possible. Transfer to a bowl and set aside.

2. In another bowl, beat egg whites until soft peaks form. Gradually add 2 tbsp sugar, beating until stiff peaks form. Fold in vanilla. Fold into ground nut mixture until blended. Drop by teaspoonfuls onto prepared baking sheet. If desired, sprinkle with a few sliced almonds.

3. Bake for 25 minutes or until golden.

Makes 30 cookies (3 cookies per serving)

DIETITIAN'S NOTE *When separating the eggs, be careful not to allow any egg yolk to escape into the whites. If it does, they will not beat properly.*

SESAME SEED COOKIES

Preheat oven to 350°F
Lightly greased cookie sheet

1½	cups whole wheat flour
1	tsp baking powder
¼	tsp salt
¼	cup softened margarine or butter
¼	cup liquid honey
¼	cup sesame paste (tahini)
½	tsp almond extract
½	cup sesame seeds, toasted

1. In a bowl, mix together flour, baking powder and salt.

2. In another bowl, beat margarine, honey, sesame paste and almond extract until smooth. Add flour mixture and mix well. Stir in sesame seeds.

3. Shape dough into 1-inch balls and place about 2 inches apart on prepared cookie sheet. Using the tines of a fork dipped in flour, flatten, or using your hands, mold into crescent shapes. (Wet your hands first, if using to mold the dough.) Bake in preheated oven for 10 to 12 minutes or until lightly browned. Immediately transfer to wire racks to cool.

Makes about 2 dozen cookies (1 per serving)

NUTRIENTS PER SERVING

Calories	87
Carbohydrate	10 g
Fiber	2 g
Protein	2 g
Fat, total	5 g
Fat, saturated	1 g
Sodium	61 mg
Cholesterol	0 mg

EXCHANGES PER SERVING (1 COOKIE)

½	Starch
1	Fat

SESAME SNAP WAFERS

116

COOKIES

VARIATION Try with half black sesame seeds or flaxseeds and half white sesame seeds.

NUTRIENTS PER SERVING

Calories	43
Carbohydrate	5 g
Fiber	1 g
Protein	1 g
Fat, total	3 g
Fat, saturated	0 g
Sodium	20 mg
Cholesterol	3 mg

EXCHANGES PER SERVING

⅔ Other Carbohydrate

1 Fat

Preheat oven to 350°F
Cookie sheet, lined with parchment paper or lightly greased foil

⅔	cup all-purpose flour
¼	tsp baking powder
½	cup margarine or butter, softened
1	cup packed brown sugar
1	egg
1	tsp vanilla
1¼	cups sesame seeds, toasted

1. Combine flour and baking powder.

2. Cream margarine, sugar, egg and vanilla. Add flour mixture. Mix until combined. Stir in seeds.

3. Drop by teaspoonfuls about 2 inches apart onto prepared cookie sheet. Bake for 6 to 9 minutes or until lightly browned. Cool for 5 minutes on sheet, then transfer to rack and cool completely.

Makes 6 dozen cookies (1 per serving)

DICED RHUBARB COOKIES

Preheat oven to 350°F
Greased cookie sheet

2	cups all-purpose flour or whole wheat flour or a combination of both
2	tsp baking powder
	Pinch salt
1	tsp ground cinnamon
½	tsp ground nutmeg
½	tsp ground cloves
½	cup softened margarine or butter
1	cup lightly packed brown sugar
1	egg
¼	cup milk
1	cup diced rhubarb
1	cup chopped walnuts

1. In a bowl, combine flour, baking powder, salt, cinnamon, nutmeg and cloves.

2. In another bowl, beat margarine and sugar until smooth and creamy. Beat in egg until well incorporated. Mix in milk. Add flour mixture and beat until smooth. Fold in rhubarb and walnuts until well combined.

3. Drop by rounded teaspoonfuls, 2 inches apart, onto prepared cookie sheet. Bake in preheated oven for 18 to 20 minutes or until crisp and lightly browned. Immediately transfer to wire racks to cool.

Makes about 3½ dozen cookies (1 per serving)

TIP If you are lactose intolerant, use lactose-reduced milk in baking. It can be substituted for regular milk and will not affect the results.

NUTRIENTS PER SERVING

Calories	83
Carbohydrate	11 g
Fiber	0 g
Protein	1 g
Fat, total	4 g
Fat, saturated	2 g
Sodium	48 mg
Cholesterol	11 mg

EXCHANGES PER SERVING

⅔	Other Carbohydrate
1	Fat

CHARLIE & EMMA'S FAVORITE CARROT COOKIES

TIP When using margarine, choose a non-hydrogenated version to limit consumption of trans fats.

NUTRIENTS PER SERVING

Calories	103
Carbohydrate	13 g
Fiber	2 g
Protein	2 g
Fat, total	5 g
Fat, saturated	1 g
Cholesterol	8 mg
Sodium	86 mg

EXCHANGES PER SERVING

1 Other Carbohydrates
1 Fat

Preheat oven to 350°F
Baking sheets, lightly greased

1	cup whole wheat flour
¾	cup quick-cooking rolled oats
½	cup ground flaxseed
1	tsp ground cinnamon
½	tsp baking soda
1	egg
¾	cup lightly packed brown sugar
½	cup margarine
1	tsp vanilla
1	cup grated carrots

1. In a medium bowl, combine flour, oats, flaxseed, cinnamon and baking soda.

2. In a large bowl, using an electric mixer, beat egg, brown sugar, margarine and vanilla until smooth. Fold in flour mixture. Stir in carrots.

3. Drop dough by heaping tablespoonfuls, about 2 inches apart, onto prepared baking sheets.

4. Bake in preheated oven for 10 to 15 minutes or until lightly browned. Let cool on baking sheet on a wire rack for 5 minutes.

Makes 24 cookies (1 cookie per serving)

MERINGUE CANDY CANES

Preheat oven to 200°F
2 baking sheets, lined with parchment paper
Large pastry bag with ½-inch plain tip
Medium pastry bag with ¼-inch plain tip

4	large egg whites, at room temperature
½	tsp cream of tartar
¼	tsp salt
⅔	cup granulated sugar
½	tsp peppermint extract
	Red food coloring

1. Using a pencil, lightly draw 48 candy cane shapes on the parchment paper; flip the paper over.

2. Position oven racks in the center of the oven.

3. In a large bowl, using an electric mixer, beat egg whites, cream of tartar and salt at medium speed until foamy. Continue beating, adding sugar 2 tbsp at a time, until stiff, glossy peaks form, then beat in peppermint extract. Transfer ½ cup to a small bowl and stir in a few drops of red food coloring to tint pink.

4. Fill the large pastry bag with the white meringue and pipe onto the candy cane shapes on the parchment paper. Fill the medium pastry bag with the pink meringue and pipe into diagonal stripes across the candy canes.

5. Bake in preheated oven for 1¼ hours, or until firm. Turn heat off and leave meringues to dry in oven for 1 hour. Peel meringues off parchment paper and transfer to a rack to cool completely.

Makes 48 candy canes (2 per serving)

TIPS Eggs separate more easily when cold, but egg whites gain more volume when beaten at room temperature. To warm to room temperature, place bowl of egg whites in a larger bowl of hot water and let stand for 5 minutes.

For best results when making meringues, use a clean stainless steel or glass bowl to beat the egg whites.

NUTRIENTS PER SERVING

Calories	25
Carbohydrate	6 g
Fiber	0 g
Protein	1 g
Fat, total	0 g
Fat, saturated	0 g
Cholesterol	0 mg
Sodium	32 mg

EXCHANGES PER SERVING
½ Other Carbohydrate

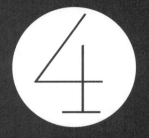

BARS, SQUARES & BROWNIES

121	Mixed Fruit Bran Bars
122	Apple Cinnamon Bars
124	Pick-Me-Up Bars
125	Apricot Seed Bars
126	Apricot Coconut Bars
128	Date Nut Bars
129	Granola Bars
130	Peanut Butter–Coconut-Raisin Granola Bars
131	Nutty Shortbread Bars
132	Chocolate Shortbread Bars
133	Hazelnut Shortbread Bars
134	Chocolate Hazelnut Bars
135	Toffee Bars
136	Berry Cheesecake Bars
137	Date Oatmeal Squares
138	Raisin & Applesauce Squares
139	Lemon Poppy Seed Squares
140	Almond Shortbread Squares
141	Coconut Seeds Cereal Squares
142	Almond Butter Cereal Squares
143	Crispy Granola Squares
144	Christmas Brownies
145	Moist 'n' Chewy Chocolate Brownies
146	Chocolate Chunk Banana Brownies
147	Triple Chocolate Brownies
148	White Chocolate Brownies
149	Sour Cream Brownies
150	Cream Cheese–Filled Brownies
151	Chocolate Brownies
152	Orange Cream Cheese Brownies

MIXED FRUIT
BRAN BARS

Preheat oven to 375°F
13- by 9-inch cake pan, greased

2	cups bran flakes cereal
1	cup unbleached all-purpose flour
⅔	cup packed brown sugar
2	tsp baking soda
¼	tsp salt
1	cup buttermilk
2	tbsp vegetable oil
2	eggs
1	tbsp grated lemon zest
¾	cup chopped dried apricots
½	cup chopped dried apples
½	cup chopped dates
½	cup dried cranberries
⅓	cup chopped pecans

1. In a food processor fitted with a metal blade, combine cereal, flour, brown sugar, baking soda and salt. Pulse until coarsely chopped, about 1 minute. Add buttermilk, vegetable oil, eggs and lemon zest and process until cereal is crushed and mixture is blended. Stir in apricots, apples, dates, cranberries and pecans. Spread evenly in prepared pan.

2. Bake in preheated oven until set and golden, 20 to 25 minutes. Let cool completely in pan on rack. Cut into bars.

Makes 36 bars (1 bar per serving)

TIP For added fiber, substitute whole wheat flour for all or half of the all-purpose.

VARIATIONS Replace lemon zest with orange or tangerine zest.

Replace dried cranberries with chopped dried cherries or raisins.

NUTRIENTS
PER SERVING

Calories	79
Carbohydrate	15 g
Fiber	1 g
Protein	1 g
Fat, total	2 g
Fat, saturated	0 g
Cholesterol	11 mg
Sodium	114 mg

EXCHANGES
PER SERVING

½ Fruit
½ Other Carbohydrate
½ Fat

APPLE CINNAMON BARS

TIP Dust lightly with confectioner's sugar if desired.

VARIATION Decrease apples to 5 cups and add 1 cup fresh cranberries.

Preheat oven to 350°F
9-inch square cake pan, greased

Crust
1	cup unbleached all-purpose flour
1	cup whole wheat flour
½	cup granulated sugar
½	tsp baking powder
¼	tsp salt
⅔	cup cold butter, cubed
1	egg, beaten

Filling
⅓	cup granulated sugar
2	tbsp all-purpose flour
1	tsp ground cinnamon
2	lb tart cooking apples, peeled, cored and thinly sliced (5 ½ cups)
1	tbsp freshly squeezed lemon juice

1. *Crust:* In a bowl, combine all-purpose and whole wheat flours, sugar, baking powder and salt. Using a pastry blender, 2 knives or your fingers, cut in butter until mixture resembles coarse crumbs. Add egg and, using a fork, mix until thoroughly blended. Press half of the mixture (about 2 cups) evenly into prepared pan. Set aside remainder.

2. *Filling:* In a large bowl, combine sugar, flour, cinnamon, apples and lemon juice, mixing well. Layer evenly over crust. Sprinkle remaining crumble mixture over top.

3. Bake in preheated oven until apples are tender and crust is golden, 45 to 50 minutes. Let cool completely in pan on rack. Cut into bars.

Makes 36 bars (1 bar per serving)

DIETITIAN'S NOTE *Fashion affects not only clothing and footwear, but also food—and in both instances, the fashion may not always be good for us. No one knows when we first began to mill wheat into flour, but the product certainly did not resemble the white all-purpose flour most people now have in their kitchens. Like today's whole wheat flour, the original contained the bran and germ portions of the grain.*

About 150 years ago, millers started to produce a "higher-quality" flour by sifting out the bran and germ. These nutritious leftovers, rich in fiber and important nutrients, became animal feed. White flour became a culinary status symbol, and whole-grain flour was scorned as "peasant food." Later, a bleaching process (which destroys any remaining vitamin E) was added to make the flour even whiter.

As more and more people used white flour, they began to experience nutritional deficiencies. Today, white flour, whether bleached or not, must by law be enriched—some of the vitamins and iron are added back, but the fiber is not.

NUTRIENTS PER SERVING

Calories	87
Carbohydrate	13 g
Fiber	1 g
Protein	1 g
Fat, total	4 g
Fat, saturated	2 g
Cholesterol	14 mg
Sodium	57 mg

EXCHANGES PER SERVING

1 Other Carbohydrates
1 Fat

PICK-ME-UP BARS

TIP When baking, you can usually use 1 whole egg in place of 2 egg whites or vice versa. However, in desserts like custards, where the yolk is needed for thickening, this rule doesn't apply.

VARIATIONS Replace whole wheat flour with all-purpose, but be aware that you'll lose some of the health benefits, such as added fiber.

Replace sunflower seeds with a mixture of sesame and flaxseeds.

NUTRIENTS PER SERVING

Calories	97
Carbohydrate	15 g
Fiber	1 g
Protein	2 g
Fat, total	3 g
Fat, saturated	1 g
Cholesterol	0 mg
Sodium	44 mg

EXCHANGES PER SERVING

1 Other Carbohydrates
½ Fat

Preheat oven to 350°F
8-inch square cake pan, greased

1	cup graham wafer crumbs
⅔	cup packed brown sugar
½	cup whole wheat flour
½	cup butterscotch chips
⅓	cup quick-cooking rolled oats
⅓	cup sunflower seeds
1	tsp baking powder
2	egg whites (see Tip)
1	tbsp vegetable oil
1½	tsp vanilla

1. In a bowl, combine graham wafer crumbs, brown sugar, flour, butterscotch chips, oats, sunflower seeds and baking powder.

2. In a separate bowl, whisk egg whites, oil and vanilla until blended. Stir into dry ingredients, mixing well. Press evenly into prepared pan.

3. Bake in preheated oven until top is golden, about 20 minutes. Let cool completely in pan on rack. Cut into bars.

Makes 24 bars (1 bar per serving)

APRICOT SEED BARS

Preheat oven to 350°F
13- by 9-inch cake pan, greased

¾	cup butter, softened
¾	cup packed brown sugar
1	egg
1	cup unbleached all-purpose flour
½	tsp baking soda
¼	tsp salt
¾	tsp ground cinnamon
1	cup quick-cooking rolled oats
¾	cup finely chopped dried apricots
¾	cup dried cranberries
¼	cup sesame seeds
¼	cup flaxseeds
¼	cup sunflower seeds

1. In a bowl, using an electric mixer on medium speed, beat butter, brown sugar and egg until smooth and creamy. Combine flour, baking soda, salt and cinnamon. Stir into creamed mixture, mixing well. Stir in rolled oats, apricots, cranberries, sesame seeds, flaxseeds and sunflower seeds. Spread evenly in prepared pan.

2. Bake in preheated oven until top is set and golden, 25 to 30 minutes. Let cool completely in pan on rack. Cut into bars.

Makes 36 bars (1 bar per serving)

TIPS To prevent sticking, use cooking spray to get a light, even coating of grease on baking pans.

To ease cleanup, rather than combining the dry ingredients in a bowl (in Step 1), place a large piece of waxed paper on the counter. Spread the flour on the paper and sprinkle the baking soda, salt and cinnamon over it. Using the paper as a funnel, transfer the dry ingredients to the egg mixture.

VARIATION Replace cranberries with chopped dried figs or raisins.

NUTRIENTS PER SERVING

Calories	111
Carbohydrate	14 g
Fiber	1 g
Protein	2 g
Fat, total	6 g
Fat, saturated	3 g
Cholesterol	16 mg
Sodium	77 mg

EXCHANGES PER SERVING

1 Other Carbohydrates
1 Fat

APRICOT COCONUT BARS

Preheat oven to 350°F
13- by 9-inch baking pan, greased

2	cups	whole wheat flour
1½	cups	quick-cooking rolled oats
1⅓	cups	lightly packed brown sugar
½	cup	oat bran
½	cup	natural wheat bran
½	tsp	baking soda
½	cup	margarine or butter, softened
½	cup	vegetable oil
2	cups	chopped dried apricots
1½	cups	water
½	cup	granulated sugar
2	tbsp	all-purpose flour
1	cup	unsweetened shredded coconut

1. In a large bowl, combine flour, oats, brown sugar, oat bran, wheat bran and baking soda.

2. In a small bowl, combine margarine and oil. Stir into flour mixture until mixture resembles coarse crumbs. Reserve 1 cup crumb mixture. Press remaining crumb mixture into bottom of prepared pan. Set aside.

3. In a large saucepan, over medium high heat, combine apricots and water; bring to a boil. Reduce heat, cover and simmer for 5 minutes, until softened.

4. Meanwhile, combine sugar and flour. Stir into apricot mixture. Cook, stirring, for 1 minute or until thick. Stir in coconut.

5. Spread apricot mixture over crumbs in the pan and sprinkle evenly with reserved crumb mixture.

6. Bake for 35 minutes or until golden brown on top. Let cool completely in pan on a wire rack, then cut into bars.

Makes 36 bars (1 bar per serving)

DIETITIAN'S NOTE *When planning what to eat, we need to take into account both the type of food and the portion size. Getting the correct portion size (in other words, the right number of bars or squares) from a cake baked in a rectangular or square pan is easy: just look at how many bars are specified in the yield and cut the cake into that many portions. For example, this recipe makes 36 bars. To get that number, you would cut the cake lengthwise 3 times and crosswise 8 times. Make sure all your bars are the same size, or the Nutrients per Serving and Exchanges will not be accurate.*

NUTRIENTS PER SERVING

Calories	173
Carbohydrate	27 g
Fiber	3 g
Protein	2 g
Fat, total	7 g
Fat, saturated	2 g
Cholesterol	0 mg
Sodium	57 mg

EXCHANGES PER SERVING

½ Starch
½ Fruit
½ Other Carbohydrate
1½ Fat

DATE NUT BARS

**NUTRIENTS
PER SERVING**

Calories	80
Carbohydrate	14 g
Fiber	2 g
Protein	1 g
Fat, total	3 g
Fat, saturated	0 g
Cholesterol	0 mg
Sodium	4 mg

**EXCHANGES
PER SERVING**

1 Fruit
½ Fat

8-inch square baking dish

- 1⅓ cups chopped dates
- ¼ cup walnut pieces
- ¼ cup whole almonds
- ½ cup granola

1. In a food processor, combine dates, walnuts and almonds; process until mixture begins to come together.

2. Sprinkle half of granola over bottom of baking dish. Press date mixture firmly and evenly over granola. Top with remaining granola, pressing down slightly to embed in date mixture. Chill.

3. Cut into squares.

Makes 16 bars (1 bar per serving)

DIETITIAN'S NOTE *Cut dried fruit into small pieces to spread its flavor through a batter or dough.*

GRANOLA BARS

Preheat oven to 350°F
13- by 9-inch metal baking pan, lined with foil, sprayed with nonstick spray, then lined with parchment paper

⅓	cup unsalted butter, softened
¾	cup honey
½	cup packed brown sugar
2	cups old-fashioned rolled oats
1	cup natural bran
1	cup sunflower seeds
1	cup dates, pitted and chopped
½	cup pecans, toasted and chopped
¼	cup sesame seeds
2	tsp ground cinnamon

1. In a small saucepan over medium heat, melt butter. Stir in honey and brown sugar. Bring to a boil, about 3 minutes. Simmer over low heat for 5 minutes. Let cool slightly.

2. In a large bowl, combine rolled oats, bran, sunflower seeds, dates, pecans, sesame seeds and cinnamon. Gradually stir in sugar mixture. Firmly press into prepared baking pan. Bake in preheated oven until golden brown, 15 to 18 minutes. Let cool completely in baking pan before cutting into bars.

Makes 18 bars (1 bar per serving)

TIP After cutting into bars, wrap each bar in its own plastic wrap and store in a cool, dry place or a cookie jar for easy serving.

VARIATION You can replace dates with any dried fruit.

NUTRIENTS PER SERVING

Calories	250
Carbohydrate	37 g
Fiber	5 g
Protein	5 g
Fat, total	12 g
Fat, saturated	3 g
Cholesterol	9 mg
Sodium	5 mg

EXCHANGES PER SERVING

1	Starch
½	Fruit
1	Other Carbohydrates
2½	Fat

PEANUT BUTTER–COCONUT-RAISIN GRANOLA BARS

TIPS Corn flakes can replace bran flakes. Chopped dates can replace raisins.

When using margarine, choose a soft (non-hydrogenated) version to limit consumption of trans fats.

Prepare these up to 2 days ahead and keep tightly closed in a cookie tin. These freeze for up to 2 weeks.

NUTRIENTS PER SERVING

Calories	99
Carbohydrate	14 g
Fiber	1 g
Protein	2 g
Fat, total	5 g
Fat, saturated	1 g
Cholesterol	0 mg
Sodium	92 mg

EXCHANGES PER SERVING

1 Other Carbohydrates

1 Fat

Preheat oven to 350°F
9-inch square pan sprayed with vegetable spray

1⅓	cups rolled oats
⅔	cup raisins
½	cup bran flakes cereal
⅓	cup unsweetened shredded coconut
3	tbsp chocolate chips
2	tbsp chopped pecans
1	tsp baking soda
¼	cup peanut butter
¼	cup brown sugar
3	tbsp margarine or butter
3	tbsp honey
1	tsp vanilla

1. Put oats, raisins, bran flakes, coconut, chocolate chips, pecans and baking soda in bowl. Combine until well mixed.

2. In a small saucepan, whisk together peanut butter, brown sugar, margarine, honey and vanilla over medium heat for approximately 30 seconds or just until sugar dissolves and mixture is smooth. Pour over dry ingredients and stir to combine. Press into prepared pan and bake for 15 to 20 minutes or until browned. Let cool completely before cutting into bars.

Makes 24 bars (1 bar per serving)

NUTTY SHORTBREAD BARS

Preheat oven to 300°F
9-inch square cake pan, ungreased

1	cup	butter, softened
⅓	cup	granulated sugar
2	tbsp	cornstarch
1	tsp	vanilla
2	cups	all-purpose flour
⅓	cup	finely chopped walnuts
⅓	cup	finely chopped pecans

1. In a bowl, using an electric mixer on medium speed, beat butter, sugar, cornstarch and vanilla until light and creamy. Stir in flour, walnuts and pecans, mixing well. Using your hands, knead to form a smooth dough. Press evenly into pan.

2. Bake in preheated oven until light golden around edges, 40 to 45 minutes. Cut into bars just as the pan comes out of the oven, then let cool completely in pan on rack. Recut.

Makes 48 bars (1 bar per serving)

NUTRIENTS PER SERVING

Calories	71
Carbohydrate	6 g
Fiber	0 g
Protein	1 g
Fat, total	5 g
Fat, saturated	2 g
Cholesterol	10 mg
Sodium	39 mg

EXCHANGES PER SERVING

½ Starch
1 Fat

CHOCOLATE SHORTBREAD BARS

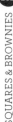
NUTRIENTS PER SERVING

Calories	112
Carbohydrate	11 g
Fiber	1 g
Protein	1 g
Fat, total	7 g
Fat, saturated	4 g
Cholesterol	14 mg
Sodium	52 mg

EXCHANGES PER SERVING

1 Other Carbohydrates
1½ Fat

Preheat oven to 300°F
13- by 9-inch cake pan, ungreased

1	cup butter, softened
½	cup granulated sugar
2	cups all-purpose flour
2	squares (1 oz each) semisweet chocolate, melted and cooled

1. In a bowl, using an electric mixer on medium speed, beat butter and sugar until light and creamy, about 3 minutes. Stir in flour, mixing well. Stir in melted chocolate, mixing well. Using your hands, knead to form a smooth dough. Press evenly into pan.

2. Bake in preheated oven until firm and dry, 35 to 40 minutes. Cut into bars just as the pan comes out of the oven, then let cool completely in pan on rack. Recut.

Makes 36 bars (1 bar per serving)

HAZELNUT SHORTBREAD BARS

Preheat oven to 300°F
9-inch square cake pan, ungreased

1	cup butter, softened
½	cup superfine granulated sugar
1½	cups all-purpose flour
¾	cup cornstarch
½	cup finely chopped hazelnuts

1. In a bowl, using an electric mixer on medium speed, beat butter and sugar until light and creamy, about 3 minutes. Stir in flour, cornstarch and hazelnuts, mixing well. Using your hands, knead to form a smooth dough. Press evenly into pan. Prick surface all over with a fork.

2. Bake in preheated oven until lightly browned, 30 to 35 minutes. Cut into bars just as the pan comes out of the oven, then let cool completely in pan on rack. Recut.

Makes 25 bars (1 bar per serving)

NUTRIENTS PER SERVING

Calories	137
Carbohydrate	14 g
Fiber	0 g
Protein	1 g
Fat, total	9 g
Fat, saturated	5 g
Cholesterol	20 mg
Sodium	76 mg

EXCHANGES PER SERVING

½ Starch
½ Other Carbohydrate
2 Fat

DIETITIAN'S NOTE *Shortbread recipes all have three basic ingredients: flour, sugar and butter. Other fats will not produce the typical shortbread texture. Do remember, however, that butter is high in saturated fat.*

CHOCOLATE HAZELNUT BARS

TIPS For a softer cookie, prepare these bars the day before you intend to serve them.

Hazelnuts are also called filberts. If you prefer, remove the outer brown skin before using them in baking. Toast the nuts on a rimmed baking sheet at 350°F for about 5 minutes. Transfer the warm nuts to a towel and rub together. The skins should come off in the towel.

VARIATION Macadamia nuts make a wonderful substitution for the hazelnuts in this bar.

NUTRIENTS PER SERVING

Calories	114
Carbohydrate	13 g
Fiber	1 g
Protein	2 g
Fat, total	7 g
Fat, saturated	3 g
Cholesterol	14 mg
Sodium	66 mg

EXCHANGES PER SERVING

1 Other Carbohydrates
1½ Fat

Preheat oven to 375°F
17- by 11- by 1-inch jelly-roll pan, greased

1	cup butter, softened
1	cup packed brown sugar
½	cup granulated sugar
2	eggs
1	tsp vanilla
1¾	cups all-purpose flour
1	cup quick-cooking rolled oats
1	tsp baking soda
¼	tsp salt
2	cups semisweet chocolate chips
1½	cups coarsely chopped hazelnuts

1. In a bowl, using an electric mixer on medium speed, beat butter and brown and granulated sugars until light and creamy, about 3 minutes. Add eggs, one at a time, beating well after each addition. Beat in vanilla. Stir in flour, oats, baking soda and salt, mixing well. Stir in chocolate chips and hazelnuts. Spread dough evenly in prepared pan.

2. Bake in preheated oven until golden, about 15 minutes. Let cool completely in pan on rack. Cut into bars.

Makes 60 bars (1 bar per serving)

TOFFEE BARS

Preheat oven to 350°F
13- by 9-inch baking pan, lined with parchment paper

2	cups quick-cooking rolled oats
½	cup lightly packed brown sugar
⅓	cup melted butter or margarine
¼	cup liquid honey or corn syrup
1½	tsp vanilla
½	tsp salt
1	cup semisweet chocolate chips
½	cup finely chopped nuts (pecans, walnuts, peanuts, etc.) or unsweetened shredded coconut

1. In a large bowl, combine oats, brown sugar, butter, honey, vanilla and salt; mix thoroughly. Stir in chocolate chips and nuts until evenly mixed.

2. Pour mixture into prepared pan. Press down with clean, damp hands to compact evenly.

3. Bake in preheated oven for 25 minutes or until brown and crisp. Let cool in pan on a wire rack for 5 minutes. Remove from pan by lifting parchment and transfer to a cutting board. Remove parchment and cut into bars.

Makes 24 bars (1 bar per serving)

TIP When using margarine, choose a non-hydrogenated version to limit consumption of trans fats.

VARIATION You can substitute any kind of chip for the chocolate chips—white chocolate, butterscotch, peanut butter, etc.

NUTRIENTS PER SERVING

Calories	131
Carbohydrate	18 g
Fiber	1 g
Protein	2 g
Fat, total	7 g
Fat, saturated	3 g
Cholesterol	7 mg
Sodium	78 mg

EXCHANGES PER SERVING

1	Other Carbohydrates
1½	Fat

BERRY CHEESECAKE BARS

TIPS When lining the baking pan, make sure the foil extends 1 inch beyond the edge for easy removal.

We tested these bars with raspberries, blueberries and mixed berries. All versions tasted great.

VARIATION If you prefer, replace the almond extract with vanilla and the orange zest with lemon.

NUTRIENTS PER SERVING

Calories	171
Carbohydrate	26 g
Fiber	1 g
Protein	3 g
Fat, total	6 g
Fat, saturated	3 g
Cholesterol	32 g
Sodium	121 mg

EXCHANGES PER SERVING

½ Starch
1 Other Carbohydrates
1 Fat

Preheat oven to 350°F
13- by 9-inch baking pan, lined with greased foil

Crumb Mixture

1	cup all-purpose flour
1	cup packed brown sugar
½	cup ground almonds
¼	cup melted butter
2	tbsp cold water

Filling

2	eggs
1	egg white
1	package (8 oz) light cream cheese, softened
¾	cup granulated sugar
½	cup low-fat plain yogurt
1½	tsp almond extract
1	tsp grated orange zest
1½	cups fresh or frozen berries (see Tip)

1. *Crumb Mixture:* In a medium bowl, combine flour, brown sugar, almonds, butter and water.

2. *Filling:* In a large bowl, using an electric mixer on high speed, beat eggs, egg white, cream cheese, sugar, yogurt, almond extract and orange zest until fluffy.

3. Press half of the crumb mixture into prepared pan. Pour in filling and spread evenly. Sprinkle with berries. Drop remaining crumb mixture by tablespoonfuls over berries. Using a knife, swirl filling, berries and crumb mixture.

4. Bake in preheated oven for 35 minutes or until a tester inserted in the center comes out clean. Let cool completely in pan on a wire rack. Remove from pan by lifting foil and transfer to a cutting board. Remove foil and cut into bars.

Makes 20 bars (1 bar per serving)

DATE OATMEAL SQUARES

Preheat oven to 350°F
8-inch square cake pan, sprayed with nonstick vegetable spray

½	lb pitted dates, chopped
1	cup water or orange juice
1	cup all-purpose flour
1	cup rolled oats
⅔	cup brown sugar
½	cup bran cereal*
½	tsp baking powder
½	tsp baking soda
½	cup soft margarine

* Use a wheat bran breakfast cereal.

1. In a saucepan, cover and cook dates and water over low heat, stirring often, for approximately 15 minutes or until dates are soft and liquid absorbed. Set aside.

2. In a bowl, combine flour, rolled oats, brown sugar, cereal, baking powder and baking soda; cut in margarine until crumbly.

3. Pat half onto bottom of cake pan; spoon date mixture over top. Pat remaining crumb mixture over date mixture. Bake for 20 to 25 minutes or until golden.

Makes 16 squares (1 square per serving)

TIPS For easier preparation, use scissors to cut the dates. Try half dates and half pitted, chopped prunes for a change.

When using margarine, choose a soft (non-hydrogenated) version.

NUTRIENTS PER SERVING

Calories	181
Carbohydrate	31 g
Fiber	3 g
Protein	2 g
Fat, total	6 g
Fat, saturated	1 g
Cholesterol	0 mg
Sodium	147 mg

EXCHANGES PER SERVING

1	Starch
½	Fruit
½	Other Carbohydrate
1	Fat

RAISIN & APPLESAUCE SQUARES

TIP To ease cleanup, rather than combining the dry ingredients in a bowl (Step 2), place a large piece of waxed paper on the counter. Spread the flours on the paper. Sprinkle with the baking powder, baking soda, cinnamon and cloves. Using the paper as a funnel, transfer the dry ingredients to the butter mixture.

VARIATIONS Replace orange zest with lemon zest.

Replace raisins with dried cranberries or cherries.

NUTRIENTS PER SERVING

Calories	82
Carbohydrate	15 g
Fiber	1 g
Protein	1 g
Fat, total	2 g
Fat, saturated	1 g
Cholesterol	12 mg
Sodium	54 mg

EXCHANGES PER SERVING

½ Fruit

½ Other Carbohydrate

½ Fat

Preheat oven to 350°F
8-inch square cake pan, greased

¼	cup butter, softened
½	cup packed brown sugar
1	egg
1	tbsp grated orange zest
1	tsp vanilla
1	cup unbleached all-purpose flour
½	cup whole wheat flour
½	tsp baking powder
½	tsp baking soda
1	tsp ground cinnamon
¼	tsp ground cloves
1	cup unsweetened applesauce
¾	cup raisins

1. In a large bowl, using an electric mixer on low speed, beat butter, brown sugar, egg, orange zest and vanilla until blended, about 3 minutes.

2. Combine all-purpose and whole wheat flours, baking powder, baking soda, cinnamon and cloves. Stir into creamed mixture alternately with applesauce, making 3 additions and mixing lightly after each addition. Stir in raisins. Spread evenly in prepared pan.

3. Bake in preheated oven until a toothpick inserted in center comes out clean, 25 to 30 minutes. Let cool completely in pan on rack. Cut into squares.

Makes 25 squares (1 square per serving)

LEMON POPPY SEED SQUARES

Preheat oven to 350°F
8-inch square baking pan, sprayed with vegetable spray

Cake

½	cup granulated sugar
1	tbsp margarine or butter
2	tsp poppy seeds
1½	tsp grated lemon zest
1	egg
¾	cup cake and pastry flour

Topping

⅔	cup granulated sugar
2	tsp grated lemon zest
⅓	cup freshly squeezed lemon juice
1	tbsp cornstarch
1	egg
1	egg white

1. *Cake:* In a bowl, whisk together sugar, margarine, poppy seeds, lemon zest and egg until smooth. Add wet ingredients to flour and stir just until mixed. Pat into prepared pan; set aside.

2. *Topping:* In a bowl, stir together sugar, lemon zest, lemon juice, cornstarch, whole egg and egg white. Pour over cake batter in pan.

3. Bake 20 to 25 minutes or until set with center still slightly soft. Cool to room temperature on a wire rack.

Makes 20 squares (1 square per serving)

TIPS Try substituting lime juice and zest for the lemon.

When using margarine, choose a soft (non-hydrogenated) version.

NUTRIENTS PER SERVING

Calories	77
Carbohydrate	16 g
Fiber	0 g
Protein	1 g
Fat, total	1 g
Fat, saturated	0 g
Cholesterol	19 mg
Sodium	17 mg

EXCHANGES PER SERVING

1 Other Carbohydrates

ALMOND SHORTBREAD SQUARES

NUTRIENTS PER SERVING

Calories	151
Carbohydrate	15 g
Fiber	1 g
Protein	2 g
Fat, total	9 g
Fat, saturated	5 g
Cholesterol	21 mg
Sodium	79 mg

EXCHANGES PER SERVING

1 Other Carbohydrates

2 Fat

Preheat oven to 325°F
13- by 9-inch cake pan, ungreased

¾	cup sliced almonds, toasted
2	cups all-purpose flour
1	cup cold butter, cubed
½	cup granulated sugar
½	cup cornstarch
2	tbsp grated orange zest
¾	tsp almond extract

1. In a food processor, pulse almonds until coarsely chopped. Add flour, butter, sugar, cornstarch, orange zest and almond extract and pulse until crumbly. Press evenly into pan.

2. Bake in preheated oven until lightly browned around edges, 30 to 35 minutes. Cut into squares just as the pan comes out of the oven, then let cool completely in pan on rack. Recut.

Makes 24 squares (1 square per serving)

COCONUT SEEDS CEREAL SQUARES

Preheat oven to 375°F
15- by 10- by 1-inch jelly-roll pan, greased

¾	cup butter
1¼	cups packed brown sugar
1	tsp vanilla
2¼	cups quick-cooking rolled oats
¼	cup sesame seeds
¼	cup flaxseeds
¼	cup sunflower seeds
¼	cup unsweetened flaked coconut
¾	tsp baking powder
¼	tsp salt

1. In a large saucepan, melt butter over medium heat. Stir in brown sugar and vanilla. Cook, stirring often, until mixture is bubbly, about 2 minutes. Remove from heat. Stir in rolled oats, sesame seeds, flaxseeds, sunflower seeds, coconut, baking powder and salt, mixing well until all ingredients are moistened. Press evenly into prepared pan.

2. Bake in preheated oven until light golden, about 10 minutes. Let cool completely in pan on rack. Cut into squares.

Makes 24 squares (1 square per serving)

TIP Teach kids how to measure brown sugar properly. Unlike granulated sugar, which is simply scooped into a dry measuring cup, then leveled off, brown sugar is packed into the cup. To test if they did it right, turn the cup upside down on a piece of waxed paper. When you remove the cup, the sugar should hold its shape.

VARIATION Use other kinds of seeds. Pumpkin seeds add an interesting appearance, texture and flavor.

NUTRIENTS PER SERVING

Calories	160
Carbohydrate	19 g
Fiber	2 g
Protein	2 g
Fat, total	9 g
Fat, saturated	4 g
Cholesterol	16 mg
Sodium	97 mg

EXCHANGES PER SERVING

1 Other Carbohydrates
2 Fat

ALMOND BUTTER CEREAL SQUARES

TIP Brown rice syrup is available in the natural food section of your supermarket or from health food stores. If you cannot find it, use fancy molasses instead.

VARIATION Instead of apricots, substitute another dried fruit. Raisins, cranberries, cherries, chopped pitted dates and figs all work well.

NUTRIENTS PER SERVING

Calories	241
Carbohydrate	37 g
Fiber	4 g
Protein	5 g
Fat, total	10 g
Fat, saturated	1 g
Cholesterol	0 mg
Sodium	90 mg

EXCHANGES PER SERVING

½ Starch
½ Fruit
1½ Other Carbohydrates
2 Fat

9-inch square baking pan, lightly greased

½	cup crunchy almond butter
½	cup brown rice syrup
½	cup liquid honey
1	tsp vanilla
1	cup chopped dried apricots
½	cup sliced almonds
¼	cup sesame seeds
¼	cup ground flaxseed
¼	cup sunflower seeds
2½	cups high-fiber cereal, such as bran flakes
1¼	cups old-fashioned rolled oats

1. In a large saucepan, over low heat, cook almond butter, rice syrup, honey and vanilla until blended. Add apricots, almonds, sesame seeds, flaxseed and sunflower seeds; mix well. Add cereal and oats; mix well.

2. Pour mixture into prepared pan. Press down with clean, damp hands to compact evenly. Let stand for 30 minutes, until firm, then cut into squares.

Makes 16 squares (1 square per serving)

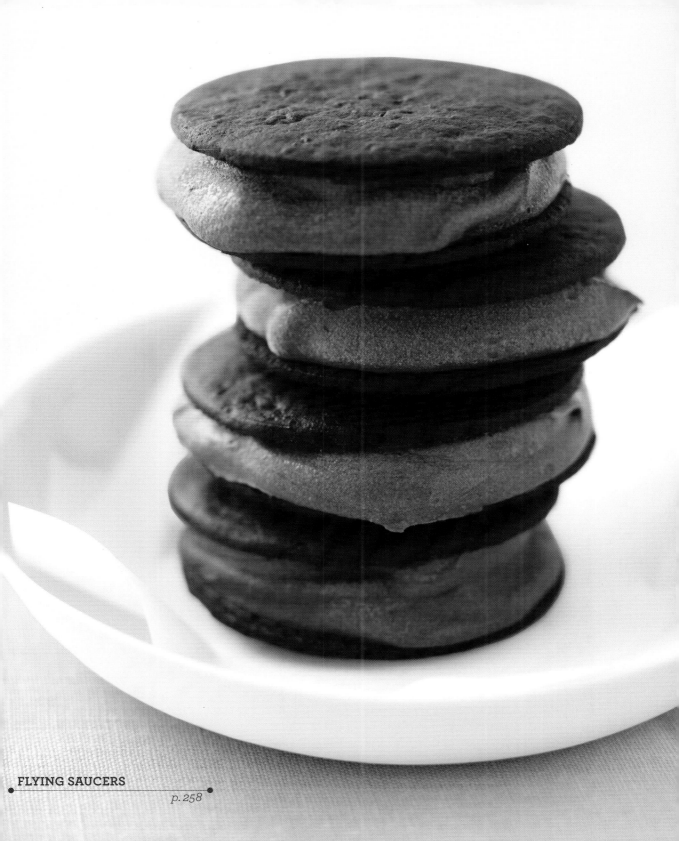

FLYING SAUCERS

p. 258

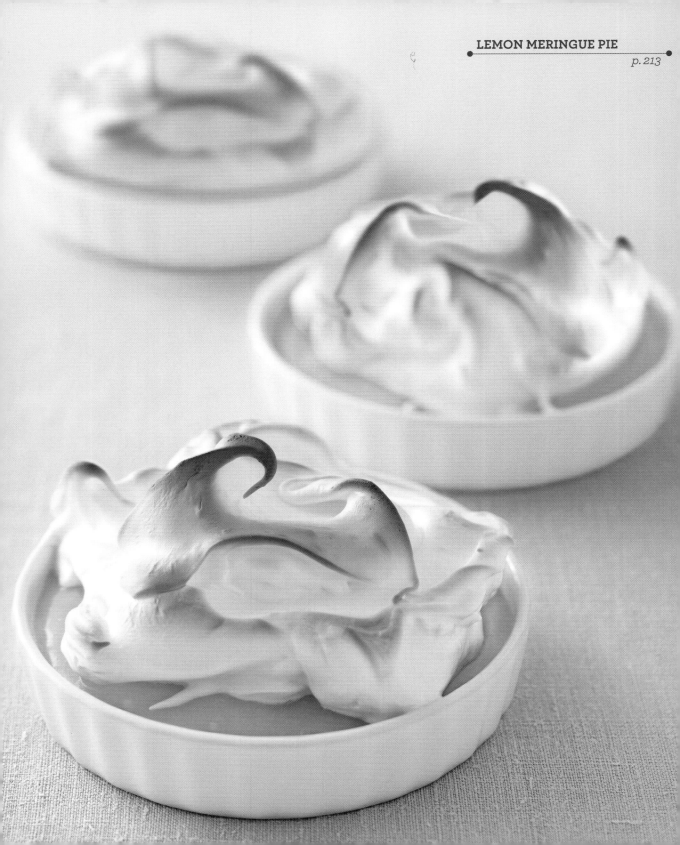

LEMON MERINGUE PIE

p. 213

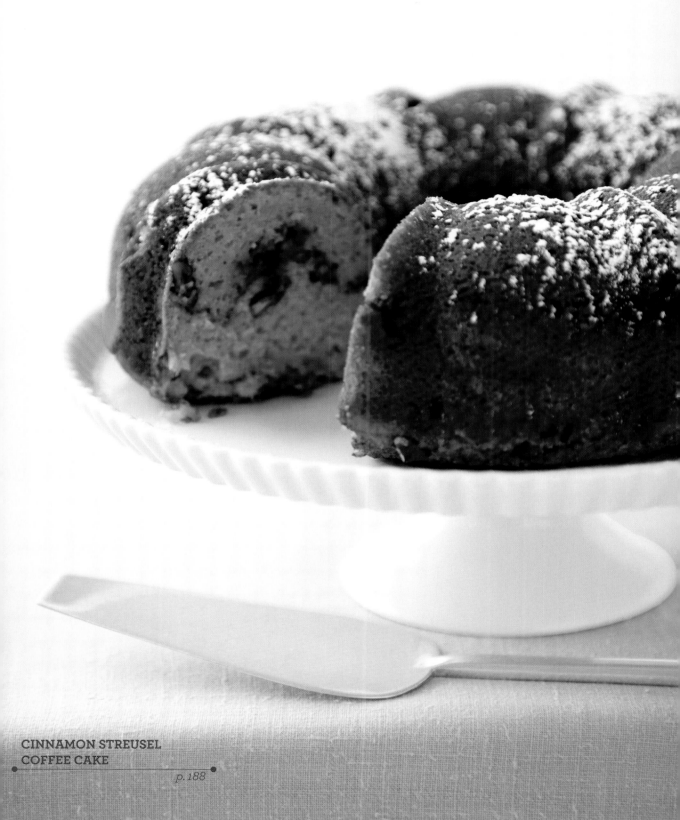

CINNAMON STREUSEL
COFFEE CAKE
p. 188

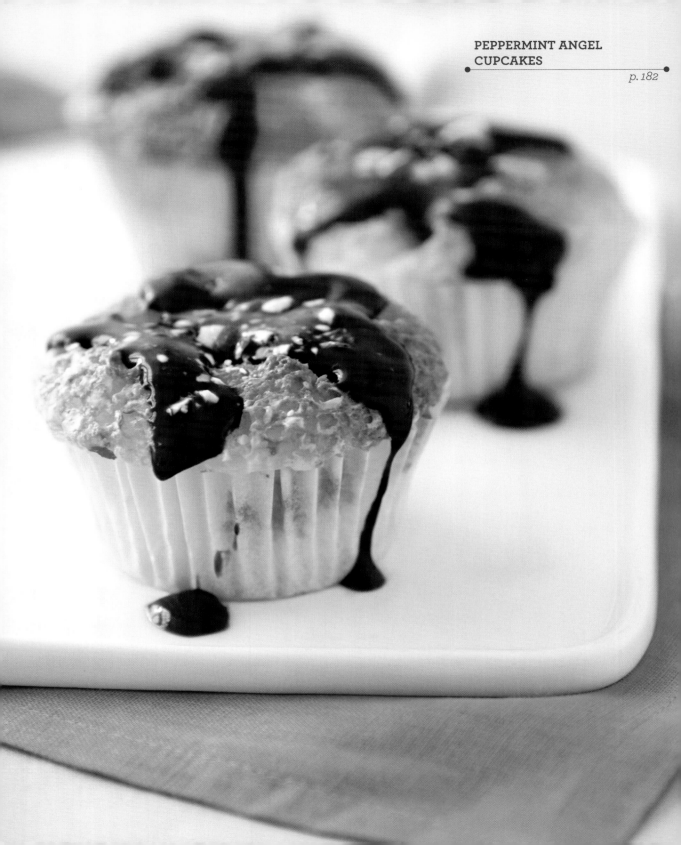

PEPPERMINT ANGEL
CUPCAKES

p. 182

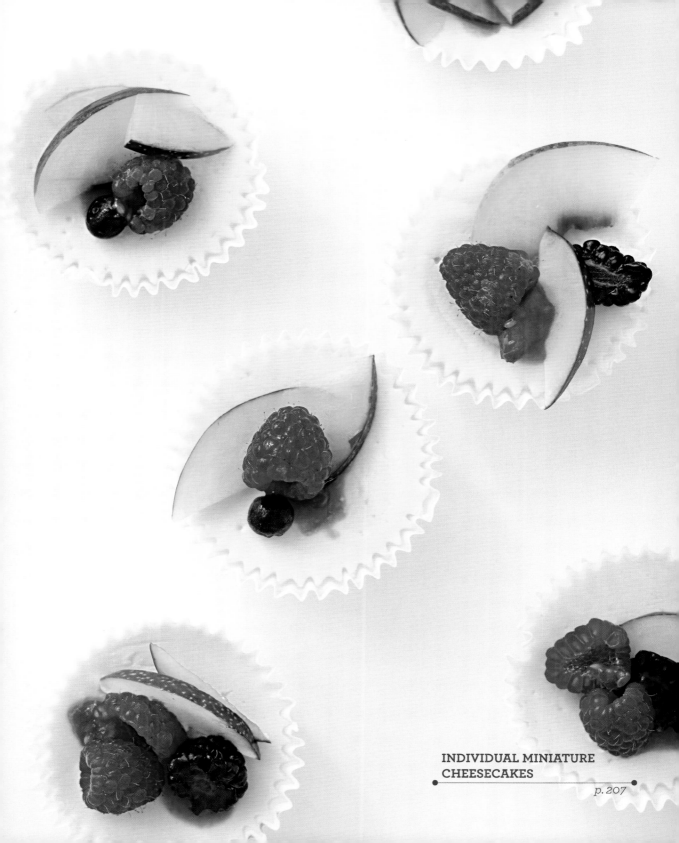

INDIVIDUAL MINIATURE
CHEESECAKES

p. 207

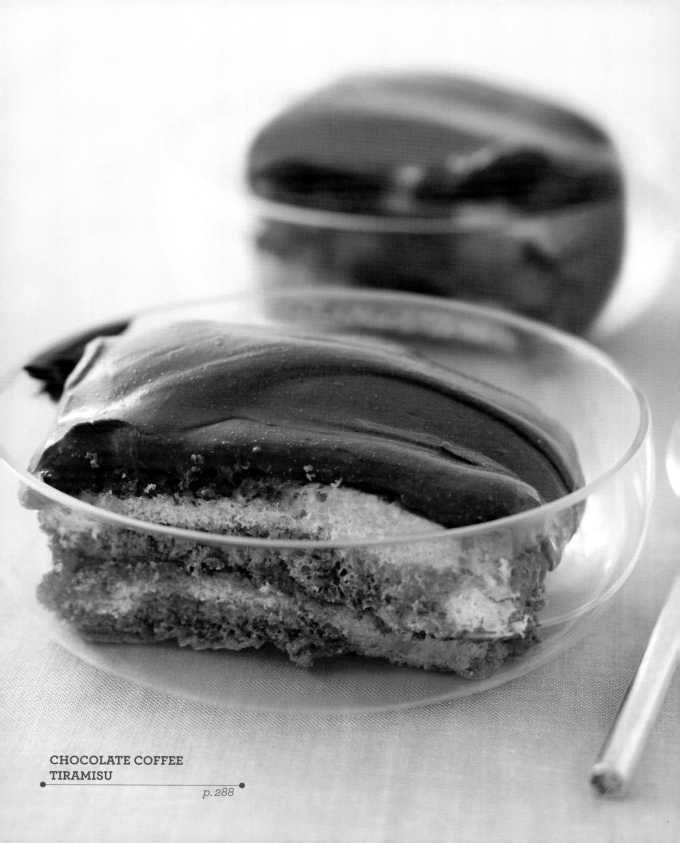

**CHOCOLATE COFFEE
TIRAMISU**

p. 288

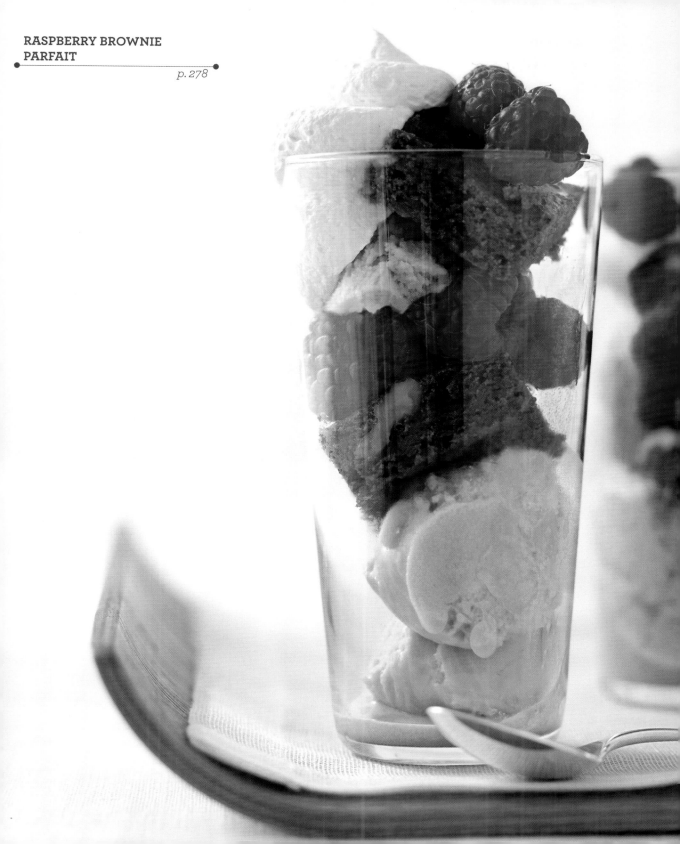

CHOCOLATE ZUCCHINI CAKE
p. 181

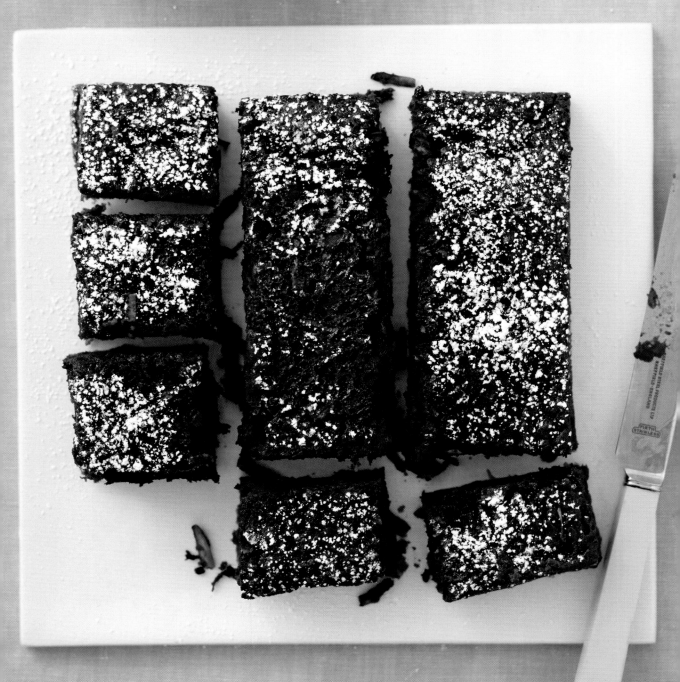

CRISPY GRANOLA SQUARES

13- by 9-inch baking pan, lined with foil and sprayed with vegetable spray

¼	cup soft margarine
3	cups mini marshmallows
5	cups crisp rice cereal
¼	cup unsweetened cocoa powder, sifted
1	tsp vanilla
⅓	cup quick-cooking rolled oats
⅓	cup unsweetened flaked coconut
¼	cup raisins
¼	cup semisweet chocolate chips

1. In a large, heavy saucepan, over low heat, melt margarine. Add marshmallows and stir constantly until marshmallows are melted, about 10 minutes. Remove from heat, stir in rice cereal, cocoa and vanilla and mix until evenly coated. Add oats, coconut, raisins and chocolate chips and mix until evenly coated.

2. Press evenly into prepared baking pan. Refrigerate for 30 minutes to 1 hour, until firm. Using foil, lift the bars out of the pan and cut into 24 squares.

Makes 24 squares (1 per serving)

TIPS So you can get the squares out of the pan easily, allow the foil to extend over the edges of the pan.

To cut easily into neat squares, dip your knife in hot water before each cut.

NUTRIENTS PER SERVING

Calories	94
Carbohydrate	15 g
Fiber	1 g
Protein	1 g
Fat, total	4 g
Fat, saturated	2 g
Cholesterol	0 mg
Sodium	84 mg

EXCHANGES PER SERVING

1 Other Carbohydrates
1 Fat

DIETITIAN'S NOTE *Crisp rice cereal is fortified with B vitamins, and the carbohydrate from the marshmallows, raisins and chocolate chips can readily fit into the meal plan of active children. School-age kids will love finding these squares as a surprise in their lunch.*

CHRISTMAS BROWNIES

TIP Because it is easy to overcook the brownies, always bake bars in the center of the oven and check for doneness at the minimum suggested baking time.

NUTRIENTS PER SERVING

Calories	124
Carbohydrate	18 g
Fiber	1 g
Protein	2 g
Fat, total	6 g
Fat, saturated	2 g
Cholesterol	27 mg
Sodium	24 mg

EXCHANGES PER SERVING

1 Other Carbohydrates

1 Fat

Preheat oven to 300°F
9-inch square baking pan, sprayed with vegetable spray

24	lower-fat graham wafers
2	tbsp unsweetened cocoa powder
½	tsp salt
2	large eggs
1	large egg white
⅓	cup packed brown sugar
¼	cup granulated sugar
2	tsp vanilla
½	cup white chocolate chips
½	cup slivered almonds
⅓	cup coarsely chopped dried cranberries

1. In a food processor, pulse wafers into coarse crumbs. (Or place wafers on a large sheet of waxed paper, cover with another sheet of waxed paper and crush with a rolling pin.) Add cocoa and salt and process until combined.

2. In a large bowl, using an electric mixer or wooden spoon, beat eggs, egg white, brown sugar, granulated sugar and vanilla until well blended and thickened. Stir in crumb mixture.

3. Spread batter evenly in prepared pan and sprinkle with chocolate chips, almonds and cranberries. Press toppings gently into the batter so they will adhere when baked.

4. Bake in preheated oven for 25 to 30 minutes, or until knife inserted in the center comes out clean. Let cool completely in pan on a rack and cut into 16 squares.

Makes 16 brownies (1 per serving)

MOIST 'N' CHEWY CHOCOLATE BROWNIES

Preheat oven to 375°F
9-inch square cake pan, greased

½	cup butter
3	squares (1 oz each) unsweetened chocolate, chopped
1¼	cups granulated sugar
1½	tsp vanilla
3	eggs
⅔	cup all-purpose flour
½	tsp baking powder
¼	tsp salt

1. In a saucepan over low heat, melt butter and chocolate, stirring constantly, until smooth. Remove from heat. Stir in sugar and vanilla, mixing well. Whisk in eggs, one at a time, beating lightly after each addition.

2. Combine flour, baking powder and salt. Stir into chocolate mixture until well blended. Spread evenly in prepared pan.

3. Bake in preheated oven just until set, 25 to 30 minutes. Let cool completely in pan on rack. Cut into bars.

Makes 24 brownies (1 brownie per serving)

TIPS These brownies are quite dense and chewy. If you prefer them more cake-like, add an egg.

Instead of greasing pans, line them with parchment paper that extends up the sides and over the edges so you can lift out the brownies in a block. Spraying the pan lightly with cooking spray or greasing it lightly before adding the parchment helps the paper to stick, preventing it from shifting.

NUTRIENTS PER SERVING

Calories	113
Carbohydrate	16 g
Fiber	0 g
Protein	1 g
Fat, total	5 g
Fat, saturated	3 g
Cholesterol	34 mg
Sodium	77 mg

EXCHANGES PER SERVING

1 Other Carbohydrates
1 Fat

CHOCOLATE CHUNK BANANA BROWNIES

TIPS These brownies are nice plain or dusted with confectioner's sugar.

For recipes calling for chopped chocolate, I like to buy large bittersweet chocolate bars and chop them to the size of chips.

VARIATIONS Replace chocolate chunks with chocolate chips.

Substitute peanut butter chips for the chopped chocolate and coarsely chopped peanuts for the walnuts.

NUTRIENTS PER SERVING

Calories	128
Carbohydrate	16 g
Fiber	1 g
Protein	2 g
Fat, total	7 g
Fat, saturated	2 g
Cholesterol	10 mg
Sodium	46 mg

EXCHANGES PER SERVING

1 Other Carbohydrates
1½ Fat

Preheat oven to 350°F
13- by 9-inch cake pan, greased

1	cup granulated sugar
⅓	cup vegetable oil
2	eggs
1	cup mashed ripe banana (2 large bananas)
¾	cup unsweetened cocoa powder, sifted
1	cup all-purpose flour
1	tsp baking powder
½	tsp baking soda
¼	tsp salt
1½	cups chopped semisweet chocolate
1⅓	cups coarsely chopped walnuts

1. In a large bowl, using an electric mixer on medium speed, beat sugar, oil and eggs until thick and light, about 2 minutes. Add banana and cocoa and beat on low speed.

2. Combine flour, baking powder, baking soda and salt. Add to cocoa mixture, beating on low speed just to blend. Stir in chopped chocolate and walnuts. Spread evenly in prepared pan.

3. Bake in preheated oven just until set, 25 to 30 minutes. Let cool completely in pan on rack. Cut into bars or squares.

Makes 36 brownies (1 brownie per serving)

TRIPLE CHOCOLATE BROWNIES

Preheat oven to 350°F
8-inch square cake pan sprayed with vegetable spray

½	cup granulated sugar
⅓	cup margarine or butter
1	egg
1	tsp vanilla
½	cup all-purpose flour
⅓	cup unsweetened cocoa powder
1	tsp baking powder
¼	cup 2% milk
¼	cup chocolate chips

Icing

¼	cup confectioner's sugar
1½	tbsp unsweetened cocoa powder
1	tbsp milk

1. In a bowl, beat together sugar and margarine. Beat in egg and vanilla, mixing well.

2. In another bowl, combine flour, cocoa and baking powder; stir into sugar and butter mixture just until blended. Stir in milk and chocolate chips. Pour into prepared pan and bake approximately 18 minutes or until edges start to pull away from pan and center is still a little wet. Let cool slightly before glazing.

3. *Icing:* In small bowl, whisk together confectioner's sugar, cocoa and milk; pour over brownies in pan.

Makes 16 brownies (1 brownie per serving)

DIETITIAN'S NOTE *Enjoy these brownies with or without the icing, which supplies about 2 grams of carbohydrate per brownie.*

TIP When using margarine, choose a soft (non-hydrogenated) version to limit consumption of trans fats.

NUTRIENTS PER SERVING

Calories	105
Carbohydrate	14 g
Fiber	1 g
Protein	2 g
Fat, total	5 g
Fat, saturated	1 g
Cholesterol	12 mg
Sodium	74 mg

EXCHANGES PER SERVING

1 Other Carbohydrates
1 Fat

WHITE CHOCOLATE BROWNIES

TIPS These make a nice holiday gift. Pack them in a decorative airtight cookie tin or box, tie with a festive ribbon and add the recipe with your gift tag.

If you can find orange-flavored dried cranberries, try them in this recipe. They taste particularly delicious in this brownie.

NUTRIENTS PER SERVING

Calories	72
Carbohydrate	9 g
Fiber	0 g
Protein	1 g
Fat, total	4 g
Fat, saturated	2 g
Cholesterol	11 mg
Sodium	23 mg

EXCHANGES PER SERVING

½ Other Carbohydrate

1 Fat

Preheat oven to 375°F
8-inch square cake pan, greased

6	squares (1 oz each) white chocolate, chopped
¾	cup granulated sugar
2	eggs
⅓	cup butter, melted
1	tsp vanilla
1¼	cups all-purpose flour
¾	tsp baking powder
¾	cup coarsely chopped hazelnuts
⅓	cup dried cranberries

1. In a small saucepan over low heat, melt white chocolate, stirring constantly, until smooth. Remove from heat and set aside.

2. In a bowl, whisk sugar and eggs until blended. Whisk in melted butter and vanilla. Combine flour and baking powder. Stir into egg mixture alternately with melted chocolate, making 2 additions of each and mixing until smooth. Stir in hazelnuts and cranberries. Spread evenly in prepared pan.

3. Bake in preheated oven just until set and golden, 25 to 30 minutes. Let cool completely in pan on rack. Cut into bars or squares.

Makes 48 brownies (1 brownie per serving)

SOUR CREAM BROWNIES

Preheat oven to 350°F
8-inch square cake pan, sprayed with nonstick vegetable spray

⅔	cup granulated sugar	
⅓	cup soft margarine	
1	egg	
1	tsp vanilla	
⅓	cup unsweetened cocoa powder	
⅓	cup all-purpose flour	
1	tsp baking powder	
¼	cup light sour cream	

1. In a bowl, beat together sugar and margarine until smooth. Beat in egg and vanilla, mixing well.

2. Combine cocoa, flour and baking powder; stir into bowl just until blended. Stir in sour cream. Pour into prepared pan.

3. Bake for 20 to 25 minutes or until edges start to pull away from pan and center is still slightly soft.

Makes 16 brownies (1 brownie per serving)

TIPS If desired, sprinkle 2 tbsp chopped nuts over the batter before baking.

Garnish with a sprinkling of confectioner's sugar after baking.

When using margarine, choose a soft (non-hydrogenated) version to limit consumption of trans fats.

Bake a day before or freeze for up to 6 weeks.

NUTRIENTS PER SERVING

Calories	89
Carbohydrate	12 g
Fiber	1 g
Protein	1 g
Fat, total	5 g
Fat, saturated	1 g
Cholesterol	12 mg
Sodium	76 mg

EXCHANGES PER SERVING

1	Other Carbohydrates
1	Fat

CREAM CHEESE-FILLED BROWNIES

TIP Prepare up to 2 days in advance. Freeze for up to 4 weeks.

NUTRIENTS PER SERVING

Calories	145
Carbohydrate	22 g
Fiber	1 g
Protein	3 g
Fat, total	6 g
Fat, saturated	1 g
Cholesterol	17 mg
Sodium	91 mg

EXCHANGES PER SERVING

1½ Other Carbohydrates
1 Fat

Preheat oven to 350°F
8-inch square baking dish, sprayed with vegetable spray

Filling

4	oz light cream cheese, softened
2	tbsp granulated sugar
2	tbsp 2% milk
1	tsp vanilla

Cake

1	cup packed brown sugar
⅓	cup light sour cream
¼	cup vegetable oil
1	egg
1	egg white
¾	cup all-purpose flour
½	cup unsweetened cocoa powder
1	tsp baking powder

1. *Filling:* In a food processor or in a bowl with an electric mixer, beat together cream cheese, sugar, milk and vanilla until smooth. Set aside.

2. *Cake:* In a large bowl, whisk together brown sugar, sour cream, oil, whole egg and egg white. In a separate bowl, stir together flour, cocoa and baking powder. Add liquid ingredients to dry, blending just until mixed.

3. Pour half the cake batter into prepared pan. Spoon filling on top; spread with a wet knife. Pour remaining batter into pan. Bake for 20 to 25 minutes or until just barely loose at center.

Makes 16 brownies (1 brownie per serving)

CHOCOLATE BROWNIES

Preheat oven to 350°F
8-inch square baking pan, sprayed with vegetable spray

⅔	cup all-purpose flour
½	cup granulated sugar
⅓	cup unsweetened cocoa powder, sifted
1	tsp baking powder
¼	tsp salt
⅓	cup chopped walnuts
2	large eggs
⅓	cup soft margarine
1	tsp vanilla
½	cup unsweetened applesauce

1. In a medium bowl, stir together flour, sugar, cocoa, baking powder and salt. Stir in walnuts.

2. In a large bowl, using an electric mixer, beat eggs, margarine and vanilla at high speed for 1 minute, until well mixed. Add applesauce and beat just until blended. Add flour mixture and mix at low speed just until blended.

3. Spread batter evenly in prepared pan and bake in preheated oven for 15 minutes, or until a knife inserted in the center comes out clean. Let cool completely in pan on a rack and cut into 16 squares.

Makes 16 brownies (1 per serving)

NUTRIENTS PER SERVING

Calories	111
Carbohydrate	13 g
Fiber	1 g
Protein	2 g
Fat, total	6 g
Fat, saturated	1 g
Cholesterol	27 mg
Sodium	106 mg

EXCHANGES PER SERVING

½	Starch
½	Other Carbohydrate
1	Fat

DIETITIAN'S NOTE *Unsweetened cocoa powder has only 115 calories and 4 grams of fat per ⅓ cup, whereas 1 oz of unsweetened baking chocolate has 139 calories and 14 grams of fat. Cocoa has just as much rich chocolate flavor as baking chocolate, so substituting cocoa is a good way to cut fat.*

ORANGE CREAM CHEESE BROWNIES

TIP To ease cleanup, rather than combining the dry ingredients in a bowl (in Step 2), place a large piece of waxed paper on the counter. Spread the flour on the paper and sift the cocoa powder and baking powder over it. Using the paper as a funnel, transfer the dry ingredients to the egg mixture.

VARIATIONS For thinner, less cake-like bars, bake these in a 9-inch square cake pan for 20 to 25 minutes.

Replace yogurt with light sour cream.

Preheat oven to 350°F
8-inch square cake pan, greased

Filling

4	oz	light cream cheese, softened
2	tbsp	granulated sugar
2	tbsp	2% milk
1	tbsp	grated orange zest

Batter

1	cup	packed brown sugar
⅓	cup	2% plain yogurt
¼	cup	vegetable oil
1		egg
1		egg white
¾	cup	unbleached all-purpose flour
½	cup	unsweetened cocoa powder, sifted
1	tsp	baking powder

1. *Filling:* In a small bowl, using an electric mixer on low speed, beat cream cheese and sugar until blended, about 3 minutes. Add milk and orange zest, beating until smooth. Set aside.

2. *Batter:* In a bowl, whisk brown sugar, yogurt, oil, egg and egg white until blended. Combine flour, cocoa and baking powder. Stir into egg mixture, mixing well.

3. Spread half of the brownie batter in prepared pan. Spread filling evenly over top. Drop remaining batter by spoonfuls over filling. Swirl batters together lightly with small spatula or knife to make a marbled effect.

4. Bake in preheated oven until set, 25 to 30 minutes. Let cool completely in pan on rack. Cut into bars or squares.

Makes 24 brownies (1 brownie per serving)

DIETITIAN'S NOTE *You can reduce the amount of sugar in some recipes by using a low-calorie sweetener (also known as a sugar substitute or artificial sweetener). These products contain intensely sweet ingredients that typically replace 150 to 300 times their weight in sugar. Such minuscule amounts would be impossible to measure, so the sweetening agent is combined with carriers such as dextrose and maltodextrin. These carriers are carbohydrates, but only a very small amount is required to deliver a lot of sweetness.*

Typically, about ¼ tsp of a powdered low-calorie sweetener—containing only a few milligrams of the sweetening ingredient—is equivalent to 2 tsp of sugar.

Low-calorie sweeteners vary considerably. For example, some are affected by cooking temperatures, while others are not. Some are sold as sachets to add to beverages and foods at the table, while others come in a granular form that "measures like sugar." Some manufacturers make both types.

Because low-calorie sweeteners vary so much, and because sugar is often an important part of a food's structure, you often can't make a simple substitution on the basis of equal sweetness. If you want to try one of these products, first try it in recipes specifically developed for that product.

You can find out more about low-calorie sweeteners, including recommendations for their use, from the American Diabetes Association (www.diabetes.org).

NUTRIENTS PER SERVING

Calories	95
Carbohydrate	14 g
Fiber	1 g
Protein	2 g
Fat, total	4 g
Fat, saturated	1 g
Cholesterol	11 mg
Sodium	59 mg

EXCHANGES PER SERVING

1 Other Carbohydrates

1 Fat

5

CAKES, COFFEE CAKES & CHEESECAKES

155   Perfect Angel Food Cake

156   Chocolate Angel Food Cake

157   Spiced Angel Food Cake

158   Angel Tunnel Cake

159   Fruit-Filled Angel Tunnel Cake

160   Chiffon Cake

161   Striped Strawberry Cake

162   Chocolate Espresso Cake

163   Blueberry Honey Cake

164   Blueberry Peach Cake

165   Orange Pumpkin Snacking Cake

166   Sour Cream Orange Apple Cake

168   Banana Cake with Lemon Cream Frosting

170   Date Cake with Coconut Topping

172   Prune Orange Spice Cake

174   Banana Spice Cake

176   Banana Date Cake

177   Carrot Cake

178   Applesauce Carrot Cake

180   Piña Colada Snacking Cake

181   Chocolate Zucchini Cake

182   Peppermint Angel Cupcakes

183   Spicy Apple Cupcakes

184   Apple Pecan Streusel Cake

186   Apricot Date Streusel Cake

188   Cinnamon Streusel Coffee Cake

190   Mennonite Streusel Cake

192   Orange-Glazed Coffee Cake

193   Orange Coffee Cake

194   Cinnamon Date Coffee Cake

196   Chocolate Chunk Coffee Cake

198   Chocolate Marble Coffee Cake

199   La Costa Cheesecake with Strawberry Sauce

200   Raspberry Cheesecake

201   Tangy Banana Cheesecake

202   Marble Mocha Cheesecake

204   Chocolate Cheesecake

206   Chocolate Marble Vanilla Cheesecake

207   Individual Miniature Cheesecakes

PERFECT ANGEL FOOD CAKE

Preheat oven to 375°F
10-inch tube pan, ungreased

1	cup cake flour
1½	cups granulated sugar, divided
12	egg whites, very cold (about 1¼ cups)
1½	tsp cream of tartar
1½	tsp vanilla
1	tsp almond extract
½	tsp salt

1. Make sure all tools, including tube pan, mixer and whip attachment, are free of any oil, very clean and dry. If any traces of oil are on any of your tools, your cake will not work.

2. Sift cake flour together with ¾ cup of the granulated sugar. Set aside.

3. In a mixer bowl fitted with whip attachment, whip egg whites, cream of tartar, vanilla, almond extract and salt on high speed until soft peaks form, about 4 minutes. With mixer running, gradually sprinkle in remaining sugar, beating until stiff, glossy peaks form. Using a rubber spatula, gradually fold in flour mixture just until incorporated.

4. Pour batter into pan, smoothing top and gently removing any large bubbles. Bake in preheated oven until golden brown and top springs back when lightly touched, 40 to 45 minutes. Invert pan, balancing on tube, and let cake cool completely. The cake should fall out of pan when cool. If it needs a little help, run a rubber spatula around the sides of pan to loosen.

Makes 12 slices (1 slice per serving)

NUTRIENTS PER SERVING

Calories	149
Carbohydrate	33 g
Fiber	0 g
Protein	4 g
Fat, total	0 g
Fat, saturated	0 g
Cholesterol	0 mg
Sodium	152 mg

EXCHANGES PER SERVING

½ Starch
1½ Other Carbohydrates
½ Very Lean Meat

CHOCOLATE ANGEL FOOD CAKE

TIP Eggs separate more easily when cold. Use 3 bowls—one to separate eggs over, one for the yolks and one to which perfectly clean whites are transferred. Make sure there's not a speck of yolk in the whites or they won't beat properly. Egg whites beat to a greater volume when at room temperature.

NUTRIENTS PER SERVING

Calories	141
Carbohydrate	31 g
Fiber	1 g
Protein	5 g
Fat, total	0 g
Fat, saturated	0 g
Cholesterol	0 mg
Sodium	55 mg

EXCHANGES PER SERVING

½ Starch
1½ Other Carbohydrates
½ Very Lean Meat

Preheat oven to 375°F
10-inch tube pan, sprayed with baking spray

1	cup cake and pastry flour
¼	cup unsweetened cocoa powder
1⅓	cups granulated sugar, divided
12	egg whites, at room temperature
½	tsp cream of tartar
1	tsp vanilla
½	tsp almond extract
	Strawberry purée or sliced strawberries

1. Into a bowl, sift together flour, cocoa and ⅓ cup of the sugar; set aside.

2. In a large bowl, beat egg whites until foamy. Add cream of tartar; beat until soft peaks form. Gradually add remaining sugar, beating until stiff peaks form. In 2 additions, gently fold cocoa mixture into egg whites until well blended. Fold in vanilla and almond extract. Pour batter into prepared pan.

3. Bake for 35 to 40 minutes or until cake springs back when lightly touched. Turn pan upside down and place over a bottle or an inverted funnel. Cool cake completely before removing from pan. Serve with strawberry purée or sliced strawberries.

Makes 12 slices (1 slice per serving)

DIETITIAN'S NOTE *Strawberries and chocolate are a great combination. Two strawberries, or 2 tbsp strawberry purée without sugar, adds only 1 gram of carbohydrate.*

SPICED ANGEL FOOD CAKE

Preheat oven to 325°F
10-inch tube pan, ungreased

1	package (1 lb) vanilla angel food cake mix
1	tsp ground cinnamon
1	tsp ground ginger
½	tsp ground nutmeg

Cran-Apple Topping

4	red apples (e.g., Macintosh), cored and thinly sliced
½	cup freshly squeezed orange juice
⅓	cup lightly packed brown sugar
2	tsp cornstarch
1	tsp ground cinnamon
1	cup cranberries, fresh or frozen

1. To the dry cake mix, add cinnamon, ginger and nutmeg, then bake according to package instructions. Let cool in the pan, inverted on a wire rack.

2. *Cran-Apple Topping:* Put the apples in a large skillet. In a small bowl, stir together orange juice, brown sugar and cornstarch until smooth. Add cinnamon and ¼ cup water. Pour orange juice mixture over the apples and cook over medium heat, stirring occasionally, for 5 to 8 minutes, until juice starts to bubble. Reduce heat to low and add cranberries; simmer for 10 to 15 minutes, or until berries pop.

3. Serve the warm topping over slices of cake.

Makes 16 servings

TIP Because heat rises, oven temperatures are not even throughout. For best results, bake cakes in the very center of the oven. If baking more than one item at a time, stagger them on the same rack so they don't touch the walls of the oven or each other.

NUTRIENTS PER SERVING

Calories	143
Carbohydrate	34 g
Fiber	1 g
Protein	2 g
Fat, total	0 g
Fat, saturated	0 g
Cholesterol	0 mg
Sodium	182 mg

EXCHANGES PER SERVING

½	Starch
½	Fruit
1	Other Carbohydrates

ANGEL TUNNEL CAKE

TIP It's hard to cut an angel food cake because it is sticky. Try using a wet knife with a serrated edge, and use your fingers to help hollow out the trench.

NUTRIENTS PER SERVING

Calories	171
Carbohydrate	36 g
Fiber	0 g
Protein	5 g
Fat, total	2 g
Fat, saturated	1 g
Cholesterol	6 mg
Sodium	268 mg

EXCHANGES PER SERVING

1	Starch
1½	Other Carbohydrates

1	prepared vanilla or chocolate angel food cake (from mix, store-bought or homemade)
1	package (1½ oz) fat-free instant chocolate pudding mix, sweetened with aspartame
1½	cups 1% milk
3	cups lower-fat non-dairy whipped topping, divided
2	tbsp unsweetened cocoa powder

1. Slice a 1-inch layer off the top of the cake. Gently hollow out a trench 1½ inches wide and 2 inches deep from the bottom piece. Cut the cake removed from the trench into small pieces.

2. In a large bowl, beat pudding mix and milk for 2 minutes, until thickened and smooth. Stir in 1 cup of the whipped topping and the reserved cake pieces. Fill the trench with the pudding mixture and replace the top of the cake.

3. In a medium bowl, sift cocoa into the remaining 2 cups whipped topping and stir gently until smooth. Frost cake with chocolate whipped topping and chill for at least 4 hours, until set, or overnight.

Makes 12 servings

DIETITIAN'S NOTE *Angel food cake is low in calories because it is made primarily with egg whites.*

FRUIT-FILLED ANGEL TUNNEL CAKE

- 1 prepared vanilla or lemon angel food cake (from mix, store-bought or homemade)
- 1 package (1⅓ oz) reduced-calorie vanilla mousse mix
- 1½ cups 1% milk
- 2 cups lower-fat non-dairy whipped topping, divided
- 1 cup diced fresh fruit (such as strawberries, blueberries, kiwi)
- 1 tbsp grated lemon zest

1. Slice a 1-inch layer off the top of the cake. Gently hollow out a trench 1½ inches wide and 2 inches deep from the bottom piece. Cut the cake removed from the trench into small pieces.

2. In a medium bowl, beat vanilla mousse mix and milk for 3 minutes, until thickened. Fold in ½ cup of the whipped topping, fresh fruit, lemon zest and cake pieces. Fill the trench with the fruit mixture and replace the top of the cake.

3. Frost with the remaining 1½ cups whipped topping and chill for at least 4 hours, until set, or overnight. Garnish with lemon slices just before serving.

Makes 12 servings

NUTRIENTS PER SERVING

Calories	164
Carbohydrate	35 g
Fiber	0 g
Protein	5 g
Fat, total	1 g
Fat, saturated	1 g
Cholesterol	4 mg
Sodium	263 mg

EXCHANGES PER SERVING

- 1 Starch
- 1 Other Carbohydrates

CHIFFON CAKE

TIP Eggs separate more easily when cold. Use 3 bowls—one to separate eggs over, one for the yolks and one to hold the perfectly clean whites. Make sure there's not a speck of yolk in the whites or they won't beat properly.

NUTRIENTS PER SERVING

Calories	108
Carbohydrate	19 g
Fiber	0 g
Protein	4 g
Fat, total	1 g
Fat, saturated	0 g
Cholesterol	49 mg
Sodium	84 mg

EXCHANGES PER SERVING

½ Starch
½ Other Carbohydrate
½ Lean Meat

Preheat oven to 350°F
9-inch springform pan, sprayed with baking spray

1	cup cake and pastry flour
½	cup granulated sugar
1½	tsp baking powder
3	medium eggs
2	medium egg whites
⅓	cup water
1	tsp grated lemon zest
1	tsp grated orange zest
½	tsp vanilla
½	cup egg whites (from about 4 medium eggs)
¼	tsp cream of tartar
	Sliced fresh fruit

1. Sift flour, sugar and baking powder into a bowl. In another bowl, beat together whole eggs, 2 egg whites, water, lemon zest, orange zest and vanilla until well mixed. Slowly add wet ingredients to dry ingredients, mixing until combined. Set aside.

2. In a separate bowl, beat egg whites until foamy. Add cream of tartar; beat until stiff peaks form. Gently fold egg whites into batter. Pour into prepared pan. Bake for 25 to 30 minutes or until tester inserted in center comes out clean. Cool on wire rack.

3. Serve garnished with sliced fresh fruit.

Makes 10 slices (1 slice per serving)

DIETITIAN'S NOTE *Count 2 tbsp sliced banana or ¼ cup of most other unsweetened fresh fruits as a Free Food or Extra.*

STRIPED STRAWBERRY CAKE

Preheat oven to 350°F
13- by 9-inch baking pan, sprayed with vegetable spray

1	package (18¼ oz) white cake mix
1	package (⅓ oz) no-sugar-added strawberry-flavored gelatin
1	cup boiling water
½	cup cold water
2	cups lower-fat non-dairy whipped topping
20	strawberries

1. Bake the cake in the prepared pan according to package instructions. Let cool in the pan for 10 minutes. Remove from the pan and let cool completely on a rack. Wash the pan.

2. In a medium bowl, dissolve gelatin in boiling water. Add cold water and let gelatin cool to room temperature, but do not let it begin to set.

3. When cake is cool, return it to the clean pan and prick it with a large serving fork at ½-inch intervals.

4. Pour cooled gelatin evenly over the cake, cover and refrigerate for 3 to 4 hours, until gelatin is set.

5. Dip the pan in warm water, invert onto a serving plate and remove the pan.

6. Frost the top and sides of the cake with whipped topping. Mark 20 even pieces in the frosting and garnish each square with a sliced and fanned strawberry.

Makes 20 servings

VARIATION Make seasonal striped cakes: pink hearts for Valentine's Day; green trees for Christmas. Use a shaped cake pan and gelatin that is the appropriate color, and add food coloring to the whipped topping.

NUTRIENTS PER SERVING

Calories	130
Carbohydrate	23 g
Fiber	0 g
Protein	2 g
Fat, total	3 g
Fat, saturated	1 g
Cholesterol	2 mg
Sodium	185 mg

EXCHANGES PER SERVING

½	Starch
1	Other Carbohydrates
½	Fat

CHOCOLATE ESPRESSO CAKE

TIPS To make cutting easier, dip knife in hot water before slicing.

For a chocolate liqueur flavor, try using half coffee and half chocolate liqueur.

This cake seems so dense and rich you'll never believe it is light. A small piece goes a long way.

Decorate with fresh berries.

Prepare up to 2 days in advance or freeze for up to 6 weeks.

NUTRIENTS PER SERVING

Calories	137
Carbohydrate	25 g
Fiber	1 g
Protein	3 g
Fat, total	4 g
Fat, saturated	2 g
Cholesterol	32 mg
Sodium	30 mg

EXCHANGES PER SERVING

1½ Other Carbohydrates
1 Fat

Preheat oven to 350°F
8-inch springform pan, sprayed with vegetable spray

½	cup semisweet chocolate chips
¼	cup espresso or strong brewed coffee
2	eggs, separated
¾	cup granulated sugar
¾	cup 2% evaporated milk
½	cup unsweetened cocoa powder
3	tbsp all-purpose flour
1	tsp vanilla
3	tbsp granulated sugar

1. Melt chocolate chips with coffee; stir until smooth. Allow to cool.

2. In a large bowl, beat together egg yolks, ¾ cup sugar, evaporated milk, cocoa, flour and vanilla until smooth. Beat in chocolate-coffee mixture.

3. With an electric mixer, in a separate bowl, beat egg whites until soft peaks form. Gradually add 3 tbsp sugar and continue beating until stiff peaks form.

4. Stir one-quarter of egg whites into chocolate batter. Gently fold in remaining egg whites. Spoon into prepared pan. Bake 30 to 35 minutes or until cake is set at the center. Chill before serving.

Makes 12 slices (1 slice per serving)

BLUEBERRY HONEY CAKE

Preheat oven to 350°F
9-inch round cake pan, sprayed with baking spray

1	cup fresh or frozen blueberries
⅓	cup liquid honey
⅓	cup water
1	tbsp cornstarch or arrowroot
1	tbsp water
1½	cups whole wheat flour
1	tsp baking powder
1	cup 2% milk
⅓	cup honey
1	tbsp vegetable oil

1. In a saucepan, combine blueberries, honey and ⅓ cup water; bring to a boil over medium heat. Stir together cornstarch and 1 tbsp water; add to simmering blueberry mixture. Cook, stirring constantly, until thickened. Remove from heat; set aside.

2. In a large bowl, stir together flour and baking powder. In another bowl, whisk together milk, honey and oil until smooth; add to flour mixture, stirring to combine. Pour into prepared pan. Pour blueberry mixture on top of batter. Bake for 25 to 35 minutes or until a tester inserted in center comes out clean.

Makes 10 slices (1 slice per serving)

NUTRIENTS PER SERVING

Calories	165
Carbohydrate	36 g
Fiber	3 g
Protein	3 g
Fat, total	2 g
Fat, saturated	0 g
Cholesterol	2 mg
Sodium	41 mg

EXCHANGES PER SERVING

1	Starch
1½	Other Carbohydrates
½	Fat

CAKES, COFFEE CAKES & CHEESECAKES

DIETITIAN'S NOTE *Honey is high in fructose, which makes up half the sucrose molecules in ordinary table sugar. Although fructose tastes sweeter than sucrose, it does not raise blood sugar as much. Like sucrose, 1 tbsp fructose is an Other Carbohydrate Exchange.*

BLUEBERRY PEACH CAKE

TIPS If using frozen blueberries, thaw first, then drain off the excess liquid.

Bake a day before or freeze for up to 6 weeks.

NUTRIENTS PER SERVING

Calories	165
Carbohydrate	29 g
Fiber	2 g
Protein	3 g
Fat, total	4 g
Fat, saturated	1 g
Cholesterol	24 mg
Sodium	118 mg

EXCHANGES PER SERVING

1 Starch

1 Other Carbohydrates

1 Fat

Preheat oven to 350°F
9-inch Bundt pan, sprayed with nonstick vegetable spray

1	cup granulated sugar
¾	cup applesauce
¼	cup vegetable oil
2	eggs
1	tsp vanilla
1½	cups all-purpose flour
½	cup whole wheat flour
2	tsp ground cinnamon
1½	tsp baking powder
1	tsp baking soda
½	cup 2% yogurt
1	cup sliced peeled peaches
1	cup blueberries
	Confectioner's (icing) sugar

1. In a large bowl, beat together sugar, applesauce, oil, eggs and vanilla, mixing well.

2. Combine all-purpose and whole wheat flours, cinnamon, baking powder and baking soda; stir into bowl just until blended. Stir in yogurt; fold in peaches and blueberries. Pour into prepared pan.

3. Bake for 40 to 45 minutes or until cake tester inserted into center comes out clean. Let cool; dust with confectioner's sugar.

Makes 16 slices (1 slice per serving)

DIETITIAN'S NOTE *To dust a cake with confectioner's sugar, use a fine sieve. One tablespoon will add only ½ gram of carbohydrate to a serving of this cake.*

ORANGE PUMPKIN SNACKING CAKE

Preheat oven to 350°F
9-inch springform pan, lightly greased

1	cup whole wheat flour
2	cups all-purpose flour
¾	cup packed brown sugar
1	tbsp grated orange zest
1	tbsp baking powder
1	tsp baking soda
1	tsp ground cinnamon
½	tsp ground allspice
½	tsp ground ginger
½	tsp ground nutmeg
¼	tsp ground cloves
½	cup vegetable oil
3	eggs
1¼	cups canned pumpkin puree (not pie filling)
½	cup orange juice
1	cup chopped pecans

1. In a large bowl, stir together whole wheat flour, flour, brown sugar, zest, baking powder, baking soda, cinnamon, allspice, ginger, nutmeg and cloves; set aside.

2. In a separate bowl, using an electric mixer, beat oil, eggs, pumpkin puree and orange juice until combined. Pour mixture over dry ingredients and stir just until combined. Stir in pecans. Spoon into prepared pan.

3. Bake in preheated oven for 60 to 70 minutes or until a cake tester inserted in the center comes out clean. Immediately invert on a cooling rack. Remove pan and let cool completely.

Makes 1 cake or 16 slices (1 per serving)

TIP Be sure to buy pumpkin puree, not pumpkin pie filling, which is too sweet and contains too much moisture for this snacking cake.

VARIATION Substitute 2 to 3 tsp pumpkin pie spice for the individual spices.

NUTRIENTS PER SERVING

Calories	253
Carbohydrate	32 g
Fiber	2 g
Protein	5 g
Fat, total	13 g
Fat, saturated	1 g
Cholesterol	30 mg
Sodium	139 mg

EXCHANGES PER SERVING

1	Starch
1	Other Carbohydrates
2½	Fat

SOUR CREAM ORANGE APPLE CAKE

TIPS Try chopped pears or peaches instead of apples.

To increase fiber, use ⅔ cup whole wheat and 1 cup all-purpose flour.

Makes two 9- by 5-inch loaves. Bake approximately 35 minutes or until tester comes out clean.

If you don't want to layer the cake, just mix apples with batter, then add topping.

When using margarine, choose a soft (non-hydrogenated) version to limit consumption of trans fats.

Prepare up to 2 days in advance.

Freeze for up to 6 weeks.

Preheat oven to 350°F
10-inch springform pan, sprayed with vegetable spray

Topping
⅓	cup packed brown sugar
3	tbsp chopped pecans
1½	tbsp all-purpose flour
2	tsp margarine or butter
½	tsp ground cinnamon

Filling
2	cups chopped peeled apples
½	cup raisins
1	tbsp granulated sugar
1	tsp ground cinnamon

Cake
⅔	cup packed brown sugar
½	cup granulated sugar
⅓	cup vegetable oil
2	eggs
1	tbsp grated orange zest
2	tsp vanilla
1⅔	cups all-purpose flour
2	tsp baking powder
1	tsp baking soda
½	cup orange juice
½	cup light sour cream

1. *Topping:* In a small bowl, combine brown sugar, pecans, flour, margarine and cinnamon. Set aside.

2. *Filling:* In a bowl, mix together apples, raisins, sugar and cinnamon. Set aside.

3. *Cake:* In a food processor or in a large bowl with an electric mixer, beat together brown sugar, granulated sugar and oil. Add eggs, one at a time, beating well after each. Mix in orange zest and vanilla.

4. In a separate bowl, stir together flour, baking powder and baking soda. In another bowl, stir together orange juice and sour cream. Add flour mixture and sour cream mixture alternately to beaten sugar mixture, mixing just until blended. Spoon half of batter into prepared pan. Top with half of apple mixture. Spoon remaining batter into pan. Top with remaining apple mixture; sprinkle with topping.

5. Bake 45 to 50 minutes or until a cake tester inserted in center comes out clean. Cool on a wire rack.

Makes 20 slices (1 slice per serving)

DIETITIAN'S NOTES *To create a pretty pattern on the top of a cake, cover it with a paper doily and sift confectioner's sugar over it. Then carefully lift the doily straight up.*

A little bit of confectioner's sugar (also called icing sugar or powdered sugar) can make a plain cake look elegant while adding almost no carbohydrate. One tablespoon—plenty for most cakes—contains only 8 grams of carbohydrate. Use a fine sieve to distribute it evenly.

You may wonder why 1 tbsp of confectioner's sugar contains only 8 grams of carbohydrate when other sugars contain 15 grams. Confectioner's sugar is made from finely ground granulated sugar combined with a small amount of cornstarch, which makes it fluffy. Thus, 1 tbsp contains only half the amount of carbohydrate found in the same amount of granulated sugar.

NUTRIENTS PER SERVING

Calories	185
Carbohydrate	32 g
Fiber	1 g
Protein	2 g
Fat, total	6 g
Fat, saturated	1 g
Cholesterol	19 mg
Sodium	113 mg

EXCHANGES PER SERVING

½ Starch
½ Fruit
1 Other Carbohydrates
1 Fat

CAKES, COFFEE CAKES & CHEESECAKES

BANANA CAKE WITH LEMON CREAM FROSTING

TIPS For the smoothest frosting, use extra-smooth ricotta cheese.

For the most intense walnut flavor, use walnut oil in the cake and toast the walnuts for garnishing the cake.

Preheat oven to 350°F
13- by 9-inch cake pan, sprayed with baking spray

Cake

1¾	cups	whole wheat flour
2	tsp	baking powder
¾	tsp	baking soda
½	cup	buttermilk
½	cup	liquid honey
¼	cup	walnut oil or vegetable oil
3		ripe bananas
4		egg whites

Lemon Cream Frosting

1	cup	5% ricotta cheese
1½	tbsp	honey
1	tbsp	grated lemon zest
1	tbsp	lemon juice
1½	tsp	cornstarch or arrowroot
¼	cup	chopped walnuts
		Lemon zest, cut into thin strips

1. *Cake:* In a bowl, stir together flour, baking powder and baking soda; set aside. In a food processor or blender, purée buttermilk, honey, oil and bananas until smooth; stir into flour mixture just until mixed. In another bowl, beat egg whites until stiff peaks form; fold into batter. Pour into prepared pan. Bake for 20 to 30 minutes or until a tester inserted in center comes out clean. Cool in pan on wire rack.

2. *Frosting:* In a food processor, purée ricotta, honey, lemon zest, lemon juice and cornstarch until smooth. Transfer to a saucepan. Cook over medium heat, stirring constantly, until steaming hot. Remove from heat. Chill.

3. Spread cold frosting over cooled cake. Sprinkle with walnuts and strips of lemon zest.

Makes 25 slices (1 slice per serving)

DIETITIAN'S NOTES *If a recipe contains both oil and a sticky ingredient such as honey or molasses, measure the oil first. The small amount of oil left in the cup or spoon will help the honey slide out smoothly.*

The fat found in nuts and seeds is primarily the desirable monounsaturated type. Like other fats, however, it also contributes calories. To get the most out of nuts when using them in baking, finely chop them to distribute their flavor and texture throughout the dough or batter.

Nuts and seeds are even more flavorful when they are lightly toasted before they are combined with other ingredients. Spread them evenly in a pie plate or cake pan and toast in a 350°F oven for 7 to 10 minutes, or until lightly toasted and fragrant. The timing varies depending on the type of nuts or seeds, so watch them carefully to make sure they don't burn.

NUTRIENTS PER SERVING

Calories	109
Carbohydrate	17 g
Fiber	1 g
Protein	3 g
Fat, total	4 g
Fat, saturated	1 g
Cholesterol	2 mg
Sodium	86 mg

EXCHANGES PER SERVING

½ Starch
½ Other Carbohydrate
1 Fat

169

CAKES, COFFEE CAKES & CHEESECAKES

DATE CAKE WITH COCONUT TOPPING

TIPS To chop dates easily, use kitchen shears. Whole pitted dates can be used, but then use a food processor to finely chop dates after they are cooked.

Chopped pitted prunes can replace dates.

When using margarine, choose a soft (non-hydrogenated) version to limit consumption of trans fats.

Prepare up to 2 days ahead or freeze for up to 6 weeks. The dates keep this cake moist.

Preheat oven to 350°F
9-inch square cake pan, sprayed with vegetable spray

Cake

12	oz chopped pitted dates
1¾	cups water
¼	cup margarine or butter
1	cup granulated sugar
2	eggs
1½	cups all-purpose flour
1½	tsp baking powder
1	tsp baking soda

Topping

⅓	cup unsweetened coconut
¼	cup brown sugar
3	tbsp 2% milk
2	tbsp margarine or butter

1. *Cake:* Put dates and water in saucepan; bring to a boil, cover and reduce heat to low. Cook for 10 minutes, stirring often, or until dates are soft and most of the liquid has been absorbed. Set aside to cool for 10 minutes.

2. In a large bowl or food processor, beat together margarine and sugar. Add eggs and mix well. Add cooled date mixture and mix well.

3. In a bowl, combine flour, baking powder and baking soda. Stir into date mixture just until blended. Pour into prepared cake pan and bake for 35 to 40 minutes or until a cake tester inserted in center comes out dry.

4. *Topping:* In a small saucepan, combine coconut, brown sugar, milk and margarine; cook over medium heat, stirring, for 2 minutes, or until sugar dissolves. Pour over cake.

Makes 20 slices (1 slice per serving)

DIETITIAN'S NOTE *When planning what to eat, we need to take into account both the type of food and the portion size. Getting the correct portion size (in other words, the right number of slices) from a cake baked in a rectangular or square pan is easy: just look at how many slices are specified in the yield and cut the cake into that many portions. For example, this recipe makes 20 slices. To get that number, you would cut the cake lengthwise 3 times and crosswise 4 times. Make sure all your slices are the same size, or the Nutrients per Serving and Exchanges will not be accurate.*

NUTRIENTS PER SERVING

Calories	177
Carbohydrate	33 g
Fiber	2 g
Protein	2 g
Fat, total	5 g
Fat, saturated	1 g
Cholesterol	19 mg
Sodium	138 mg

EXCHANGES PER SERVING

1 Fruit

1 Other Carbohydrates

1 Fat

PRUNE ORANGE SPICE CAKE

TIPS To cut prunes easily, use kitchen shears, or you can use whole pitted prunes, but you'll need to finely chop prunes in a food processor after they are cooked.

Chopped pitted dates can replace prunes.

When using margarine, choose a soft (non-hydrogenated) version to limit consumption of trans fats.

Bake up to 2 days ahead or freeze for up to 6 weeks. The dried fruit keeps this cake very moist.

Preheat oven to 350°F
9-inch square baking dish, sprayed with vegetable spray

Cake

8	oz chopped pitted prunes
1	cup orange juice
⅓	cup margarine or butter
¾	cup granulated sugar
2	eggs
2	tsp grated orange zest
1	tsp vanilla
1	cup all-purpose flour
½	cup whole wheat flour
1	tsp baking powder
¾	tsp ground cinnamon
½	tsp baking soda
⅛	tsp ground nutmeg
⅓	cup 2% yogurt

Icing

4	tsp orange juice
½	cup confectioner's sugar

1. *Cake:* Put prunes and orange juice in a saucepan; bring to a boil, cover and reduce heat to low. Cook for 10 to 12 minutes, stirring often, or until prunes are soft and most of the liquid has been absorbed. Set aside.

2. In a large bowl, cream together margarine and sugar; add eggs, orange zest and vanilla and mix well. Stir in prune mixture and mix well.

3. In a bowl, combine flour, whole wheat flour, baking powder, cinnamon, baking soda and nutmeg. Add to wet ingredients alternately with yogurt. Pour into prepared cake pan and bake for 30 to 35 minutes or until a cake tester inserted in center comes out clean.

4. *Icing:* In a small bowl, combine orange juice and confectioner's sugar until well mixed. Pour over cake.

Makes 16 slices (1 slice per serving)

DIETITIAN'S NOTES *The icing (which is included in the calculations) contributes 4 grams of carbohydrate and 15 calories.*

It's important to measure ingredients accurately. This is especially true for cakes and cookies, which may not turn out properly if ingredient quantities are changed. Also, if the amounts are incorrect, the nutrients and Exchanges per serving will not be accurate.

To measure correctly, be sure to use standard measuring cups and spoons. There are different measuring cups for dry and liquid ingredients. Dry ingredient measures, usually made of metal or plastic, come in measures of ¼ cup, ⅓ cup, ½ cup and 1 cup.

Liquid measures are usually made of glass, with the measures marked on the outside and extra space below the rim so you can measure the full amount without spilling. The most common sizes are 1 cup and 2 cups.

Standard measuring spoons may be used for either liquid or dry ingredients. The standard set includes ¼ tsp, ½ tsp, 1 tsp and 1 tbsp.

See page 53 for more information on measuring accurately.

NUTRIENTS PER SERVING

Calories	181
Carbohydrate	33 g
Fiber	2 g
Protein	3 g
Fat, total	5 g
Fat, saturated	1 g
Cholesterol	24 mg
Sodium	119 mg

EXCHANGES PER SERVING

1 Fruit

1 Other Carbohydrates

1 Fat

BANANA SPICE CAKE

TIPS Increase amount of spices to your taste— or omit any not on hand.

Freeze overripe bananas in their skins for up to 3 months. Defrost and use mashed in baking.

Use as a muffin batter. Bake 15 to 20 minutes or until tester comes out clean.

When using margarine, choose a soft (non-hydrogenated) version to limit consumption of trans fats.

Bake up to 2 days in advance. Freeze for up to 6 weeks.

Preheat oven to 350°F
10-inch Bundt pan, sprayed with vegetable spray

Cake

⅓	cup margarine or butter
¾	cup granulated sugar
½	cup packed brown sugar
2	eggs
¾	cup light sour cream
2	tsp vanilla
1	medium ripe banana, mashed
1½	cups all-purpose flour
2	tsp baking powder
1½	tsp ground cinnamon
1	tsp baking soda
⅛	tsp ground allspice
⅛	tsp ground ginger
⅛	tsp ground nutmeg

Icing

⅓	cup light cream cheese, softened
⅔	cup confectioner's sugar
1	tbsp 2% milk

1. *Cake:* In a food processor or in a bowl with an electric mixer, cream together margarine, sugar and brown sugar. Add eggs one at a time, beating well after each; beat in sour cream, vanilla and banana. In a separate bowl, stir together flour, baking powder, cinnamon, baking soda, allspice, ginger and nutmeg. Add liquid ingredients to dry ingredients, blending just until mixed. Pour into prepared pan.

2. Bake for 35 minutes or until a cake tester inserted in center comes out clean. Cool in pan on wire rack.

3. *Icing:* In a bowl or food processor, beat together cream cheese, confectioner's sugar and milk until smooth.

4. Invert cake and drizzle icing over top.

Makes 16 slices (1 slice per serving)

DIETITIAN'S NOTE *Because we are surrounded by "jumbo" and "super-size" items and ever-larger plates, it's easy to lose track of what a reasonable serving is. (Even dietitians can fall into this trap!) The information included with the recipes in this book can teach you a lot about portion sizes. It will help you learn what ingredients are in different desserts and will give you an idea of what Exchanges a reasonable serving might contain.*

NUTRIENTS PER SERVING

Calories	200
Carbohydrate	33 g
Fiber	1 g
Protein	3 g
Fat, total	6 g
Fat, saturated	1 g
Cholesterol	26 mg
Sodium	221 mg

EXCHANGES PER SERVING

½	Starch
1½	Other Carbohydrates
1	Fat

BANANA DATE CAKE

TIPS For easier preparation, use scissors to cut dates. Be sure to buy pitted dates.

When using margarine, choose a soft (non-hydrogenated) version.

Prepare up to 2 days in advance or freeze for up to 6 weeks.

Use a wheat bran breakfast cereal.

NUTRIENTS PER SERVING

Calories	150
Carbohydrate	30 g
Fiber	3 g
Protein	2 g
Fat, total	4 g
Fat, saturated	0 g
Cholesterol	9 mg
Sodium	123 mg

EXCHANGES PER SERVING

1 Fruit
1 Other Carbohydrates
1 Fat

Preheat oven to 350°F
9-inch square cake pan, sprayed with nonstick vegetable spray

1	tsp baking soda
1	cup boiling water
2	cups chopped dates (about 10 oz)
½	cup brown sugar
3	tbsp margarine
1	egg
1	ripe banana, mashed
1½	cups all-purpose flour
1	cup bran cereal
⅓	cup chopped pecans or walnuts
2	tsp ground cinnamon

1. In a bowl, stir baking soda into water; add dates and let stand for 10 minutes.

2. In a large bowl or food processor, beat together sugar, margarine, egg and banana until well blended.

3. Combine flour, cereal, pecans and cinnamon; add to banana mixture alternately with soaked dates, mixing well. Pour into cake pan; bake for 25 to 30 minutes or until a cake tester comes out dry.

Makes 20 slices (1 slice per serving)

CARROT CAKE

Preheat oven to 350°F
13- by 9-inch baking pan, lightly greased

¾	cup all-purpose flour
½	cup whole wheat flour
1¼	tsp baking powder
1¼	tsp baking soda
1	tsp ground cinnamon
½	tsp salt
3	eggs
½	cup vegetable oil
1	cup lightly packed brown sugar
2	tsp vanilla
2	cups grated carrots

1. In a small bowl, combine all-purpose flour, whole wheat flour, baking powder, baking soda, cinnamon and salt.

2. In a large bowl, beat eggs, oil, brown sugar and vanilla until well combined. Fold in dry ingredients. Stir in carrots. Pour into prepared pan.

3. Bake in preheated oven for 30 to 35 minutes or until a tester inserted in the center comes out clean. Let cool completely in pan on a wire rack. Cut cake into slices and lift servings out with a flat lifter.

Makes 20 slices (1 slice per serving)

TIP Dust with confectioner's sugar for a pretty presentation.

NUTRIENTS PER SERVING

Calories	134
Carbohydrate	18 g
Fiber	1 g
Protein	2 g
Fat, total	6 g
Fat, saturated	1 g
Cholesterol	28 mg
Sodium	174 mg

EXCHANGES PER SERVING

1 Other Carbohydrates

1 Fat

APPLESAUCE CARROT CAKE

Preheat oven to 350°F
8-inch Bundt pan, sprayed with baking spray

2⅓	cups whole wheat flour
4	tsp ground cinnamon
2	tsp baking powder
1	tsp baking soda
½	tsp ground nutmeg
¼	tsp ground allspice
¼	tsp salt
1	cup unsweetened applesauce
¾	cup liquid honey
⅓	cup corn oil
3	eggs
2	cups grated carrots
	Lemon Cream Frosting (optional) (see recipe, page 168)
	Lemon, orange and/or lime zest cut into thin strips (optional)

1. In a large bowl, stir together flour, cinnamon, baking powder, baking soda, nutmeg, allspice and salt. In another bowl, beat together applesauce, honey, oil and eggs; gradually stir into flour mixture until well mixed. Stir in grated carrots. Pour into prepared pan.

2. Bake for 35 minutes or until a tester inserted in center comes out clean. Cool in pan for 5 minutes; invert and cool completely on wire rack. Ice with Lemon Cream Frosting and garnish with zest, if desired. Store in refrigerator.

Makes 16 slices (1 slice per serving)

DIETITIAN'S NOTES *Use whole wheat flour to boost fiber in your baking. Along with fiber, the germ of the wheat is retained in the milling and gives it a slightly nutty flavor. Buy it in small quantities and keep it tightly covered in a cool place.*

If you use the Lemon Cream Frosting, use only half the recipe and count the quantity on 1 slice of cake as a Free Food or Extra.

NUTRIENTS PER SERVING

Calories	176
Carbohydrate	29 g
Fiber	3 g
Protein	4 g
Fat, total	6 g
Fat, saturated	1 g
Cholesterol	35 mg
Sodium	169 mg

EXCHANGES PER SERVING

2	Other Carbohydrates
1	Fat

179

PIÑA COLADA SNACKING CAKE

NUTRIENTS PER SERVING

Calories	136
Carbohydrate	27 g
Fiber	1 g
Protein	3 g
Fat, total	2 g
Fat, saturated	2 g
Cholesterol	27 mg
Sodium	80 mg

EXCHANGES PER SERVING

1 Starch
½ Other Carbohydrate

Preheat oven to 350°F
13- by 9-inch baking pan, sprayed with vegetable spray

2	cups all-purpose flour
½	cup packed brown sugar
½	cup shredded unsweetened coconut
1	tsp ground cinnamon
½	tsp ground ginger
½	tsp salt
2	large eggs
1	can (19 oz) crushed pineapple, in juice
¼	cup confectioner's sugar, sifted

1. In a large bowl, combine flour, brown sugar, coconut, cinnamon, ginger and salt.

2. In a small bowl, mix eggs well with a fork. Add pineapple and juice and stir to combine. Add to flour mixture and stir until blended.

3. Pour batter into prepared pan and bake in preheated oven for 25 to 30 minutes, or until a knife inserted in the center comes out clean. Let cool completely in pan on a rack and cut into 16 squares.

4. In a small bowl, mix confectioner's sugar with about 1 tbsp water to make a thin glaze. Transfer to an icing bag and drizzle onto cooled squares.

Makes 16 squares (1 per serving)

DIETITIAN'S NOTE *Kids can easily prepare this recipe with a little supervision—and there's little cleanup involved. Supervise the portioning, though, as the cake tastes great!*

CHOCOLATE ZUCCHINI CAKE

Preheat oven to 350°F
8-inch square baking pan, lightly greased

1	cup self-rising flour
⅓	cup unsweetened cocoa powder
1	tsp baking soda
1	tsp ground cinnamon
6	egg whites
1⅓	cups firmly packed brown sugar
1	cup buttermilk
2	tsp vanilla
¼	tsp almond extract
2	cups shredded zucchini
	Confectioner's sugar (optional)

1. In a small bowl, sift flour, cocoa powder, baking soda and cinnamon.

2. In a large bowl, beat egg whites, brown sugar, buttermilk, vanilla and almond extract until well blended. Fold in flour mixture until evenly moistened. Stir in zucchini. Pour batter into prepared pan.

3. Bake in preheated oven for 30 to 40 minutes or until center of cake springs back when lightly pressed and a tester inserted in the center comes out clean. Let cool on a wire rack for 10 minutes before removing from pan. Turn out onto rack to cool completely. Just before serving, dust with confectioner's sugar, if desired.

Makes 12 slices (1 slice per serving)

TIPS If you don't have self-rising flour, substitute 1 cup all-purpose flour and add 1½ tsp baking powder and ½ tsp salt.

If you prefer, use commercial liquid egg whites. You'll need about ¾ cup for this recipe.

NUTRIENTS PER SERVING

Calories	155
Carbohydrate	35 g
Fiber	1 g
Protein	4 g
Fat, total	1 g
Fat, saturated	0 g
Cholesterol	1 mg
Sodium	297 mg

EXCHANGES PER SERVING

½	Starch
1½	Other Carbohydrates
1	Free Food

Recipe photo in color insert.

PEPPERMINT ANGEL CUPCAKES

TIP As a general rule, cake and muffin batter should fill a pan about ⅔ full. If you don't fill pans enough, your cakes will be flat; if you fill them too much, they will overflow and make a mess!

NUTRIENTS PER SERVING

Calories	103
Carbohydrate	25 g
Fiber	0 g
Protein	2 g
Fat, total	0 g
Fat, saturated	0 g
Cholesterol	0 mg
Sodium	129 mg

EXCHANGES PER SERVING

½ Starch
1 Other Carbohydrates

Preheat oven to 350°F
24 muffin cups, lined with paper liners

½	cup red, green and white peppermint candies
1	package (1 lb) white angel food cake mix
½	cup Chocolate Sauce (see recipe, page 293)

1. Crush candies in a food processor or by placing them between tea towels or in a resealable freezer bag and smashing them with a hammer.

2. Prepare cake batter according to package instructions, then stir in ½ of the crushed candies. Pour into prepared muffin cups.

3. Bake in preheated oven for 30 minutes, rotating pans halfway, until tops are golden and firm. Immediately remove from the pan to cool on a rack.

4. Drizzle chocolate sauce on top of the cupcakes and sprinkle with the remaining candies.

Makes 24 cupcakes (1 per serving)

Recipe photo in color insert.

SPICY APPLE CUPCAKES

Preheat oven to 350°F
10 muffin cups, lined with paper cups or sprayed with vegetable spray

1	cup all-purpose flour
1	tsp pumpkin pie spice
½	tsp baking powder
½	tsp baking soda
½	tsp salt
½	cup granulated sugar
¼	cup lightly packed brown sugar
¼	cup soft margarine
1	large egg
½	tsp vanilla
½	cup unsweetened applesauce

1. In a small bowl, combine flour, pumpkin pie spice, baking powder, baking soda and salt.

2. In a medium bowl, using an electric mixer or wooden spoon, cream granulated sugar, brown sugar and margarine until fluffy. Beat in egg and vanilla. Stir in flour mixture until blended. Stir in applesauce.

3. Divide batter among the muffin cups, filling them ½ full. Bake in pre-heated oven for 20 to 25 minutes, or until a toothpick inserted in the center comes out clean. Let cool in pan on a rack for 10 minutes. Transfer to rack to cool completely.

Makes 10 cupcakes (1 per serving)

VARIATION If you wish, mix a simple glaze of ½ cup confectioner's sugar, sifted, and 2 tbsp water or unsweetened apple juice to drizzle on these cupcakes.

NUTRIENTS PER SERVING

Calories	160
Carbohydrate	27 g
Fiber	1 g
Protein	2 g
Fat, total	5 g
Fat, saturated	1 g
Cholesterol	22 mg
Sodium	189 mg

EXCHANGES PER SERVING

½	Starch
1	Other Carbohydrates
1	Fat

APPLE PECAN STREUSEL CAKE

184

TIPS Try substituting pears for the apples and chopped dates for the raisins.

When measuring flour, fill a dry measure to overflowing, then level off with a knife.

When using margarine, choose a soft (non-hydrogenated) version to limit consumption of trans fats.

Bake a day before or freeze for up to 6 weeks.

Preheat oven to 350°F
10-inch Bundt pan, sprayed with nonstick vegetable spray

Topping

¼	cup chopped pecans
¼	cup all-purpose flour
3	tbsp brown sugar
1	tbsp margarine, melted
1½	tsp ground cinnamon

Cake

¼	cup soft margarine
1	cup brown sugar
2	eggs
2	tsp vanilla
1¼	cups all-purpose flour
¾	cup whole wheat flour
2½	tsp ground cinnamon
1½	tsp baking powder
1	tsp baking soda
1	cup 2% yogurt or light sour cream
2¾	cups diced peeled apples
¼	cup raisins

1. *Topping:* In a small bowl, combine pecans, flour, brown sugar, margarine and cinnamon until crumbly. Set aside.

2. *Cake:* In a large bowl or food processor, cream together margarine and brown sugar. Beat in eggs and vanilla until well blended.

3. Combine all-purpose and whole wheat flours, cinnamon, baking powder and baking soda; add to bowl alternately with yogurt, mixing just until blended. Fold in apples and raisins. Pour into prepared pan.

4. Sprinkle with topping; bake for 40 to 45 minutes or until a cake tester inserted into center comes out clean.

Makes 16 slices (1 slice per serving)

DIETITIAN'S NOTE *With a few changes, many recipes can be made healthier. Here are some suggestions.*

Increase fiber by substituting whole wheat flour for all-purpose flour. Start with one-quarter of the amount; you can usually replace up to half the all-purpose flour in a recipe with whole wheat.

Lower saturated fat by replacing butter with non-hydrogenated margarine. (Avoid solid margarines, which are high in saturated and/or trans fats.) You can also replace a small proportion of the vegetable shortening or lard in a recipe with non-hydrogenated margarine.

Reduce the total amount of fat by replacing one-quarter to half of the oil in a recipe with applesauce or plain yogurt.

Boost vitamins and minerals by replacing chocolate chips with an equal quantity of chopped dried fruit.

See the worksheet on pages 314–315 to calculate the Exchanges for your favorite recipes.

NUTRIENTS PER SERVING

Calories	209
Carbohydrate	36 g
Fiber	2 g
Protein	4 g
Fat, total	6 g
Fat, saturated	1 g
Cholesterol	24 mg
Sodium	176 mg

EXCHANGES PER SERVING

1 Starch
½ Fruit
1 Other Carbohydrates
1 Fat

CAKES, COFFEE CAKES & CHEESECAKES

APRICOT DATE STREUSEL CAKE

TIPS It's easy to chop dried fruit when you use scissors.

Feel free to use all dates or all apricots. Dried prunes are delicious.

When using margarine, choose a soft (non-hydrogenated) version to limit consumption of trans fats.

Bake up to a day before or freeze for up to 6 weeks.

Preheat oven to 350°F
10-inch Bundt pan, sprayed with nonstick vegetable spray

Topping

¼	cup brown sugar
2	tbsp all-purpose flour
2	tbsp wheat bran cereal, crushed
1	tsp ground cinnamon
1	tbsp margarine

Cake

3	tbsp margarine
¾	cup granulated sugar
1	egg
2	egg whites
3	tbsp lemon juice
1	tsp vanilla
1¾	cups all-purpose flour
½	cup wheat bran cereal
1	tsp ground cinnamon
1	tsp baking powder
1	tsp baking soda
1⅓	cups 2% yogurt
⅓	cup finely chopped dates
⅓	cup finely chopped dried apricots

1. *Topping:* In a small bowl, combine brown sugar, flour, cereal and cinnamon; cut in margarine until crumbly. Set aside.

2. *Cake:* In a large bowl or food processor, cream together margarine and sugar; beat in egg, egg whites, lemon juice and vanilla until well mixed.

3. Combine flour, cereal, cinnamon, baking powder and baking soda; stir into bowl just until incorporated. Stir in yogurt; fold in dates and apricots.

4. Pour half of batter into pan. Sprinkle with half of topping. Pour remaining batter over top; sprinkle with remaining topping. Bake for 35 to 45 minutes or until a tester inserted into center comes out clean.

Makes 16 slices (1 slice per serving)

DIETITIAN'S NOTE *For help in planning your meals, ask your doctor to refer you to a diabetes education center or a dietitian. Local hospitals may also have referral services. On the Internet, look for the "Find a Nutrition Professional" feature at www.eatright.org.*

NUTRIENTS PER SERVING

Calories	177
Carbohydrate	33 g
Fiber	2 g
Protein	4 g
Fat, total	4 g
Fat, saturated	1 g
Cholesterol	13 mg
Sodium	184 mg

EXCHANGES PER SERVING

½	Fruit
1½	Other Carbohydrates
1	Fat

187

CINNAMON STREUSEL COFFEE CAKE

TIP When using margarine, choose a non-hydrogenated version to limit consumption of trans fats.

Preheat oven to 350°F
10-inch Bundt or 10-inch tube pan, lightly greased and floured

Streusel
½	cup lightly packed brown sugar
½	cup finely chopped pecans (optional)
1	tbsp ground cinnamon

Cake
1	cup all-purpose flour
1	cup whole wheat flour
1	tsp baking powder
¼	tsp salt
1	cup low-fat or fat-free plain yogurt
1	tsp baking soda
¾	cup granulated sugar
¾	cup unsweetened applesauce
¼	cup margarine
2	eggs
1	tsp vanilla

1. *Streusel:* In a small bowl, combine brown sugar, pecans (if using) and cinnamon. Set aside.

2. *Cake:* In a medium bowl, combine all-purpose flour, whole wheat flour, baking powder and salt. Set aside.

3. In another bowl, combine yogurt and baking soda. (Be prepared, yogurt will foam up!)

Recipe photo in color insert.

4. In a large bowl, using an electric mixer, cream sugar, applesauce and margarine until well mixed (it may look curdled). Beat in eggs, one at a time, then stir in vanilla. Stir in flour mixture alternately with yogurt, making 3 additions of flour and 2 of yogurt mixture.

5. Spoon half of the batter into prepared Bundt pan. Sprinkle with three-quarters of the streusel. Cover with remaining batter and sprinkle with remaining streusel. With the back of a small spoon, pat streusel lightly into batter (to prevent streusel from falling off when cake is inverted and removed from pan).

6. Bake in preheated oven for 40 to 50 minutes or until a tester inserted in the center comes out clean. Let cool on a wire rack for 10 minutes before removing from pan. Turn out onto rack to cool completely.

Makes 16 slices (1 slice per serving)

DIETITIAN'S NOTES *The pecans in the streusel are optional. If you use them, add ½ Fat Exchange per serving.*

As you prepare the recipes in this book, you will become familiar with the appropriate portion sizes for different types of desserts and the approximate Exchanges assigned to them. Use this knowledge to help you choose wisely when you're eating away from home.

NUTRIENTS PER SERVING

Calories	167
Carbohydrate	30 g
Fiber	1 g
Protein	3 g
Fat, total	4 g
Fat, saturated	1 g
Cholesterol	24 mg
Sodium	192 mg

EXCHANGES PER SERVING

1 Starch
1 Other Carbohydrates
1 Fat

MENNONITE STREUSEL CAKE

TIPS For a smaller-size cake to serve 6, halve the ingredients and bake in a buttered 8-inch square pan for 35 to 40 minutes.

In baking, always use large eggs, not medium or extra large, either of which can affect the baking result.

To soften butter, microwave on Defrost and check at 15-second intervals.

Preheat oven to 350°F
13- by 9-inch baking pan, sprayed with vegetable cooking spray

Cake

2	cups all-purpose flour
½	cup granulated sugar
1	tbsp baking powder
¼	tsp salt
⅓	cup butter, softened
1	egg
1	cup half-and-half (10%) cream
1½	tsp vanilla or grated lemon zest
4	cups fresh or frozen blueberries or other seasonal sliced fruits

Crumb Topping

¼	cup all-purpose flour
¼	cup packed brown sugar
1	tbsp butter, softened

1. *Cake:* In a large bowl, combine flour, sugar, baking powder and salt. Cut in butter using a pastry blender or two knives to make coarse crumbs.

2. In another bowl, beat egg with cream and vanilla. Stir into flour mixture to make a thick batter.

3. Drop tablespoonfuls of batter into prepared baking dish and spread evenly. Top with blueberries in a single layer.

4. *Crumb Topping:* In a bowl, combine flour and brown sugar. Cut in butter using a pastry blender or two knives to make coarse crumbs. Sprinkle evenly over fruit.

5. Bake on middle rack in preheated oven for 45 to 50 minutes or until crumb topping is golden. Place on a rack and let cool. Cut into squares and serve.

Serves 12

NUTRIENTS PER SERVING

Calories	248
Carbohydrate	39 g
Fiber	2 g
Protein	4 g
Fat, total	9 g
Fat, saturated	5 g
Sodium	195 mg
Cholesterol	38 mg

EXCHANGES PER SERVING

1	Starch
½	Fruit
1	Other Carbohydrates
1½	Fat

ORANGE-GLAZED COFFEE CAKE

TIP If you pierce the cake with a fork when warm and pour glaze over the top, the icing will filter through the cake.

NUTRIENTS PER SERVING

Calories	166
Carbohydrate	31 g
Fiber	1 g
Protein	3 g
Fat, total	4 g
Fat, saturated	1 g
Cholesterol	23 mg
Sodium	146 mg

EXCHANGES PER SERVING

1 Starch

1 Other Carbohydrates

1 Fat

Preheat oven to 350°F
10-inch Bundt pan, sprayed with nonstick vegetable spray

¼	cup soft margarine
1	cup granulated sugar
2	eggs
1	egg white
1½	cups orange juice
1½	tsp grated orange zest
1	cup whole wheat flour
1	cup all-purpose flour
1	tsp ground cinnamon
1	tsp baking powder
1	tsp baking soda

Glaze

½	cup confectioner's sugar
4	tsp frozen orange juice concentrate, thawed

1. In large bowl or food processor, cream together margarine and sugar. Beat in eggs, egg white, orange juice and zest until well blended.

2. Combine whole wheat and all-purpose flours, cinnamon, baking powder and baking soda; add to creamed mixture and mix until well blended. Pour into pan. Bake for 35 to 40 minutes or until cake tester inserted into center comes out clean. Let cool.

3. *Glaze:* Mix confectioner's sugar with orange juice concentrate; pour over cake, allowing to drip down sides.

Makes 16 slices (1 slice per serving)

DIETITIAN'S NOTE *The glaze on this coffee cake contributes about 4 grams of carbohydrate per serving.*

ORANGE COFFEE CAKE

Preheat oven to 350°F
8-inch Bundt pan, sprayed with baking spray

2	cups orange juice
2	tsp grated orange zest
1	cup granulated sugar
¼	cup butter
3	medium eggs
1	cup all-purpose flour
1	cup whole wheat flour
2	tsp baking soda
	Confectioner's sugar
	Sliced fresh strawberries

1. In a saucepan, combine orange juice and orange zest; bring to a boil. Remove from heat, transfer to a bowl and refrigerate until cool.

2. In a bowl, cream sugar with butter; add eggs, one at a time, beating well after each. In another bowl, stir together flour, whole wheat flour and baking soda. Add to creamed mixture alternately with orange juice, making 3 additions of flour and 2 of orange juice. Pour into prepared pan. Bake for 35 to 40 minutes or until a tester inserted in center comes out clean. Cool in pan for 5 minutes; invert and cool completely on wire rack.

3. Serve dusted with sifted confectioner's sugar and garnished with sliced strawberries.

Makes 12 slices (1 slice per serving)

NUTRIENTS PER SERVING

Calories	205
Carbohydrate	36 g
Fiber	2 g
Protein	4 g
Fat, total	5 g
Fat, saturated	3 g
Cholesterol	51 mg
Sodium	265 mg

EXCHANGES PER SERVING

1	Starch
1½	Other Carbohydrates
1	Fat

DIETITIAN'S NOTE *Fresh unsweetened fruit makes an attractive low-carbohydrate garnish. One strawberry or 4 raspberries add only 1 gram of carbohydrate.*

CINNAMON DATE COFFEE CAKE

Preheat oven to 350°F
8-inch Bundt pan, sprayed with baking spray

¾	cup granulated sugar
3	tbsp softened butter
2	egg whites
1	egg
1⅓	cups low-fat yogurt
3	tbsp lemon juice
1	tsp vanilla
2	cups all-purpose flour
1	tsp baking powder
1	tsp baking soda
1	tsp ground cinnamon
⅛	tsp ground nutmeg
¼	cup packed brown sugar
⅔	cup chopped dates
	Confectioner's sugar
	Extra sliced dates (optional)

1. In a bowl, beat together sugar, butter, egg whites and egg until smooth. Beat in yogurt, lemon juice and vanilla. In another bowl, sift together flour, baking powder, baking soda, cinnamon and nutmeg; stir into yogurt mixture just until combined.

2. In a small bowl, stir together brown sugar and dates. Pour half of cake batter into prepared pan and sprinkle with half of date mixture. Repeat. Bake for 40 minutes or until a tester inserted in center comes out clean. Cool in pan for 5 minutes; invert and cool completely on wire rack. Serve dusted with sifted confectioner's sugar and garnished with sliced dates, if desired.

Makes 16 slices (1 slice per serving)

DIETITIAN'S NOTES *Dried fruits are concentrated sources of carbohydrate. If you use dates to garnish this cake, remember that 2 to 3 dates (about ⅔ oz) count as a Fruit Exchange.*

Cut dried fruit into small pieces to spread its flavor through a batter or dough.

For added fiber, use whole wheat flour whenever possible. In most recipes, you can substitute whole wheat flour for up to half the all-purpose flour without significantly altering the finished product. First, try replacing one-quarter of the all-purpose flour, then increase the amount each time you make the recipe.

Because whole wheat flour contains the germ of the wheat, it can become rancid if kept for a long time. Buy it in small quantities and store in a cool place.

NUTRIENTS PER SERVING

Calories	166
Carbohydrate	32 g
Fiber	1 g
Protein	4 g
Fat, total	3 g
Fat, saturated	2 g
Cholesterol	18 mg
Sodium	144 mg

EXCHANGES PER SERVING

1 Starch
1 Other Carbohydrates
½ Fat

CHOCOLATE CHUNK COFFEE CAKE

Preheat oven to 350°F
10-inch Bundt or 10-inch tube pan, lightly greased and floured

2	cups all-purpose flour
1	cup whole wheat flour
1½	tsp baking powder
¼	tsp salt
2	cups plain yogurt or light sour cream
1	tsp baking soda
2	oz semisweet chocolate
2	oz white chocolate
1¼	cups granulated sugar
½	cup unsalted butter, at room temperature
2	egg whites
2	whole eggs
2	tsp vanilla
⅓	cup unsweetened cocoa powder
¼	cup water

1. In a large bowl, using a fork, combine all-purpose flour, whole wheat flour, baking powder and salt until evenly blended. Set aside.

2. In a medium bowl, combine yogurt and baking soda. (Be prepared, yogurt will foam up!) Set aside.

3. Coarsely chop semisweet chocolate until pieces are about the size of chocolate chips. Repeat with white chocolate, keeping the two separate. Set aside.

4. In a large bowl, using an electric mixer, cream sugar and butter. Add egg whites and eggs, one at a time, beating well after each addition. Stir in vanilla. Stir in flour mixture alternately with yogurt mixture, making 3 additions of flour and 2 of yogurt.

5. To make the chocolate batter, sift cocoa powder into a medium bowl. Stir in water until a smooth paste forms. Stir in one-third of the white batter.

6. Add the white chocolate pieces to the chocolate batter and the semisweet chocolate pieces to the white batter.

7. Pour white batter into prepared Bundt pan, then pour chocolate batter on top. Using a spatula, swirl the two mixtures together to create a ribbon effect.

8. Bake in the lower third of preheated oven for 60 to 65 minutes or until a tester inserted in the center comes out clean. Let cool on a wire rack for 10 minutes before removing from pan. Turn out onto rack to cool completely.

Makes 18 slices (1 slice per serving)

DIETITIAN'S NOTES *If you buy butter in sticks, one stick is equivalent to ½ cup.*

To create a pretty pattern on the top of a cake, cover it with a paper doily and sift confectioner's sugar over it. Then carefully lift the doily straight up.

NUTRIENTS PER SERVING

Calories	236
Carbohydrate	36 g
Fiber	2 g
Protein	6 g
Fat, total	8 g
Fat, saturated	5 g
Cholesterol	36 g
Sodium	161 mg

EXCHANGES PER SERVING

1	Starch
1½	Other Carbohydrates
1½	Fat

CHOCOLATE MARBLE COFFEE CAKE

TIPS One ounce of unsweetened cocoa has 3 grams of fat, compared to 1 oz of semisweet chocolate, which has 9 grams of fat.

Sift confectioner's sugar over top of cooled cake to decorate.

Bake a day before or freeze for up to 6 weeks.

NUTRIENTS PER SERVING

Calories	131
Carbohydrate	22 g
Fiber	1 g
Protein	3 g
Fat, total	4 g
Fat, saturated	1 g
Cholesterol	13 mg
Sodium	122 mg

EXCHANGES PER SERVING

1½ Other Carbohydrates
1 Fat

Preheat oven to 350°F
8-inch square cake pan, sprayed with nonstick vegetable spray

¼	cup margarine
¾	cup granulated sugar
1	egg
1	egg white
1½	tsp vanilla
1¼	cups all-purpose flour
1½	tsp baking powder
1	tsp ground cinnamon
½	tsp baking soda
1	cup 2% yogurt

Chocolate Marble

¼	cup granulated sugar
3	tbsp sifted unsweetened cocoa powder
3	tbsp 2% milk

1. In a large bowl or food processor, cream together margarine and sugar. Beat in egg, egg white and vanilla.

2. Combine flour, baking powder, cinnamon and baking soda; add to bowl alternately with yogurt, mixing just until blended. Do not overmix. Pour all but 1 cup into cake pan.

3. *Chocolate Marble:* In a small bowl, stir together sugar, cocoa and milk until blended. Add to reserved batter, mixing well. Pour over batter in pan; draw knife through mixture to create marbled effect. Bake for 35 to 40 minutes or until a cake tester inserted into center comes out clean.

Makes 16 slices (1 slice per serving)

DIETITIAN'S NOTE *If preparing the cake in advance, don't dust with confectioner's sugar until ready to serve. A little confectioner's sugar goes a long way. One tablespoon is enough for this cake, adding less than ½ gram of carbohydrate per serving.*

LA COSTA CHEESECAKE WITH STRAWBERRY SAUCE

Preheat oven to 325°F
9-inch pie plate

Cheesecake

2	cups low-fat cottage cheese
3	tbsp fructose
2	tbsp lemon juice
2	tsp vanilla
2	eggs
2	tbsp low-fat milk powder

Strawberry Sauce

2	cups strawberries
1	ripe banana
	Fresh strawberries (optional)

1. *Cheesecake:* In a blender or food processor, combine cottage cheese, fructose, lemon juice, vanilla and eggs; purée until smooth. Add milk powder; blend just until mixed. Pour into pie plate. Set pie plate in larger pan; pour in enough hot water to come halfway up sides. Bake for 30 to 35 minutes. Remove from water bath; cool on wire rack. Chill.

2. *Strawberry Sauce:* In a blender or food processor, purée strawberries with banana until smooth.

3. To serve, drizzle 2 tbsp strawberry sauce over each slice of cheese-cake. Garnish with strawberries, if desired.

Makes 8 slices (1 slice with 2 tbsp sauce per serving)

DIETITIAN'S NOTE *You will have about ½ cup of sauce left over. It goes well with pancakes or French toast. Count 3 tbsp as ½ Fruit Exchange.*

TIPS Thaw unsweetened frozen strawberries for sauce or use fresh ripe berries; if using frozen, drain excess liquid before puréeing.

The milk powder gives an extra calcium boost to this cheesecake.

NUTRIENTS PER SERVING

Calories	118
Carbohydrate	14 g
Fiber	1 g
Protein	10 g
Fat, total	3 g
Fat, saturated	1 g
Cholesterol	51 mg
Sodium	251 mg

EXCHANGES PER SERVING

1 Other Carbohydrates
1 Meat and Alternatives

RASPBERRY CHEESECAKE

TIP You can substitute whole frozen raspberries for fresh. Thaw and drain before using.

NUTRIENTS PER SERVING

Calories	87
Carbohydrate	9 g
Fiber	1 g
Protein	6 g
Fat, total	2 g
Fat, saturated	1 g
Cholesterol	36 mg
Sodium	118 mg

EXCHANGES PER SERVING

½ Other Carbohydrate

1 Lean Meat

Preheat oven to 350°F
8-inch springform pan, sprayed with baking spray

1	cup 5% ricotta cheese
1	cup low-fat cottage cheese
⅓	cup granulated sugar or ¼ cup fructose
⅓	cup low-fat yogurt
2	eggs
1	tsp grated lemon zest
½	tsp vanilla
1	tbsp all-purpose flour
1½	tsp cornstarch
1	cup raspberries
	Raspberry purée (optional)

1. In a food processor, beat together ricotta cheese, cottage cheese, sugar, yogurt, eggs, lemon zest and vanilla until smooth. Beat in flour and cornstarch. Transfer to a bowl; gently fold in raspberries. Pour into prepared pan.

2. Bake for 35 minutes or until a tester inserted in center comes out clean. Cool on a wire rack. Chill. Serve plain or, if desired, with raspberry purée.

Makes 12 slices (1 slice per serving)

DIETITIAN'S NOTES *Remember that the Nutrients per Serving and Exchanges do not include optional ingredients.*

To make about ½ cup raspberry purée, place 2 cups fresh or thawed frozen unsweetened raspberries in a blender and process until smooth. If you want to remove the seeds, pass the purée through a fine-mesh sieve. Count 2 tbsp as a Free Food or Extra.

CAKES, COFFEE CAKES & CHEESECAKES

TANGY BANANA CHEESECAKE

Preheat oven to 375°F
9-inch pie plate, sprayed with baking spray

1	cup low-fat cottage cheese
1	cup low-fat yogurt
2	egg whites
2	tbsp lemon juice
1	tsp vanilla
⅓	cup whole wheat flour
¼	cup honey
2	ripe bananas
	Berries or sliced bananas

1. In a blender or food processor, combine cottage cheese, yogurt, egg whites, lemon juice and vanilla; purée until smooth. Add flour; blend until well mixed. With motor running, add honey through feed tube; process until smooth. Add bananas; blend until smooth. Pour into prepared pie plate.

2. Bake for 30 to 40 minutes or until firm to the touch. Cool on wire rack. Chill at least 1 hour. Serve garnished with berries or sliced bananas.

Makes 8 slices (1 slice per serving)

TIP For a very nutritious dessert with a nutty flavor, coat pie plate with wheat germ after spraying with baking spray.

NUTRIENTS PER SERVING

Calories	126
Carbohydrate	23 g
Fiber	1 g
Protein	7 g
Fat, total	1 g
Fat, saturated	1 g
Cholesterol	4 mg
Sodium	151 mg

EXCHANGES PER SERVING

½ Fruit
1 Other Carbohydrates
1 Lean Meat

DIETITIAN'S NOTE *Count 2 tbsp sliced banana or ¼ cup of most unsweetened berries as a Free Food or Extra.*

MARBLE MOCHA CHEESECAKE

TIPS Graham crackers can also be used for the crust.

Melt chocolate in microwave on Defrost or in a double boiler.

If instant coffee is unavailable, use 2 tsp prepared strong coffee.

When using margarine, choose a soft (non-hydrogenated) version to limit consumption of trans fats.

Bake up to 2 days ahead and keep refrigerated.

Freeze for up to 6 weeks.

Preheat oven to 350°F
8-inch springform pan, sprayed with vegetable spray

Crust

1½	cups	chocolate wafer crumbs
2	tbsp	granulated sugar
2	tbsp	water
1	tbsp	margarine or butter

Filling

1⅔	cups	5% ricotta cheese
⅓	cup	light cream cheese, softened
¾	cup	granulated sugar
1		egg
⅓	cup	light sour cream or 2% yogurt
1	tbsp	all-purpose flour
1	tsp	vanilla
1½	tsp	instant coffee granules
1½	tsp	hot water
3	tbsp	semisweet chocolate chips, melted

1. *Crust:* Combine chocolate crumbs, sugar, water and margarine; mix thoroughly. Press into bottom and up sides of springform pan.

2. *Filling:* In a large bowl or food processor, beat together ricotta cheese, cream cheese, sugar, egg, sour cream, flour and vanilla until well blended. Dissolve coffee granules in hot water; add to batter and mix until incorporated.

3. Pour batter into springform pan and smooth top. Drizzle melted chocolate on top. Draw knife or spatula through the chocolate and batter several times to create marbling. Bake for 35 to 40 minutes; center will be slightly loose. Let cool and refrigerate several hours before serving.

Makes 12 slices (1 slice per serving)

DIETITIAN'S NOTE *When people hear the word "cheesecake," they usually think "high fat." While this is still true of many cheesecake recipes, there are now some that call for reduced-fat ingredients. This recipe calls for 5% ricotta cheese, light cream cheese and light sour cream, all of which have lower fat levels than their traditional counterparts. If this recipe were prepared with regular ricotta, cream cheese and sour cream, the total fat in each serving would increase from 8 grams to 14 grams.*

Keep in mind, though, that substituting lower-fat ingredients in a recipe doesn't always produce the same results, so if you have a favorite recipe, it's often a good idea to look for a lower-fat version that has already been tested.

Fat-free versions of cream cheese, sour cream and other dairy products are also available; however, recipe developers have discovered that, in general, they are not acceptable substitutes in recipes developed for regular-fat items, likely because they are higher in moisture.

When replacing regular cream cheese with a reduced-fat variety, be sure to use the solid type that comes in a bar, not the one in the tub.

NUTRIENTS PER SERVING

Calories	209
Carbohydrate	29 g
Fiber	1 g
Protein	7 g
Fat, total	8 g
Fat, saturated	3 g
Cholesterol	25 mg
Sodium	196 mg

EXCHANGES PER SERVING

1	Starch
1	Other Carbohydrates
½	Lean Meat
1	Fat

CHOCOLATE CHEESECAKE

TIPS Garnish with fresh berries or sifted cocoa.

Cooking with cocoa rather than chocolate has a major advantage. One ounce of semisweet chocolate has 140 calories and 9 grams of fat. One ounce of cocoa has 90 calories and 3 grams of fat.

When using margarine, choose a soft (non-hydrogenated) version to limit consumption of trans fats.

Prepare a day before or freeze for up to 3 weeks.

Preheat oven to 350°F
8-inch springform pan, sprayed with nonstick vegetable spray

Crust

1½	cups	graham or chocolate wafer crumbs
2	tbsp	water
1	tbsp	margarine, melted

Cake

8	oz	ricotta cheese
8	oz	2% cottage cheese
1	cup	granulated sugar
1		large egg
1	tsp	vanilla
¼	cup	sifted unsweetened cocoa powder
1	tbsp	all-purpose flour

Topping

1	cup	light sour cream
2	tbsp	granulated sugar
1	tsp	vanilla

1. *Crust:* In a bowl, combine crumbs, water and margarine; mix well. Pat onto bottom and sides of springform pan. Refrigerate.

2. *Cake:* In a food processor, combine ricotta and cottage cheeses, sugar, egg and vanilla; process until smooth. Add cocoa and flour; process just until combined. Pour into prepared pan and bake for 30 minutes or until set around edge but still slightly loose in center.

3. *Topping:* Meanwhile, stir together sour cream, sugar and vanilla; pour over cheesecake. Bake for 10 more minutes. (Topping will be loose.) Let cool and refrigerate for at least 3 hours or until set.

Makes 12 slices (1 slice per serving)

DIETITIAN'S NOTES *For the garnish, count ¼ cup of most unsweetened berries as a Free Food or Extra. You will need only a very light dusting of cocoa powder.*

We are all familiar with the expression "food for thought." It's equally important to give thought for food—not just to the nutrient values and Exchanges, but also to the experience of eating. Unfortunately, many meals today have become "refueling stops" on the run (both at and away from home), with little time to socialize and even less time to enjoy what we've chosen. Various strategies can help us be more thoughtful about what we eat:

Plan meals at least a day in advance, and make sure you have all the ingredients you need.

Involve other family members in planning and preparing meals.

When ordering from a menu, ask how foods are prepared, what comes with them and possible substitutions. At a buffet, survey everything before making your choices.

At home, you are able to serve yourself appropriate portions. Restaurant servings are often larger. Do not feel obliged to eat everything on your plate.

NUTRIENTS PER SERVING

Calories	213
Carbohydrate	32 g
Fiber	1 g
Protein	8 g
Fat, total	6 g
Fat, saturated	2 g
Cholesterol	26 mg
Sodium	212 mg

EXCHANGES PER SERVING

½	Starch
1½	Other Carbohydrates
1	Lean Meat
½	Fat

CHOCOLATE MARBLE VANILLA CHEESECAKE

TIPS For a mocha flavor, dissolve 2 tsp instant coffee in same amount of water and add to batter.

When using margarine, choose a soft (non-hydrogenated) version to limit consumption of trans fats.

Prepare up to 2 days ahead. Freeze for up to 6 weeks.

NUTRIENTS PER SERVING

Calories	222
Carbohydrate	32 g
Fiber	1 g
Protein	8 g
Fat, total	7 g
Fat, saturated	3 g
Cholesterol	31 mg
Sodium	210 mg

EXCHANGES PER SERVING

2 Other Carbohydrates

1 Lean Meat

1 Fat

Preheat oven to 350°F

9-inch springform pan, sprayed with vegetable spray

Crust

2	cups chocolate wafer crumbs
3	tbsp water
1½	tbsp margarine or butter, melted

Filling

2	cups ricotta cheese
2	cups 2% cottage cheese
1¾	cups granulated sugar
2	large eggs
⅓	cup all-purpose flour
⅔	cup light sour cream
2	tsp vanilla
2	oz semisweet chocolate
2	tbsp water

1. *Crust:* In a bowl, combine crumbs, water and margarine; mix well. Press onto sides and bottom of springform pan; refrigerate.

2. *Filling:* In a food processor, combine ricotta and cottage cheeses, sugar and eggs; process until completely smooth. Add flour, sour cream and vanilla; process until well combined. Pour into pan. Melt chocolate with water and stir until smooth. Spoon onto cake in several places and swirl through lightly with a knife. Bake for 65 minutes or until set around edge but still slightly loose in center. Let cool; refrigerate until well chilled.

Makes 20 slices (1 slice per serving)

INDIVIDUAL MINIATURE CHEESECAKES

Preheat oven to 350°F
Line 10 muffin cups with muffin paper cups

1	cup 5% ricotta cheese
1	cup low-fat cottage cheese
⅓	cup granulated sugar
1	medium egg
¼	cup light sour cream
½	tsp cornstarch
⅛	tsp vanilla extract
	Fruit purée (optional)

1. In a food processor, combine ricotta cheese, cottage cheese and sugar; purée until smooth. Beat in egg. Blend in sour cream, cornstarch and vanilla until well mixed. Divide batter among muffin cups. Set muffin tin in larger pan; pour in enough hot water to come halfway up sides. Bake 30 to 35 minutes or until tester inserted in center comes out clean. Remove from water bath; cool on wire rack. Chill.

2. Serve with fruit purée, if desired.

Makes 10 miniature cheesecakes (1 per serving)

TIPS Substitute one 8-oz package of light cream cheese for the ricotta cheese.

Decorate cheesecakes with berries and sliced fresh fruit; glaze with 2 tbsp no-sugar-added apricot spread.

Count fruit topping as a Fruit Exchange.

NUTRIENTS PER SERVING

Calories	127
Carbohydrate	9 g
Fiber	0 g
Protein	6 g
Fat, total	8 g
Fat, saturated	4 g
Sodium	268 mg
Cholesterol	42 mg

EXCHANGES PER SERVING

⅔ Other Carbohydrate

1 Lean Meat

1 Fat

Recipe photo in color insert.

6

PIES, TARTS, CRISPS & FRUIT DESSERTS

209	Phyllo Apple Pie
210	Sour Cream Apple Pie
212	Sour Cream & Berry Pie
213	Lemon Meringue Pie
214	Creamy Pumpkin Cheese Pie
216	Strawberry Mousse Pie
217	Sweetheart Berry Pie
218	Fresh Fruit Tart
219	Tropical Fruit Tart
220	Blueberry Apple Crisp
221	Apple, Pear & Cranberry Crisp
222	Blueberry Strawberry Pear Crisp
223	Peach & Blueberry Crisp
224	Peanut Butter Apple Crisp
225	Cherry Cobbler
226	Strawberry Rhubarb Cobbler
228	Pear, Apple & Raisin Strudel
229	Mango Blueberry Strudel
230	Baked Granola Apples
231	Coupe Bircher
232	Fried Pineapple
233	Pears in Tosca Sauce
234	Poached Pears in Chocolate Sauce
235	Wine-Poached Pear Fans
236	Key Lime Dessert
238	Fluffy Apricot Soufflé with Raspberry Sauce
240	Melon Balls with Ginger Sauce
241	Rhubarb Bread Pudding
242	Cocoa Roll with Creamy Cheese & Berries
244	Chocolate Quesadillas
245	Dessert Nachos
246	Chocolate Fondue
247	Strawberry Delights
248	Fruit on a Cloud
250	Creamy Dreamy Fruit Salad
251	Fresh Fruit Parfait
252	Balsamic Strawberry Sauce
253	Whipped Cream & Yogurt Topping

PHYLLO
APPLE PIE

Preheat oven to 400°F
10-inch deep-dish pie plate

8	apples (Granny Smith or other cooking variety)
⅓	cup lightly packed brown sugar
⅓	cup granulated sugar
⅓	cup unsweetened apple juice
3	tbsp all-purpose flour
2	tbsp freshly squeezed lemon juice
1	tsp ground cinnamon
½	tsp ground ginger
¼	tsp ground nutmeg
4	sheets phyllo pastry
1	tbsp melted butter
1	tbsp additional granulated sugar

1. Peel, core and quarter the apples. Cut each quarter into ½-inch-thick slices and place in a heavy saucepan.

2. In a small bowl, combine brown sugar, granulated sugar, apple juice, flour, lemon juice, cinnamon, ginger and nutmeg. Add to the apples and toss gently to coat. Cover and cook over medium-low heat, stirring occasionally, for 15 to 20 minutes, or until apples are tender. Spoon into pie plate and let cool slightly.

3. Spread out one sheet of phyllo and brush with ¼ of the butter. Fold one long end over to make a square. Lay another sheet of phyllo cross-wise over the first, brush with butter and fold to make a square. Continue layering and buttering the phyllo sheets, but don't butter the top one. Place the phyllo stack on the pie filling. Dot with the remaining butter and sprinkle lightly with 1 tbsp granulated sugar.

4. Gather the edges of the phyllo to form a ruffle around the pie. Spray the ruffle with vegetable spray. Cut slits into the phyllo top.

5. Bake in preheated oven for 15 minutes, until phyllo is golden.

Makes 8 servings

TIP Phyllo pastry dries out very quickly, so work with one sheet at a time, work quickly and keep the roll covered with a damp tea towel.

VARIATION Substitute 8 cups sliced peaches or pears for the apples.

NUTRIENTS PER SERVING

Calories	198
Carbohydrate	45 g
Fiber	3 g
Protein	1 g
Fat, total	3 g
Fat, saturated	1 g
Cholesterol	4 mg
Sodium	61 mg

EXCHANGES PER SERVING

1	Starch
1	Fruit
1	Other Carbohydrates
½	Fat

SOUR CREAM APPLE PIE

TIPS For an attractive presentation, sprinkle a little confectioner's sugar over top.

Substitute vanilla wafer crumbs for the graham crumbs for a change.

When using margarine, choose a soft (non-hydrogenated) version to limit consumption of trans fats.

Prepare early in the day and warm slightly before serving. Or freeze for up to 2 weeks.

Preheat oven to 350°F
8-inch springform pan

Crust

1½	cups graham wafer crumbs
2	tbsp margarine, melted
1	tbsp brown sugar
1	tbsp water

Filling

5½	cups sliced peeled apples (5 to 6 apples)
½	cup granulated sugar
½	cup 2% yogurt
½	cup light sour cream
¼	cup raisins
2	tbsp all-purpose flour
1	tsp ground cinnamon
1	egg, lightly beaten
1	tsp vanilla

Topping

¼	cup packed brown sugar
3	tbsp all-purpose flour
2	tbsp rolled oats
½	tsp ground cinnamon
1	tbsp margarine

1. *Crust:* In a bowl, combine graham crumbs, margarine, brown sugar and water; pat onto bottom and sides of pan. Refrigerate.

2. *Filling:* In a large bowl, combine apples, sugar, yogurt, sour cream, raisins, flour, cinnamon, egg and vanilla; toss together until well mixed. Pour over crust.

3. *Topping:* In a small bowl, combine brown sugar, flour, rolled oats and cinnamon; cut in margarine until crumbly. Sprinkle over pie; bake for 30 to 40 minutes or until topping is browned and apples are tender.

Makes 12 servings

DIETITIAN'S NOTES *A little confectioner's sugar goes a long way. One tablespoon sifted over this pie adds 1 gram of carbohydrate per serving.*

For help in planning your meals, ask your doctor to refer you to a diabetes education center or a dietitian. Local hospitals may also have referral services. On the Internet, look for the "Find a Nutrition Professional" feature at www.eatright.org.

NUTRIENTS PER SERVING

Calories	204
Carbohydrate	37 g
Fiber	2 g
Protein	3 g
Fat, total	5 g
Fat, saturated	1 g
Cholesterol	16 mg
Sodium	129 mg

EXCHANGES PER SERVING

1 Starch
½ Fruit
1 Other Carbohydrates
1 Fat

SOUR CREAM & BERRY PIE

TIP Before cooking with unflavored gelatin, always allow it to soften in a cold liquid. Gently warm the mixture as the gelatin dissolves. Allowing softened gelatin to boil will destroy its ability to thicken.

NUTRIENTS PER SERVING

Calories	215
Carbohydrate	33 g
Fiber	2 g
Protein	5 g
Fat, total	7 g
Fat, saturated	1 g
Cholesterol	2 mg
Sodium	142 mg

EXCHANGES PER SERVING

½ Starch

½ Low-Fat Milk

1 Other Carbohydrates

1 Fat

1	envelope (¼ oz) unflavored gelatin
3	tbsp cornstarch
½	cup granulated sugar
1½	cups 1% milk
1	cup lower-fat sour cream
½	cup plain yogurt
1	tsp vanilla
3	cups mixed raspberries, blueberries, and sliced strawberries
	Graham Wafer Crust (see recipe, page 267)

1. In a medium saucepan, combine gelatin and cornstarch; stir in sugar. Whisk in milk. Cook, stirring, over medium heat until it begins to thicken. Lower heat and allow to simmer, stirring, for 2 minutes longer. Remove from heat and cool slightly.

2. Meanwhile, in a medium bowl, combine sour cream and yogurt. Slowly stir the warm milk mixture into the sour cream mixture and add vanilla. Cover and chill for 1 hour, stirring once or twice, until firm.

3. Wash berries and pat dry with a paper towel. Reserve ½ cup of berries for garnish and fold the rest into the sour cream mixture. Spoon into Graham Wafer Crust and garnish with reserved berries. Cover and chill for 4 to 6 hours, until set.

Makes 8 servings

LEMON MERINGUE PIE

Preheat oven to 450°F
Six ½-cup ovenproof dishes
Baking sheet

Filling

1¼	cups	water
½	cup	fructose
1	tsp	grated lemon zest
¼	cup	freshly squeezed lemon juice
¼	cup	cornstarch
¾	cup	water
1	tsp	margarine

Meringue

2		egg whites
1	tbsp	fructose

1. *Filling:* In a saucepan, combine 1¼ cups water, fructose, lemon zest and juice. Bring to a boil. In a bowl, stir together cornstarch and ¾ cup water until dissolved. Stir into boiling lemon mixture. Cook, stirring, until thickened. Remove from heat. Stir in margarine. Divide among dishes. Cool.

2. *Meringue:* In a bowl, beat egg whites until soft peaks form. Gradually add fructose, beating until stiff peaks form. Spoon over filling; transfer dishes to baking sheet. Bake for 5 minutes or until golden. Cool to room temperature. Chill before serving.

Makes 6 servings

Recipe photo in color insert.

DIETITIAN'S NOTE *Although fructose does not raise blood sugar as much as sucrose (ordinary table sugar), it is not a sugar substitute or a Free Food or Extra. As with ordinary sugar, 1 tbsp counts as an Other Carbohydrate Exchange. You'll find fructose in specialty grocery stores and some health food stores.*

TIPS Separate eggs carefully for meringue—egg whites contaminated with yolk will not beat properly. Also, make sure your bowls and beaters are perfectly clean when making meringue.

When using margarine, choose a soft (non-hydrogenated) version.

NUTRIENTS PER SERVING

Calories	102
Carbohydrate	24 g
Fiber	0 g
Protein	1 g
Fat, total	1 g
Fat, saturated	0 g
Cholesterol	0 mg
Sodium	30 mg

EXCHANGES PER SERVING

½ Starch
1 Other Carbohydrates

CREAMY PUMPKIN CHEESE PIE

TIPS In the fall use fresh pumpkin. Bake pumpkin or squash in a 400°F oven until tender, approximately 1 hour.

The topping is simple but highly decorative.

Bake up to 2 days in advance. Freeze for up to 6 weeks.

Preheat oven to 350°F
9-inch springform pan or 9-inch deep-dish pie plate

1½	cups graham cracker crumbs
2	tbsp granulated sugar
2	tbsp water
1	tbsp vegetable oil
4	oz light cream cheese
½	cup 5% ricotta cheese
⅓	cup granulated sugar
1	egg
1	tsp vanilla
1	cup canned pumpkin purée (not pie filling) or mashed cooked butternut squash
⅔	cup 2% evaporated milk
¾	cup packed brown sugar
1	tsp ground cinnamon
¼	tsp ground ginger
¼	tsp ground nutmeg
3	tbsp light sour cream
2½	tsp granulated sugar

1. In a bowl, combine graham crumbs, sugar, water and oil; press into bottom and sides of pan; set aside.

2. In a food processor, combine cream cheese, ricotta, sugar, egg and vanilla; process until smooth. Pour into prepared crust.

3. In a food processor, combine pumpkin, evaporated milk, brown sugar, cinnamon, ginger and nutmeg until well blended. Spoon carefully over cheese filling.

4. In a small bowl, stir together sour cream and sugar. Put in a squeeze bottle or in a small plastic sandwich bag with the very tip of corner cut off. Draw 4 concentric circles on top of pumpkin filling. Run a toothpick through the circles at regular intervals.

5. Bake for 50 minutes or until just slightly loose at the center. Cool on wire rack. Chill before serving.

Makes 12 servings

DIETITIAN'S NOTES *If you don't have a food processor, use a hand mixer.*

Be sure to bring cream cheese to room temperature before combining with other ingredients.

As you prepare the recipes in this book, you will become familiar with the appropriate portion sizes for different types of desserts and the approximate Exchanges assigned to them. Use this knowledge to help you choose wisely when you're eating away from home.

NUTRIENTS PER SERVING

Calories	207
Carbohydrate	35 g
Fiber	1 g
Protein	5 g
Fat, total	6 g
Fat, saturated	2 g
Cholesterol	25 mg
Sodium	182 mg

EXCHANGES PER SERVING

1 Starch
1 Other Carbohydrates
1 Fat
1 Free Food

STRAWBERRY MOUSSE PIE

VARIATION Use your favorite fruit-flavored gelatin and fruit. For example, try orange-flavored gelatin with mandarin oranges or raspberry-flavored gelatin with fresh raspberries.

NUTRIENTS PER SERVING

Calories	116
Carbohydrate	13 g
Fiber	1 g
Protein	3 g
Fat, total	6 g
Fat, saturated	1 g
Cholesterol	5 mg
Sodium	151 mg

EXCHANGES PER SERVING

½ Starch

½ Other Carbohydrate

1 Fat

1	package (⅓ oz) no-sugar-added strawberry-flavored gelatin
⅔	cup boiling water
	Ice cubes
½	cup cold water
2	cups lower-fat non-dairy whipped topping, divided
½	cup plain yogurt
1	cup sliced strawberries, divided
	Graham Wafer Crust (see recipe, page 267)

1. Pour gelatin into a medium bowl and stir in boiling water. Stir for 2 minutes, until all of the gelatin is dissolved.

2. And enough ice to the cold water to make 1 cup. Stir into the gelatin until it is slightly thickened and the ice is melted.

3. Stir in 1½ cups of the whipped topping and yogurt and mix until smooth. Fold in ½ cup of the strawberries. Cover and refrigerate for 10 to 14 minutes, or until mixture begins to set.

4. Spoon into Graham Wafer Crust. Refrigerate for 4 hours, or until firm. Garnish with the remaining ½ cup strawberries and the remaining ½ cup whipped topping.

Makes 8 servings

SWEETHEART BERRY PIE

Preheat oven to 450°F
Baking sheet, lined with foil

⅓	cup granulated sugar, divided
1	tsp ground cinnamon
	Pastry for a 9-inch pie (from a mix or homemade)
1½	cups blackberries, fresh or frozen
1½	cups raspberries, fresh or frozen
1½	cups blueberries, fresh or frozen
1	tbsp cornstarch
3	tbsp freshly squeezed orange juice

1. In a small bowl, combine 1 tsp sugar and the cinnamon; set aside.

2. On a lightly floured surface, roll out pastry to ⅛ inch thick and cut into 9 heart shapes, using a 3½-inch heart-shaped cookie cutter. Sprinkle with cinnamon mixture. Place on prepared baking sheet and bake in preheated oven for 6 to 8 minutes, or until lightly browned. Transfer to a rack and let cool.

3. In a medium saucepan, combine blackberries, raspberries and blueberries. Add the remaining sugar and cornstarch and toss to coat the fruit. Add orange juice. Bring to a boil over medium heat, stirring frequently. Reduce heat to low and simmer for 5 to 10 minutes, until mixture is slightly thickened. Let cool until just warm.

4. Divide berry mixture among 9 individual dessert plates. Top each with a pastry heart.

Makes 9 servings

DIETITIAN'S NOTE *Blackberries, blueberries and raspberries are rich in antioxidants and fiber. This mouthwatering pie is the perfect dessert for a special festive meal.*

NUTRIENTS PER SERVING

Calories	160
Carbohydrate	27 g
Fiber	3 g
Protein	2 g
Fat, total	6 g
Fat, saturated	1 g
Cholesterol	0 mg
Sodium	125 mg

EXCHANGES PER SERVING

½	Starch
½	Fruit
½	Other Carbohydrate
1	Fat

FRESH FRUIT TART

TIP To save time, use a store-bought pre-baked pastry shell.

NUTRIENTS PER SERVING

Calories	132
Carbohydrate	17 g
Fiber	0 g
Protein	3 g
Fat, total	6 g
Fat, saturated	2 g
Cholesterol	24 mg
Sodium	127 mg

EXCHANGES PER SERVING

½ Starch

½ Other Carbohydrate

1 Fat

1 8-inch pastry shell, baked

Filling

1	cup skim milk
2	tbsp granulated sugar
1	tsp grated lemon zest
1	tsp grated orange zest
½	tsp vanilla
1	egg, beaten
1	tbsp cornstarch
	Fresh berries and/or sliced fruit
2	tbsp red currant jelly

1. *Filling:* In a saucepan, heat milk over medium heat until hot. Stir in sugar, lemon zest, orange zest and vanilla. In a bowl, beat egg with cornstarch until blended. Whisk a little of the hot milk into egg mixture, then pour back into remaining milk. Whisk constantly until mixture is thick enough to coat a spoon; do not boil. Chill.

2. Spread custard over baked crust. Decorate with fruit and berries. In a saucepan, melt jelly. Brush over fruit.

Makes 8 servings

DIETITIAN'S NOTES *Remember that Nutrients per Serving and Exchanges do not include ingredients for which no quantity is specified. Topping the tart with 8 strawberries and 2 kiwifruit will add 1 Free Food or Extra per serving.*

Count 3 banana slices as 1 Free Food or Extra. For most other fruits, ¼ cup sliced counts as 1 Free Food or Extra.

The filling for this tart is a custard—a mixture of milk and egg and other ingredients that thickens when heated.

TROPICAL FRUIT TART

Preheat oven to 400°F
9-inch tart or springform pan, sprayed with nonstick vegetable spray

Crust

1¼	cups all-purpose flour
¼	cup confectioner's sugar
⅓	cup margarine
3	tbsp cold water (approx.)

Filling

1¾	cups 2% yogurt
⅔	cup granulated sugar
½	cup light sour cream
3	tbsp frozen orange juice concentrate, thawed
2	tbsp all-purpose flour
1½	tsp orange zest

Topping

3	cups sliced fruit (kiwi, mangos, papayas, star fruit)

1. *Crust:* In a bowl, combine flour with sugar; cut in margarine until crumbly. With a fork, gradually stir in water, adding 1 tbsp more if necessary to make dough hold together. Pat into pan and bake for 15 minutes or until browned. Reduce heat to 375°F.

2. *Filling:* Meanwhile, in a bowl, combine yogurt, sugar, sour cream, orange juice concentrate, flour and orange zest; mix well and pour over crust. Bake for 35 to 45 minutes or until filling is set. Let cool and refrigerate until chilled.

3. *Topping:* Decoratively arrange sliced fruit over filling.

Makes 12 servings

TIP When using margarine, choose a soft (non-hydrogenated) version to limit consumption of trans fats.

NUTRIENTS PER SERVING

Calories	218
Carbohydrate	36 g
Fiber	2 g
Protein	4 g
Fat, total	7 g
Fat, saturated	1 g
Cholesterol	3 mg
Sodium	106 mg

EXCHANGES PER SERVING

1	Starch
½	Fruit
1	Other Carbohydrates
1½	Fat

BLUEBERRY APPLE CRISP

VARIATION In season, substitute pears for the apples and use ground ginger instead of cinnamon.

NUTRIENTS PER SERVING

Calories	170
Carbohydrate	33 g
Fiber	3 g
Protein	3 g
Fat, total	4 g
Fat, saturated	2 g
Cholesterol	8 mg
Sodium	34 mg

EXCHANGES PER SERVING

1 Starch
½ Fruit
½ Other Carbohydrate
1 Fat

Preheat oven to 350°F
9-inch square baking dish

3	medium apples, peeled, cored and sliced
1	cup fresh blueberries
¼	cup apple juice
2	tbsp granulated sugar
1	tbsp lemon juice
1	tsp ground cinnamon

Topping

1	cup rolled oats
⅓	cup whole wheat flour
¼	cup packed brown sugar
2	tbsp apple juice
2	tbsp butter, softened
½	tsp ground cinnamon

1. In a bowl, mix together apples, blueberries, apple juice, sugar, lemon juice and cinnamon. Transfer to baking dish.

2. *Topping:* In a bowl, stir together rolled oats, flour, brown sugar, apple juice, butter and cinnamon until crumbly. Sprinkle over blueberry mixture.

3. Bake for 30 minutes or until golden. Serve warm or cold.

Makes 8 servings

DIETITIAN'S NOTE *Unsweetened frozen blueberries can be substituted for fresh.*

APPLE, PEAR & CRANBERRY CRISP

Preheat oven to 400°F
8-inch square baking dish, lightly greased

Topping

¾	cup all-purpose flour
¾	cup packed brown sugar
½	cup old-fashioned rolled oats
½	cup cold butter
3	apples, cored, peeled and sliced
2	pears, cored, peeled and sliced
¼	cup dried cranberries
1	tbsp all-purpose flour
1	tbsp packed brown sugar

1. *Topping:* In a medium bowl, combine flour, brown sugar and oats. Cut in butter until mixture resembles coarse meal.

2. Place apples, pears and cranberries in prepared baking dish. Sprinkle with flour and sugar and toss to coat. Top with oat mixture.

3. Bake in preheated oven for 30 to 45 minutes or until topping is golden and fruit is tender. Let cool for 5 minutes before serving.

Makes 8 servings

TIP Leftovers can be stored in an airtight container in the fridge for up to 3 days or in the freezer for up to 3 months.

VARIATION When available, use fresh or frozen cranberries instead of dried.

NUTRIENTS PER SERVING

Calories	315
Carbohydrate	51 g
Fiber	3 g
Protein	2 g
Fat, total	12 g
Fat, saturated	7 g
Cholesterol	31 mg
Sodium	127 mg

EXCHANGES PER SERVING

1	Starch
1	Fruit
1½	Other Carbohydrates
2½	Fat

DIETITIAN'S NOTE *This recipe includes a generous amount of crisp topping. If you use only half the amount, you will save 1 Other Carbohydrate Exchange and 1 Fat Exchange.*

BLUEBERRY STRAWBERRY PEAR CRISP

TIPS Other fruits can be substituted, such as peaches, apples or mangos.

Can be baked earlier in the day, but best if baked just ahead of serving.

NUTRIENTS PER SERVING

Calories	195
Carbohydrate	39 g
Fiber	2 g
Protein	2 g
Fat, total	4 g
Fat, saturated	2 g
Cholesterol	10 mg
Sodium	46 mg

EXCHANGES PER SERVING

½	Starch
½	Fruit
1½	Other Carbohydrates
1	Fat

Preheat oven to 350°F
9-inch square cake pan, sprayed with vegetable spray

1½	cups fresh blueberries (or frozen, thawed and drained)
1½	cups sliced strawberries
1½	cups chopped peeled pears
½	cup granulated sugar
2	tbsp all-purpose flour
2	tsp orange juice
1	tsp grated orange zest
½	tsp ground cinnamon

Topping

¾	cup brown sugar
¾	cup all-purpose flour
½	cup rolled oats
½	tsp ground cinnamon
¼	cup cold butter

1. In a large bowl, combine blueberries, strawberries, pears, sugar, flour, orange juice, orange zest and cinnamon; toss gently to mix. Spread in prepared cake pan.

2. *Topping:* In a small bowl, combine brown sugar, flour, oats and cinnamon; cut butter in until crumbly. Sprinkle over fruit mixture. Bake for 30 to 35 minutes or until topping is browned and fruit is tender.

Makes 12 servings

PEACH & BLUEBERRY CRISP

Preheat oven to 350°F
9-inch square cake pan, ungreased

½	cup granulated sugar
2	tbsp all-purpose flour
2	tsp freshly squeezed lemon juice
1	tsp grated lemon zest
1	tsp ground cinnamon
3	cups sliced peeled ripe peaches
2	cups blueberries

Topping

½	cup rolled oats
⅓	cup all-purpose flour
3	tbsp packed brown sugar
½	tsp ground cinnamon
3	tbsp soft margarine

1. In a large bowl, combine sugar, flour, lemon juice, zest and cinnamon; stir in peaches and blueberries until well mixed. Spread in cake pan.

2. *Topping:* In a small bowl, combine rolled oats, flour, brown sugar and cinnamon; cut in margarine until crumbly. Sprinkle over fruit. Bake for 30 to 35 minutes or until topping is browned and fruit is tender. Serve warm.

Makes 8 servings

TIPS Blueberries should be removed from their carton and placed in a moisture-proof container in the refrigerator. Do not wash until just before using.

Although best straight from the oven, crisp can be prepared early in the day and reheated slightly before serving.

NUTRIENTS PER SERVING

Calories	204
Carbohydrate	40 g
Fiber	3 g
Protein	2 g
Fat, total	5 g
Fat, saturated	1 g
Cholesterol	0 mg
Sodium	62 mg

EXCHANGES PER SERVING

½	Starch
1	Fruit
1	Other Carbohydrates
1	Fat

PEANUT BUTTER APPLE CRISP

TIPS Read the labels on peanut butter chips. Some have twice as many grams of fat as others. Choose the lower-fat version when possible.

Metal pans can discolor when fruit is baked in them, so always use a tempered glass baking dish for fruit desserts.

NUTRIENTS PER SERVING

Calories	247
Carbohydrate	40 g
Fiber	3 g
Protein	3 g
Fat, total	10 g
Fat, saturated	3 g
Cholesterol	0 mg
Sodium	69 mg

EXCHANGES PER SERVING

1 Starch
½ Fruit
1 Other Carbohydrates
2 Fat

Preheat oven to 350°F
9-inch square glass baking pan, sprayed with vegetable spray

Fruit Layer
4	cups peeled and sliced apples
⅓	cup peanut butter chips
¼	cup granulated sugar
2	tbsp all-purpose flour

Topping
1	cup quick-cooking rolled oats
⅓	cup all-purpose flour
⅓	cup lightly packed brown sugar
¼	cup soft margarine
½	tsp ground cinnamon

1. *Fruit Layer:* In a large bowl, stir together apples, peanut butter chips, sugar and flour. Spread into prepared pan.

2. *Topping:* In a medium bowl, combine oats, flour, brown sugar, margarine and cinnamon until crumbly. Sprinkle over the apple layer.

3. Bake in preheated oven for 40 to 45 minutes, or until apples are tender. Cut into 9 squares and serve warm.

Makes 9 servings

DIETITIAN'S NOTE *The addition of peanut butter chips to this recipe makes it very kid-friendly. And it's a way to sneak in some fruit!*

CHERRY COBBLER

Preheat oven to 375°F
9-inch square baking dish, sprayed with vegetable spray

Filling
¼	cup granulated sugar
1	tbsp cornstarch
3	cups pitted sweet cherries

Topping
½	cup all-purpose flour
¼	cup granulated sugar
½	tsp baking powder
¼	tsp salt
1	large egg
1	tbsp soft margarine
1	tbsp 1% milk
1	tbsp granulated sugar
½	tsp ground cinnamon

1. *Filling:* In a medium saucepan, combine sugar and cornstarch and toss with cherries. Add ¼ cup water and stir to mix. Bring to a boil over medium heat, stirring frequently. Simmer for 5 minutes, until slightly thickened.

2. *Topping:* In a small bowl, combine flour, sugar, baking powder and salt. In another small bowl, using an electric mixer, beat egg and margarine; add milk. Beat in flour mixture until smooth.

3. Spread hot fruit in prepared baking dish and drop batter by heaping tablespoonfuls evenly over top.

4. In a small bowl, combine sugar and cinnamon; sprinkle over topping.

5. Bake in preheated oven for 25 to 30 minutes, or until browned.

Makes 6 servings

VARIATION Substitute your favorite seasonal fruit for the cherries. Try blueberries, blackberries, sliced plums, sliced apricots or sliced peaches.

NUTRIENTS PER SERVING
Calories	191
Carbohydrate	38 g
Fiber	1 g
Protein	3 g
Fat, total	4 g
Fat, saturated	1 g
Cholesterol	36 mg
Sodium	148 mg

EXCHANGES PER SERVING
½	Starch
1	Fruit
1	Other Carbohydrates
½	Fat

STRAWBERRY RHUBARB COBBLER

TIPS If using frozen fruit, there's no need to defrost before using.

If you prefer to bake the cobbler earlier in the day, reheat in 350° F oven for about 15 minutes.

This dessert is high in carbohydrate. To reduce this, replace the ¾ cup sugar in the fruit portion with a sugar substitute. This will reduce the carbohydrate content by almost 20 g per serving and lower the Other Carbohydrates Exchange to ⅓.

Preheat oven to 400°F
9-inch round or square baking dish

4	cups chopped fresh rhubarb
2	cups sliced strawberries
¾	cup granulated sugar
2	tbsp cornstarch
1	tsp grated orange zest

Biscuit Topping

1	cup all-purpose flour
¼	cup granulated sugar
1½	tsp baking powder
¼	tsp salt
¼	cup cold margarine or butter, cut into pieces
½	cup milk
1	tsp vanilla
2	tsp granulated sugar

1. Place rhubarb and strawberries in baking dish. In a small bowl, combine sugar, cornstarch and orange zest; sprinkle over fruit and gently toss.

2. Bake in preheated oven for 20 to 25 minutes (increase to 30 minutes if using frozen fruit) until hot and bubbles appear around edges.

3. *Biscuit Topping:* In a bowl, combine flour, sugar, baking powder and salt. Cut in margarine using a pastry blender or fork to make coarse crumbs. In a glass measure, combine milk and vanilla; stir into dry ingredients to make a soft, sticky dough.

4. Using a large spoon, drop eight separate spoonfuls of dough onto hot fruit; sprinkle with 2 tsp sugar.

5. Bake in preheated oven for 25 to 30 minutes or until top is golden and fruit is bubbly.

Makes 8 servings

NUTRIENTS PER SERVING

Calories	246
Carbohydrate	46 g
Fiber	2 g
Protein	3 g
Fat, total	6 g
Fat, saturated	1 g
Cholesterol	0 mg
Sodium	198 mg

EXCHANGES PER SERVING

1	Starch
⅓	Fruit
1½	Other Carbohydrates
1	Fat

PEAR, APPLE & RAISIN STRUDEL

TIPS Sprinkle with confectioner's sugar for a finishing touch.

Ripen pears at room temperature in a bowl or paper bag.

NUTRIENTS PER SERVING

Calories	112
Carbohydrate	22 g
Fiber	2 g
Protein	1 g
Fat, total	3 g
Fat, saturated	0 g
Cholesterol	0 mg
Sodium	64 mg

EXCHANGES PER SERVING

½ Starch

1 Fruit

½ Fat

Preheat oven to 350°F
Baking sheet, sprayed with vegetable spray

2⅔	cups chopped peeled apples
2⅔	cups chopped peeled pears
⅓	cup raisins
2	tbsp chopped pecans or walnuts
2	tbsp packed brown sugar
1	tbsp freshly squeezed lemon juice
1	tbsp liquid honey
1	tsp ground cinnamon
6	sheets phyllo pastry (see Tip, opposite)
4	tsp margarine, melted

1. In a bowl, combine apples, pears, raisins, pecans, brown sugar, lemon juice, honey and cinnamon; mix well.

2. Lay out 2 sheets of phyllo; brush with some margarine. Place 2 more sheets over top; brush with margarine again. Top with remaining 2 sheets phyllo.

3. Spread filling over phyllo, leaving 1-inch border uncovered. Roll up like jelly roll and place, seam side down, on prepared baking sheet. Brush with remaining margarine. Bake for 40 to 50 minutes or until golden and fruit is tender.

Makes 12 servings

DIETITIAN'S NOTE *If you use confectioner's sugar, remember that you need only a small quantity. One tablespoon sifted over this strudel adds just 1 gram of carbohydrate per serving.*

MANGO BLUEBERRY STRUDEL

Preheat oven to 375°F
Baking sheet, sprayed with vegetable spray

2	cups fresh blueberries (or frozen, thawed and drained)
1	tbsp all-purpose flour
2 ½	cups peeled chopped ripe mango
¼	cup granulated sugar
1	tbsp lemon juice
½	tsp ground cinnamon
6	sheets phyllo pastry
2	tsp melted margarine or butter
	Confectioner's sugar

1. Toss blueberries with flour. In a large bowl, combine mango, blueberries, sugar, lemon juice and cinnamon.

2. Lay 2 phyllo sheets one on top of the other; brush with melted margarine. Layer another 2 phyllo sheets on top and brush with melted margarine. Layer last 2 sheets on top. Put fruit filling along long end of phyllo; gently roll over until all of filling is enclosed, fold sides in, and continue to roll. Put on prepared baking sheet, brush with remaining margarine and bake for 20 to 25 minutes or until golden. Sprinkle with confectioner's sugar.

Makes 8 servings

TIP Phyllo pastry is located in the freezer section of the supermarket. Handle quickly so the sheets do not dry out. Cover those not being used with a slightly damp cloth.

NUTRIENTS PER SERVING

Calories	167
Carbohydrate	37 g
Fiber	3 g
Protein	2 g
Fat, total	2 g
Fat, saturated	0 g
Cholesterol	0 mg
Sodium	86 mg

EXCHANGES PER SERVING

½ Starch

1½ Fruit

½ Other Carbohydrate

½ Fat

BAKED GRANOLA APPLES

TIP The best apples for baking are Spartan, Empire, Golden Delicious and Cortland, as they will keep their shape while cooking.

VARIATION These also bake quickly in the microwave. Place on a microwave-safe plate and cover with microwave-safe plastic wrap. Cook on High for 2 to 3 minutes or until apples are tender.

NUTRIENTS PER SERVING

Calories	213
Carbohydrate	43 g
Fiber	4 g
Protein	4 g
Fat, total	4 g
Fat, saturated	1 g
Cholesterol	2 mg
Sodium	75 mg

EXCHANGES PER SERVING

1	Starch
1½	Fruit
1	Fat
1	Free Food

Preheat oven to 350°F
9-inch glass pie plate, ungreased

4	apples
¾	cup low-fat granola
2	tsp margarine
½	cup low-fat plain yogurt
1	tbsp pure maple syrup

1. Core apples, creating a large hollow. Firmly pack with granola and dot with margarine. Place on pie plate.

2. Bake, uncovered, in preheated oven for 30 minutes or until apples are tender.

3. Meanwhile, in a small bowl, combine yogurt and maple syrup; set aside.

4. Place each apple in a dessert bowl and garnish with maple-flavored yogurt.

Makes 4 servings

COUPE BIRCHER

½ cup quick-cooking rolled oats
¼ cup raisins
1 tbsp each sliced hazelnuts and almonds
½ cup 1% milk
1¼ cups lower-fat plain yogurt
3 tbsp granulated sugar
2 tbsp liquid honey
1 tsp lemon juice
1 tsp vanilla
2 cups sliced strawberries
2 cups cubed peeled cantaloupe
  Mint leaves

1. In a bowl, soak oats, raisins, hazelnuts and almonds in milk for 1 hour in refrigerator. Stir in yogurt, sugar, honey, lemon juice and vanilla.

2. Reserve about ½ cup each of the strawberries and cantaloupe; fold remaining fruit into yogurt mixture. Refrigerate for several hours or overnight.

3. Serve in dessert glasses topped with reserved fruit and mint leaves, if desired.

Makes 8 servings

NUTRIENTS PER SERVING

Calories	139
Carbohydrate	27 g
Fiber	2 g
Protein	4 g
Fat, total	2 g
Fat, saturated	1 g
Cholesterol	3 mg
Sodium	39 mg

EXCHANGES PER SERVING

1 Fruit
1 Other Carbohydrates
½ Fat

DIETITIAN'S NOTES *Use a variety of fruits, such as apples, oranges, bananas, raspberries or blueberries, in this elegant muesli-based dessert.*

Oats and fruit provide soluble fiber, which can help to lower blood cholesterol levels and control blood sugar levels in people with diabetes. This delicious dessert can also be served as a breakfast alternative to hot oatmeal.

FRIED PINEAPPLE

TIP Here's a great recipe for when you need a decadent dessert but don't have time to fuss. Small amounts of unsalted butter and bittersweet chocolate add 6 g of saturated fat, so save this for special occasions.

NUTRIENTS PER SERVING

Calories	212
Carbohydrate	34 g
Fiber	3 g
Protein	2 g
Fat, total	10 g
Fat, saturated	6 g
Sodium	4 mg
Cholesterol	16 mg

EXCHANGES PER SERVING

1½ Fruit
½ Other Carbohydrate
2 Fat

1	ripe pineapple
2	tbsp sugar
2	tbsp unsalted butter
2	tbsp sultana raisins
1	oz bittersweet chocolate, shaved
4	sprigs fresh mint

1. With a sharp knife cut off top half of pineapple, reserving it for another use. Remove rind from the bottom (sweeter) half and slice pineapple into 4 rounds, each ½ inch thick. Spread sugar on a plate and dredge the pineapple slices in the sugar.

2. In a large frying pan melt butter over high heat until foaming. Add the dredged pineapple slices and fry for 2 minutes. Flip the slices and spread raisins around them; fry for another 2 to 3 minutes until pineapple has browned and raisins are swollen. Remove from heat and transfer one pineapple slice to each of 4 dessert plates, flipping them so the more attractively browned side faces upward. Spoon some raisins onto each plate and top with a bit of the sauce from the pan. Garnish with chocolate shavings and mint. Serve immediately.

Serves 4

PEARS IN TOSCA SAUCE

Preheat oven to 350°F
8-inch square glass baking dish, ungreased

½	cup sliced almonds
⅓	cup packed brown sugar
⅓	cup milk
2	tbsp unsalted butter
1	tbsp all-purpose flour
1	tsp vanilla
1	can (28 oz) pear halves, drained

1. In a small saucepan, over medium-high heat, combine almonds, brown sugar, milk, butter, flour and vanilla. Bring to a boil and cook until sauce thickens, about 5 minutes.

2. Place pears in baking dish and pour sauce over top.

3. Bake in preheated oven until browned on top, about 15 minutes.

Makes 6 servings

TIP This is a pretty dessert to serve directly from the dish, so use a glass or ceramic baking dish rather than a metal pan.

VARIATION Substitute a combination of canned peaches and fresh or frozen raspberries for the pears.

NUTRIENTS PER SERVING

Calories	188
Carbohydrate	26 g
Fiber	2 g
Protein	3 g
Fat, total	9 g
Fat, saturated	3 g
Cholesterol	11 g
Sodium	16 mg

EXCHANGES PER SERVING

½	Fruit
1	Other Carbohydrates
2	Fat
1	Free Food

DIETITIAN'S NOTE *Be sure to use pears canned in juice. They contain 20% less carbohydrate than pears canned in light syrup, and 30% less than those canned in heavy syrup.*

POACHED PEARS IN CHOCOLATE SAUCE

TIP Use a firm pear such as a Bosc.

NUTRIENTS PER SERVING

Calories	171
Carbohydrate	38 g
Fiber	5 g
Protein	1 g
Fat, total	3 g
Fat, saturated	2 g
Cholesterol	0 mg
Sodium	6 mg

EXCHANGES PER SERVING

2 Fruit
½ Other Carbohydrate
½ Fat

2	tbsp lemon juice
6	small ripe pears
1½	cups pear nectar (or other fruit nectar)
¼	cup semisweet chocolate chips
1	tbsp 2% evaporated milk

1. Put lemon juice and 6 cups water in a bowl. Peel pears, leaving whole with stems intact and dropping each in water mixture as it is peeled. Drain. In a saucepan, combine pears and pear nectar. Bring to a boil, reduce heat to medium-low, cover and cook, turning pears over halfway through, for 20 to 25 minutes or until tender when pierced with a knife. Transfer pears and syrup to a bowl; chill.

2. Before serving, drain pears, reserving syrup. Bring syrup to a boil; cook until reduced to ¼ cup. Stir in chocolate chips until melted. Beat in evaporated milk until smooth.

3. Serve chilled pears on top of a pool of hot chocolate sauce.

Makes 6 servings

WINE-POACHED PEAR FANS

2 cups red wine (or 1 cup pure cranberry juice—not cocktail—plus 1 cup water)
½ cup granulated sugar
1 cinnamon stick
3 whole cloves
2 strips (each 3 inches) orange peel
4 Bartlett pears, peeled, halved and cored
Extra-thick low-fat yogurt
Freshly grated nutmeg and fresh mint sprigs

1. In a medium saucepan, combine wine, sugar, cinnamon stick, cloves and orange peel. Bring to a boil, stirring to dissolve sugar. Add pear halves; reduce heat, cover and simmer for 15 minutes or until just tender when pierced with a knife. Remove with a slotted spoon to a dish; let cool.

2. Bring poaching liquid in saucepan to a boil over high heat; boil until reduced to ¾ cup. Strain through a sieve to remove spices; let cool and refrigerate.

3. Place pears cut side down on work surface. Beginning near the stem end, cut each pear half into ¼-inch lengthwise slices. (Do not cut through the stem itself; slices will still be attached at stem end.) Arrange a pear half on each dessert plate, pressing down gently to fan out slices. Spoon syrup over. Garnish with a dollop of yogurt and sprinkle with nutmeg. Garnish with mint sprigs.

Serves 8

TIPS Poach the pears the day before. They are best served well-chilled.

Select pears that are not overly ripe so they will hold their shape when sliced.

NUTRIENTS PER SERVING

Calories	127
Carbohydrate	27 g
Fiber	2 g
Protein	2 g
Fat, total	1 g
Fat, saturated	0 g
Sodium	25 mg
Cholesterol	1 mg

EXCHANGES PER SERVING

1 Fruit
1 Other Carbohydrates

KEY LIME DESSERT

TIPS To get the most juice from limes or other citrus fruit, bring fruit to room temperature before juicing.

Make sure the egg whites for the meringue are perfectly pure, without a speck of yolk, or they will not beat properly.

Preheat oven to 400°F
4-cup soufflé dish or eight ½-cup ramekins

Filling
¾	cup fructose
¼	cup cornstarch
1½	cups water
2	egg whites, at room temperature
1	egg, at room temperature
2	tsp grated lime zest
¼	cup freshly squeezed lime juice

Meringue
2	egg whites
¼	tsp cream of tartar
4	tsp fructose

1. *Filling:* In a saucepan, stir together fructose and cornstarch. Gradually whisk in water until smooth. Bring to a boil over medium heat, stirring constantly. Continue to boil for 1 minute, stirring constantly, or until thickened. Remove from heat.

2. In a bowl, beat egg whites with egg. Gradually whisk half of hot cornstarch mixture into egg mixture. Pour back into remaining cornstarch mixture. Return saucepan to medium heat; cook, stirring, 1 minute. Remove from heat. Stir in lime zest and juice. Pour into soufflé dish.

3. *Meringue:* In a bowl, beat egg whites until foamy. Add cream of tartar and beat until soft peaks form. Gradually add fructose, beating until stiff peaks form. Spoon over hot filling. Bake for 8 to 10 minutes or until golden brown.

Makes 8 servings

DIETITIAN'S NOTES *Gram for gram, fructose is sweeter than ordinary sugar (sucrose), but it has a lower glycemic index (it does not raise blood sugar as much). It is not, however, a sugar substitute or a Free Food or Extra. Like ordinary sugar, 1 tbsp of fructose counts as an Other Carbohydrate Exchange. Look for it in specialty grocery stores and some health food stores.*

People with type 1 diabetes do not produce insulin, the hormone required to metabolize carbohydrate (starch and sugars). Before the development of injectable insulin, they were limited to a diet consisting entirely of protein and fat. Once insulin became available, they were able to add bread and other grain products, fruit, vegetables and milk products. Experts still believed, however, that even a very small amount of sugar would seriously interfere with blood glucose control, and several generations of people with diabetes were advised to avoid it altogether. We now know that the total quantity of carbohydrate—regardless of the source—and how it's distributed throughout the day are the most important factors. With the ban on sugar lifted, people with diabetes can usually eat the same foods as everyone else. It isn't necessary to seek out special foods or recipes.

Gram for gram, sugar has the same number of calories as the carbohydrate in other foods; however, it does not provide the essential vitamins, minerals and other healthy components that they do. For this reason, high-sugar foods are often called "empty-calorie foods." And that is why only a small portion of your daily carbohydrate intake should come from sugar.

NUTRIENTS PER SERVING

Calories	110
Carbohydrate	25 g
Fiber	0 g
Protein	3 g
Fat, total	1 g
Fat, saturated	0 g
Cholesterol	23 mg
Sodium	37 mg

EXCHANGES PER SERVING

1½ Other Carbohydrates
½ Lean Meat

FLUFFY APRICOT SOUFFLÉ WITH RASPBERRY SAUCE

TIPS For a strawberry sauce, substitute strawberries for the raspberries.

Thaw unsweetened frozen berries for sauce or use fresh ripe berries; if using frozen, drain excess liquid before puréeing.

PIES, TARTS, CRISPS & FRUIT DESSERTS

Preheat oven to 300°F
8-cup soufflé dish, sprayed with baking spray

Soufflé

8	oz dried apricots
¼	cup water
¼	cup granulated sugar
¼	tsp almond extract
5	egg whites

Sauce

1	cup raspberries
½	ripe banana
1	tbsp fruit jam (any flavor)
1	tsp lemon juice

1. *Soufflé:* In a saucepan, combine apricots and water; cook over medium heat for 5 minutes or until all the water is absorbed. Transfer hot apricots to a food processor or blender; purée just until finely chopped. Add sugar and almond extract; purée until well mixed. Transfer to a bowl; cool mixture to room temperature.

2. In another bowl, beat egg whites until stiff peaks form. Stir one-third of egg whites into cooled apricot mixture until well mixed. Gently fold in remaining egg whites. Apricot pieces will still be evident. Pour into prepared dish.

3. Set soufflé dish in larger pan; pour in enough hot water to come halfway up sides. Bake for 20 minutes. Reduce oven temperature to 250°F; bake for 12 minutes longer or until light brown and no longer loose.

4. *Sauce:* In a blender or food processor, combine raspberries, banana, jam and lemon juice; purée until smooth. Strain to remove seeds.

5. Serve soufflé hot, drizzled with raspberry sauce.

Makes 6 servings

DIETITIAN'S NOTES *Be sure to choose unsweetened frozen fruit. Sweetened varieties generally contain about twice as much carbohydrate as unsweetened.*

Would you like to include a favorite dessert recipe in your meals? To estimate Exchanges for a recipe serving, use the worksheets on pages 316–317. There you will find lists of dessert ingredients and the Exchanges contained in common amounts (usually 1 cup), as well as instructions on how to use the worksheet. To calculate Exchanges, use the worksheet on pages 314–315.

NUTRIENTS PER SERVING

Calories	164
Carbohydrate	39 g
Fiber	4 g
Protein	5 g
Fat, total	0 g
Fat, saturated	0 g
Cholesterol	0 mg
Sodium	50 mg

EXCHANGES PER SERVING

2 Fruit
½ Other Carbohydrate
½ Lean Meat

MELON BALLS WITH GINGER SAUCE

TIPS If you don't have a melon baller, use a small spoon to scoop melon flesh, or cut flesh into small cubes.

Make sauce in advance and store, covered, in refrigerator for up to 2 days; reheat before serving.

NUTRIENTS PER SERVING

Calories	77
Carbohydrate	19 g
Fiber	1 g
Protein	1 g
Fat, total	0 g
Fat, saturated	0 g
Cholesterol	0 mg
Sodium	16 mg

EXCHANGES PER SERVING

1 Fruit

1	small ripe honeydew melon
2	small ripe cantaloupes

Sauce

2	cups orange juice
2	tbsp minced gingerroot or ½ tsp ground ginger
1	tbsp raspberry or red wine vinegar
1	tsp liquid honey
½	tsp lemon juice
	Fresh mint leaves

1. Cut melons in half and discard seeds. With a melon baller, scoop out flesh. Divide melon balls among 12 individual dessert dishes.

2. In a saucepan, combine orange juice, gingerroot, vinegar, honey and lemon juice. Bring to a boil; cook until reduced to ½ cup. Spoon warm sauce over melon balls and serve garnished with mint leaves.

Makes 12 servings

RHUBARB BREAD PUDDING

Preheat oven to 350°F
8-inch square baking dish, greased

2	cups chopped fresh or frozen rhubarb, thawed
3	cups torn stale white and whole wheat bread
1	can (14 oz) evaporated milk
2	eggs
¼	cup granulated sugar
1	tsp vanilla
1	tsp ground cinnamon
	Grated zest of 1 orange

1. Place rhubarb in prepared baking dish and cover with bread pieces.

2. In a medium bowl, beat evaporated milk, eggs, sugar, vanilla, cinnamon and orange zest. Pour over bread. Let stand for 10 minutes.

3. Bake in preheated oven for 40 to 45 minutes or until a tester inserted in the center comes out clean. Serve warm.

Makes 6 servings

TIP Leftovers can be stored in an airtight container in the fridge for up to 3 days or in the freezer for up to 3 months.

VARIATION Try making this pudding with another fruit, such as frozen berries or peaches.

NUTRIENTS PER SERVING

Calories	180
Carbohydrate	27 g
Fiber	2 g
Protein	9 g
Fat, total	4 g
Fat, saturated	2 g
Cholesterol	67 mg
Sodium	197 mg

EXCHANGES PER SERVING

½ Starch
1 Other Carbohydrates
½ Reduced-Fat Milk

DIETITIAN'S NOTE *If substituting frozen fruit for rhubarb in this recipe, be sure to choose those that do not contain added sugar. Add 1 Free Food or Extra per serving.*

COCOA ROLL WITH CREAMY CHEESE & BERRIES

TIPS Decorate roll with fresh berries.

Substitute other fresh berries of your choice.

Prepare cake early in day and keep covered until ready to roll with filling.

Preheat oven to 325°F
Jelly-roll pan, lined with parchment paper and sprayed with vegetable spray

5	egg whites
⅛	tsp cream of tartar
⅔	cup granulated sugar, divided
½	cup cake and pastry flour
4	tsp unsweetened cocoa powder
1½	tsp vanilla
	Confectioner's sugar

Filling

1¼	cups ricotta cheese
¼	cup light sour cream
3	tbsp confectioner's sugar
1¼	cups sliced strawberries and/or blueberries

1. In a medium bowl, beat egg whites and cream of tartar until soft peaks form. Gradually beat in ⅓ cup of sugar until stiff peaks form.

2. Sift together remaining sugar, flour and cocoa; sift over egg whites and fold in gently along with vanilla. Do not overmix. Pour onto prepared pan and spread evenly. Bake for 15 to 20 minutes or until top springs back when lightly touched.

3. *Filling:* In a bowl or food processor, mix together cheese, sour cream and confectioner's sugar until smooth. Fold in berries. Set aside.

4. Sprinkle cake lightly with confectioner's sugar. Carefully invert onto surface sprinkled with confectioner's sugar. Carefully remove parchment paper. Spread filling over cake and roll up. Place on serving dish. Sprinkle with confectioner's sugar.

Makes 10 servings

DIETITIAN'S NOTES *Berry garnishes are too good to leave on the plate. Five strawberries or 20 small raspberries (both without sugar) count as 1 Free Food or Extra.*

The quantity of confectioner's sugar to be sprinkled on the cake (Step 4) is not specified in this recipe, so it's excluded from the Nutrients per Serving and the Exchanges. You'll need about 1½ tbsp confectioner's sugar in total, which will add less than 2 grams of carbohydrate per serving.

Wheat flour contains a protein called gluten. In bread-making, the kneading process "develops" the gluten, allowing the dough to become stretchy, easy to handle and strong enough to trap the carbon dioxide generated by the yeast when it rises. High-gluten flour is desirable for bread-making, but cake and pastry flour, which is low in gluten, is required for pastry and delicate cakes.

All-purpose flour has an intermediate gluten level and, as its name implies, can be used for most baked goods. However, yeast doughs made with all-purpose flour may not rise as much, and pastry and delicate cakes may be less tender.

Too much stirring or handling of any batter or dough will develop the gluten and result in a less tender end product. For this reason, baking recipes often caution against overmixing.

NUTRIENTS PER SERVING

Calories	157
Carbohydrate	25 g
Fiber	1 g
Protein	6 g
Fat, total	4 g
Fat, saturated	2 g
Cholesterol	13 mg
Sodium	67 mg

EXCHANGES PER SERVING

½	Starch
1	Other Carbohydrates
1	Lean Meat

PIES, TARTS, CRISPS & FRUIT DESSERTS

CHOCOLATE QUESADILLAS

TIP You can double or triple this recipe.

NUTRIENTS PER SERVING

Calories	346
Carbohydrate	35 g
Fiber	3 g
Protein	5 g
Fat, total	21 g
Fat, saturated	7 g
Cholesterol	7 mg
Sodium	133 mg

EXCHANGES PER SERVING

1 Starch

1 Other Carbohydrates

4 Fat

1 Free Food

½	cup chopped pecans
1	tbsp granulated sugar
Pinch	salt
2	8-inch flour tortillas
3	oz bittersweet or semisweet chocolate, chopped
¼	cup sour cream
2	tsp packed light brown sugar

1. In a large nonstick skillet over medium-high heat, cook pecans, granulated sugar and salt, stirring with a wooden spoon, for 2 to 4 minutes or until pecans are toasted and sugar is melted and caramelized on nuts. If sugar or nuts start to burn, reduce heat. Transfer to a plate or baking sheet and let cool.

2. In a clean large nonstick skillet over medium-high heat, heat one of the tortillas until warm. Leaving tortilla in skillet, arrange half of the chocolate on one half of tortilla; fold opposite half over chocolate to cover. Cook quesadilla, turning once, for 3 to 4 minutes or until golden brown on both sides and chocolate is melted. Set aside on a plate. Repeat with remaining tortilla and chocolate.

3. In a small bowl, stir sour cream with brown sugar until smooth. Dollop over top of each quesadilla. Sprinkle candied pecans over sour cream mixture. Serve immediately.

Makes 4 servings (½ quesadilla with topping per serving)

DIETITIAN'S NOTE *Don't forget that the Nutrients per Serving and Exchanges are based on ½ quesadilla, not a whole one.*

DESSERT NACHOS

Preheat oven to 450°F
Baking sheets, lightly greased

½	cup granulated sugar
3	tbsp ground cinnamon
4	10-inch whole wheat flour tortillas
4	cups fresh fruit salsa (see Tip)
2	cups low-fat fruit-flavored yogurt

1. On a large flat plate, mix sugar and cinnamon. Dip each tortilla in water. Shake off the excess and dip one side into the sugar and cinnamon mixture. Stack tortillas on top of each other as they are dipped. When completed, cut the stack into 8 triangular wedges.

2. Spread tortilla wedges in a single layer on prepared baking sheets, without overlapping, and bake in batches in preheated oven for 4 to 5 minutes per tray or until golden and crisp.

3. Place on a large platter with a bowl of fruit salsa and another of yogurt.

Makes 8 servings

TIP Pick fruits of your choice to make the 4 cups salsa, or ask your children what they would like. Fresh or canned pineapple, fresh or frozen mango, fresh strawberries, kiwi, cantaloupe and watermelon all work well. Cut your chosen fruits into small dice and combine in a bowl.

NUTRIENTS PER SERVING

Calories	270
Carbohydrate	52 g
Fiber	4 g
Protein	7 g
Fat, total	4 g
Fat, saturated	1 g
Cholesterol	3 mg
Sodium	194 mg

EXCHANGES PER SERVING

1½	Starch
1	Fruit
1	Other Carbohydrates
1	Fat

CHOCOLATE FONDUE

VARIATION For a milder chocolate flavor, replace the semisweet with milk chocolate. Children tend to prefer milk chocolate.

NUTRIENTS PER SERVING

Calories	150
Carbohydrate	20 g
Fiber	2 g
Protein	2 g
Fat, total	9 g
Fat, saturated	5 g
Cholesterol	1 mg
Sodium	21 mg

EXCHANGES PER SERVING

1 Other Carbohydrates

2 Fat

1 Free Food

Fondue pot

8 oz semisweet chocolate, chopped
½ cup evaporated milk or whipping (35%) cream
A selection of chopped fruits for dipping (bananas, strawberries, apples, pears, etc.)

1. In fondue pot, over low heat, heat chocolate and evaporated milk, stirring with a wooden spatula, until chocolate has melted, about 5 minutes. Place fondue pot over tabletop burner.

2. Arrange fruit in a serving dish and serve with fondue.

Makes about 1½ cups chocolate fondue (3 tbsp per serving)

DIETITIAN'S NOTE *Remember that the Nutrients per Serving and Exchanges are for the fondue mixture only. You will need to count the fruit separately: ½ cup sliced fruit will add 1 Fruit Exchange.*

STRAWBERRY DELIGHTS

24	large strawberries
4	oz lower-fat cream cheese, at room temperature
2	tbsp granulated sugar
1½	tsp freshly squeezed lemon juice
¼	cup chocolate sprinkles

1. Wash strawberries and pat dry with a paper towel.

2. In a small bowl, combine cream cheese, sugar and lemon juice. Blend well.

3. Holding each strawberry by its leaf, dip the bottom half of the strawberry into the cream cheese mixture, coating it well. Then dip it in chocolate sprinkles and set on waxed paper.

4. Repeat until all strawberries are dipped. Arrange on a serving plate and serve immediately or cover and refrigerate for up to 2 hours.

Makes 8 servings

TIP On your next picnic, take along fresh strawberries, cream cheese mixture and sprinkles in separate containers. Arrange strawberries on a platter surrounding the toppings and let everyone dip berries in the cream cheese mixture and the sprinkles.

NUTRIENTS PER SERVING

Calories	62
Carbohydrate	8 g
Fiber	1 g
Protein	1 g
Fat, total	3 g
Fat, saturated	2 g
Cholesterol	7 mg
Sodium	75 mg

EXCHANGES PER SERVING

½ Other Carbohydrate
½ Fat

PIES, TARTS, CRISPS & FRUIT DESSERTS

DIETITIAN'S NOTE *It's all in the presentation! This is such a scrumptious little treat, and it's quite simple to make. The strawberries are a source of vitamin C and fiber, while the cream cheese and chocolate sprinkles add only 3 grams of fat.*

FRUIT
ON A CLOUD

TIP Use your favorite fruit and berries.

VARIATION Drizzle calorie-reduced sundae topping over the fruit. Or garnish with fresh sliced strawberries and drizzle with Chocolate Sauce (see recipe, page 293).

Baking sheet, lined with waxed paper

4	oz lower-fat cream cheese
1	cup lower-fat non-dairy whipped topping
1	cup miniature marshmallows
2	cups mixed fresh fruit, such as raspberries, blueberries, grapes, and sliced nectarines

1. In a medium bowl, using an electric mixer, beat cream cheese until light and fluffy. Add whipped topping, adjust mixer to slow setting and stir until smooth, about 2 minutes. Stir in marshmallows.

2. To make clouds, spoon cream cheese mixture in 4 mounds onto prepared baking sheet. Spread each mound into a 3-inch circle with the back of a spoon and make a deep well in the center of each circle, building up the sides. Freeze for 2 to 3 hours.

3. Remove clouds from the freezer and place on individual serving plates. Let stand at room temperature for 15 minutes.

4. Meanwhile, combine fruit in a small bowl.

5. Spoon ½ cup fruit into the center of each cloud and serve immediately.

Makes 4 servings

DIETITIAN'S NOTE *This dessert is high in carbohydrates because of the marshmallows, but it can be a good way to encourage a child who avoids eating fruit to eat some. Fruits are good sources of vitamin C, beta-carotene, antioxidants and fiber.*

NUTRIENTS PER SERVING

Calories	151
Carbohydrate	25 g
Fiber	2 g
Protein	3 g
Fat, total	5 g
Fat, Saturated	3 g
Cholesterol	18 mg
Sodium	168 mg

EXCHANGES PER SERVING

½	Fruit
1	Other Carbohydrates
½	Medium-Fat Meat
½	Fat

CREAMY DREAMY FRUIT SALAD

NUTRIENTS PER SERVING

Calories	128
Carbohydrate	31 g
Fiber	1 g
Protein	2 g
Fat, total	1 g
Fat, saturated	0 g
Cholesterol	2 mg
Sodium	18 mg

EXCHANGES PER SERVING

2 Fruit

1 apple, cored and diced
2 tsp freshly squeezed lemon juice
1 can (14 oz) pineapple tidbits, packed in juice, drained
1 can (10 oz) mandarin orange sections, drained
1 cup halved seedless grapes
1 cup mini marshmallows
¾ cup 1% or 2% orange- or pineapple-flavored yogurt
2 medium bananas

1. In a large bowl, toss diced apple with lemon juice to prevent browning. Add pineapple, mandarin oranges, grapes and marshmallows.

2. Drizzle with yogurt and toss gently until fruit and marshmallows are evenly coated. Refrigerate for at least 1 hour or for up to 8 hours to blend flavors.

3. Just before serving, slice bananas and stir into fruit mixture.

Makes 8 servings

DIETITIAN'S NOTE *This mix of fruit and yogurt makes a tasty, nutritious dessert. It can be a light finish to a heartier meal.*

FRESH FRUIT PARFAIT

2 cups vanilla ice milk
2 cups fresh fruit (chopped pineapple, chopped kiwi, sliced strawberries, blueberries or sliced oranges)
¼ cup lower-fat non-dairy whipped topping

1. In each of 4 dessert dishes or parfait glasses, layer ¼ cup ice milk and ¼ cup fruit. Repeat layers.

2. Top with 1 tbsp whipped topping.

Makes 4 servings

VARIATION TROPICAL PARFAIT: Use chopped mangoes, papayas and pineapple. Sprinkle 1 tsp toasted shredded coconut on top of each parfait.

NUTRIENTS PER SERVING

Calories	95
Carbohydrate	19 g
Fiber	2 g
Protein	3 g
Fat, total	2 g
Fat, saturated	1 g
Cholesterol	6 mg
Sodium	36 mg

EXCHANGES PER SERVING

½ Fruit
½ Other Carbohydrate
½ Medium-Fat Meat

DIETITIAN'S NOTE *In this case, having dessert ups your nutrient intake. Fruits give us vitamins, antioxidants and fiber, and fresh is always better. Including fresh fruit in an easy dessert recipe such as this one is a delicious way to add another fruit serving to the day.*

BALSAMIC STRAWBERRY SAUCE

VARIATION This well-known Italian sauce is traditionally served with a dash of freshly ground black pepper on top. It can also be prepared without cooking. An hour before serving, place sliced berries in a bowl and add sugar. Just before serving, add the balsamic vinegar.

4	cups sliced hulled strawberries
3	tbsp granulated sugar
¼	cup balsamic vinegar

1. In a medium saucepan, over medium heat, cook strawberries and sugar for 2 minutes or until sugar melts and starts to form a sauce. Add balsamic vinegar; cook for 2 minutes. Remove from heat.

2. Serve warm, or cover and refrigerate to serve cold.

Makes about 2½ cups (¼ cup per serving)

NUTRIENTS PER SERVING

Calories	38
Carbohydrate	9 g
Fiber	1 g
Protein	0 g
Fat, total	0 g
Fat, saturated	0 g
Cholesterol	0 mg
Sodium	2 mg

EXCHANGES PER SERVING

½ Fruit

PIES, TARTS, CRISPS & FRUIT DESSERTS

DIETITIAN'S NOTE *One of the simplest desserts for barbecue night is grilled fruit. Once the main meal has been cooked, clean the grill to remove any residue. Cut fruit into long pieces or chunks and skewer. Grill for a few minutes on each side, just until heated through. Serve drizzled with honey or your favorite dessert sauce over frozen yogurt. Crowd pleasers are pineapple, mango, watermelon, apple and pear.*

WHIPPED CREAM & YOGURT TOPPING

½ cup whipping (35%) cream
1 tbsp granulated sugar
½ tsp vanilla
½ cup low-fat plain yogurt

Beat whipping cream until thick. Add sugar and vanilla; beat until stiff peaks form. Gently fold yogurt until thoroughly combined.

Makes about 1 ½ cups (3 tbsp per serving)

NUTRIENTS PER SERVING

Calories	65
Carbohydrate	3 g
Fiber	0 g
Protein	1 g
Fat, total	5 g
Fat, saturated	3 g
Cholesterol	20 mg
Sodium	16 mg

EXCHANGES PER SERVING

1 Fat
1 Free Food

DIETITIAN'S NOTE *This whipped cream look-alike dresses up fruit and plain cakes.*

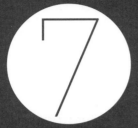

FROZEN, CHILLED & OTHER DESSERTS

255	Honey Vanilla Ice Cream
256	Mocha Ice Cream
257	Frozen Orange Cream
258	Flying Saucers
259	Ice Cream Fantasy Cake
260	Lemon Sherbet
261	Fresh Fruit Sorbet
262	Pineapple Lime Sorbet
263	Strawberry Sorbet
264	Strawberry Orange Buttermilk Sorbet
265	Tulip Cookies with Fruit Sorbet
266	Raspberry Ice with Fresh Strawberries
267	Frozen Lemon Pie
268	Frozen Vanilla Yogurt
269	Quick Chocolate Mousse
270	Frozen Jamoca Mousse
271	Rocky Road Mousse
272	Sunshine Lemon Mousse
274	Banana Strawberry Mousse
275	Mango Raspberry Fool
276	Chocolate Bavarian Pie
278	Raspberry Brownie Parfait
279	Pumpkin Custard
280	Maple Custard with Fresh Fruit
281	Orange Cappuccino Pudding Cake
282	Indian-Style Rice Pudding
283	Apple Oatmeal Pudding
284	Cornmeal Pudding
285	Lemon Blueberry Panna Cotta
286	Orange Sabayon with Fresh Berries
287	Banana Cream Tiramisu
288	Chocolate Coffee Tiramisu
289	Blueberry Flan
290	Maple Flan with Walnuts
291	Pumpkin Flan
292	Chocolate Crêpes
293	Chocolate Sauce

HONEY VANILLA
ICE CREAM

Ice Cream
- 2 cups 2% milk
- 3 tbsp liquid honey
- ⅛ tsp vanilla
- 6 egg yolks

Spiced Apple Mixture
- 3 apples
- 2 cups apple juice
- ¼ tsp ground cinnamon
- ⅛ tsp ground ginger
- ⅛ tsp ground nutmeg
- 2 tbsp cornstarch
- 1 tbsp water

1. *Ice Cream:* In a saucepan bring milk, honey and vanilla to a boil; reduce heat to low. In a bowl, beat egg yolks. Whisk a little of the hot milk into yolk mixture, then pour back into remaining milk. Whisk constantly over low heat until mixture is thick enough to coat a spoon; do not boil. Remove from heat. Chill. In an ice cream maker, freeze according to manufacturer's directions.

2. *Spiced Apple Mixture:* Peel, core and thinly slice the apples. Put in a saucepan along with apple juice, cinnamon, ginger and nutmeg. Bring to a boil, reduce heat and simmer 5 minutes. Dissolve cornstarch in water; stir into simmering apple mixture and cook 1 minute longer or until thickened. Remove from heat. Cool slightly. Serve over ice cream.

Makes 8 servings

DIETITIAN'S NOTE *A serving of the ice cream by itself counts as ½ Other Carbohydrate Exchange plus 1 Fat Exchange. The spiced apples add 1 Fruit Exchange.*

TIP Don't worry if you don't have an ice cream maker. Pour chilled ice cream mixture into a loaf pan lined with plastic wrap and freeze until solid. Break into small pieces; in a food processor, pulse on and off until smooth. Store in freezer until ready to serve.

NUTRIENTS PER SERVING

Calories	162
Carbohydrate	26 g
Fiber	1 g
Protein	4 g
Fat, total	5 g
Fat, saturated	2 g
Cholesterol	147 mg
Sodium	38 mg

EXCHANGES PER SERVING

- 1 Fruit
- ½ Other Carbohydrate
- 1 Fat

MOCHA
ICE CREAM

TIP Omit coffee if desired.

NUTRIENTS PER SERVING

Calories	121
Carbohydrate	22 g
Fiber	1 g
Protein	4 g
Fat, total	3 g
Fat, saturated	1 g
Cholesterol	37 mg
Sodium	51 mg

EXCHANGES PER SERVING

1 Other Carbohydrates
½ Reduced-Fat Milk

2	cups 2% milk
1	egg
½	cup granulated sugar
2	tbsp sifted unsweetened cocoa powder
1	tsp instant coffee granules

1. In a saucepan, heat 1 cup of the milk just until bubbles form around edge of pan.

2. Meanwhile, in a small bowl, beat egg with sugar until combined; stir in half of the warm milk. Pour egg mixture back into saucepan; stir in cocoa and coffee granules. Cook, stirring, on low heat for 4 minutes or until slightly thickened. (Do not let boil or egg will curdle.) Let cool completely.

3. Stir in remaining milk. Pour into ice cream machine and freeze according to manufacturer's instructions. (Or pour into cake pan and freeze until nearly solid. Chop into chunks and beat with electric mixer or process in food processor until smooth. Freeze again until solid.)

Makes 6 servings

FROZEN, CHILLED & OTHER DESSERTS

FROZEN ORANGE CREAM

1   tbsp grated orange zest
1⅓   cups orange juice
⅔   cup skim milk

1. In a food processor or blender, purée orange zest, orange juice and milk.

2. In an ice cream maker, freeze according to manufacturer's directions.

Makes 4 servings

DIETITIAN'S NOTE *We are all familiar with the expression "food for thought." It's equally important to give thought for food—not just to the nutrient values and Exchanges, but also to the experience of eating. Unfortunately, many meals today have become "refueling stops" on the run (both at and away from home), with little time to socialize and even less time to enjoy what we've chosen. Various strategies can help us be more thoughtful about what we eat:*

Plan meals at least a day in advance, and make sure you have all the ingredients you need.

Involve other family members in planning and preparing meals.

When ordering from a menu, ask how foods are prepared, what comes with them and possible substitutions. At a buffet, survey everything before making your choices.

At home, you are able to serve yourself appropriate portions. Restaurant servings are often larger. Do not feel obliged to eat everything on your plate.

TIP If you don't have an ice cream maker, pour into a baking dish and freeze until solid. Break into small pieces; in a food processor, pulse on and off until smooth. Store in freezer until ready to serve.

NUTRIENTS PER SERVING

Calories	52
Carbohydrate	11 g
Fiber	0 g
Protein	2 g
Fat, total	0 g
Fat, saturated	0 g
Cholesterol	1 mg
Sodium	22 mg

EXCHANGES PER SERVING

½ Fruit

FLYING SAUCERS

FROZEN, CHILLED & OTHER DESSERTS

NUTRIENTS PER SERVING

Calories	74
Carbohydrate	12 g
Fiber	0 g
Protein	2 g
Fat, total	2 g
Fat, saturated	1 g
Cholesterol	2 mg
Sodium	108 mg

EXCHANGES PER SERVING

½ Starch
½ Other Carbohydrate

Baking sheet, lined with waxed paper

1	package (1½ oz) fat-free instant chocolate pudding mix, sweetened with aspartame
1½	cups cold 1% milk
1	cup lower-fat non-dairy whipped topping
36	plain chocolate wafers

1. In a medium bowl, add chocolate pudding mix to milk. Beat for 2 minutes, until thickened and smooth. Fold in whipped topping.

2. Arrange 18 chocolate wafers in a single layer on prepared baking sheet. Spoon chocolate pudding mixture onto the wafers. Top with remaining wafers, pressing lightly and smoothing around the edges with a knife, if necessary.

3. Freeze for at least 3 hours, until firm, or in an airtight container for up to 1 month. (If they are too hard to eat, let sit at room temperature for 10 minutes before serving.)

Makes 18 servings

Recipe photo in color insert.

ICE CREAM FANTASY CAKE

9-inch springform pan

15	plain chocolate wafers
2	tbsp melted soft margarine
4	cups vanilla ice milk
	Quick Chocolate Mousse (see recipe, page 269)
4	cups raspberry-flavored frozen yogurt
1	cup lower-fat non-dairy whipped topping
½	cup calorie-reduced chocolate sundae sauce
2	tbsp chopped peanuts
14	strawberries

1. In a food processor, grind chocolate wafers into crumbs (or crush them between two sheets of waxed paper with a rolling pin). Mix chocolate crumbs with margarine and press into bottom of springform pan. Refrigerate to cool for 10 to 15 minutes.

2. Let vanilla ice milk soften slightly at room temperature, just until spreadable. Spoon onto chocolate crumb crust and spread evenly. Freeze for 30 minutes, until solid.

3. Spread chocolate mousse over frozen vanilla ice milk. Freeze for 15 minutes, until firm.

4. Scoop frozen yogurt into round balls and arrange over frozen chocolate mousse, covering it completely.

5. Pipe or spoon whipped topping decoratively around the outside edge. Freeze for at least 2 hours or overnight.

6. To serve: Drizzle cake top with chocolate sauce, sprinkle with peanuts and garnish with whole strawberries. Remove sides of the springform pan, cut cake into 14 wedges and serve.

Makes 14 servings

TIP If cake is too hard to cut, let stand at room temperature for 10 to 15 minutes before serving.

NUTRIENTS PER SERVING

Calories	263
Carbohydrate	41 g
Fiber	0 g
Protein	7 g
Fat, total	9 g
Fat, saturated	4 g
Cholesterol	17 mg
Sodium	194 mg

EXCHANGES PER SERVING

½	Starch
2	Other Carbohydrates
1	High-Fat Meat

LEMON SHERBET

TIPS This is similar to a frozen soufflé but is lighter and lower in calories.

Because of the risk of salmonella poisoning, raw eggs should be used with caution. Cracked eggs should be avoided. Recipes calling for raw eggs should be prepared as close to serving time as possible and kept well refrigerated.

This recipe courtesy of Joan Gallant, Dietitian.

NUTRIENTS PER SERVING

Calories	90
Carbohydrate	17 g
Fiber	0 g
Protein	4 g
Fat, total	1 g
Fat, saturated	0 g
Sodium	47 mg
Cholesterol	55 mg

EXCHANGES PER SERVING

1 Other Carbohydrates
½ Low-Fat Meat

8 small custard cups

½	cup granulated sugar
⅓	cup lemon juice
2	tsp grated lemon zest
2	eggs, separated
⅔	cup skim-milk powder
⅔	cup cold water

1. Whisk together sugar, lemon juice, zest and egg yolks; set aside.

2. With an electric mixer, beat egg whites, skim-milk powder and water on high speed for 3 to 5 minutes or until stiff peaks form. Fold in lemon mixture. Pour into 8 small custard cups; cover and freeze for about 3 hours or until firm. Transfer from freezer to refrigerator about 15 minutes before serving.

Serves 8

FRESH FRUIT SORBET

2 ½ cups chopped peeled soft fresh fruit (bananas, peaches, strawberries, etc.)

1. Spread fruit on baking sheet and freeze.

2. Purée frozen fruit in food processor and serve immediately.

Makes 4 servings

TIPS Try a combination of fresh fruits.

Best if served immediately. If refreezing, purée again before serving.

NUTRIENTS PER SERVING

Calories	52
Carbohydrate	13 g
Fiber	2 g
Protein	1 g
Fat, total	0 g
Fat, saturated	0 g
Cholesterol	0 mg
Sodium	1 mg

EXCHANGES PER SERVING

1 Fruit

DIETITIAN'S NOTE *The first record of sorbet dates from AD 60, when Nero served his guests a sorbet of crushed fruit, honey and snow. Is sherbet the same as sorbet? It depends who you ask. They both contain fruit and sugar. Sherbets usually contain additional ingredients, such as milk or eggs; sorbets generally do not.*

PINEAPPLE LIME SORBET

NUTRIENTS PER SERVING

Calories	60
Carbohydrate	17 g
Fiber	1 g
Protein	1 g
Fat, total	0 g
Fat, saturated	0 g
Cholesterol	0 mg
Sodium	2 mg

EXCHANGES PER SERVING

1 Fruit

1¼ cups pineapple purée
2 tsp grated lime or lemon zest
¾ cup freshly squeezed lime or lemon juice
¼ cup water
    Granulated sugar to taste (optional)
    Thin slices lime or lemon

1. In a bowl, stir together pineapple purée, lime zest and juice, water and, if desired, sugar.

2. In an ice cream maker, freeze according to manufacturer's directions.

3. Divide among 4 individual dessert dishes. Serve garnished with thin slices of lime.

Makes 4 servings

DIETITIAN'S NOTES *To make 1¼ cups puréed pineapple, you will need a fresh pineapple weighing about 1½ lbs. Peel and core it and cut it into chunks, then blend at medium speed until smooth. You can also use pineapple canned in juice. About 1¾ cups drained canned crushed pineapple or pineapple chunks will make 1¼ cups purée.*

Remember that Nutrients per Serving and Exchanges do not include optional ingredients. If you want to add sugar, 1 tbsp of sugar added to this recipe will increase the carbohydrate by 3 grams per serving. (Count as a Free Food or Extra.)

Instead of sugar, you could also use a no-calorie (artificial) sweetener, which would add neither carbohydrate nor calories. One tablespoon of a "measures like sugar" product, or 1½ sachets of a product used to sweeten beverages, is equivalent to 1 tbsp of sugar.

FROZEN, CHILLED & OTHER DESSERTS

STRAWBERRY SORBET

8-inch square pan

1½	cups fresh or frozen unsweetened strawberries
2	cups unsweetened apple juice
¼	cup granulated sugar
¼	tsp ground cinnamon
2	tbsp cold water
4	tsp cornstarch

1. Wash and hull fresh strawberries or thaw frozen strawberries. In a blender or food processor, blend strawberries and apple juice until almost smooth.

2. In a medium saucepan over medium heat, cook strawberry mixture, sugar and cinnamon, stirring frequently, for about 5 minutes or until sugar is dissolved. Combine water and cornstarch; stir into hot mixture. Cook for about 3 minutes or until thickened and clear. Chill for 1 hour. Pour into 8-inch square pan; cover and freeze for about 3 hours or until firm.

3. Break frozen mixture into chunks; beat with electric mixer at medium speed until fluffy. Transfer to an airtight container and freeze until firm. Transfer from freezer to refrigerator about 15 minutes before serving.

Serves 6

TIPS The perfect low-fat ending to any meal, this sorbet can be made with virtually any fruit. Try raspberries, peaches, blueberries, kiwifruit, cantaloupe or any other seasonal fruit.

Beating the sorbet during the freezing process helps to keep it from becoming too solid and helps to reduce the formation of ice crystals.

This recipe courtesy of Vicki McKay, Dietitian.

NUTRIENTS PER SERVING

Calories	91
Carbohydrate	23 g
Fiber	1 g
Protein	0 g
Fat, total	0 g
Fat, saturated	0 g
Sodium	3 mg
Cholesterol	0 mg

EXCHANGES PER SERVING

1	Fruit
⅓	Other Carbohydrate

STRAWBERRY ORANGE BUTTERMILK SORBET

TIPS To make soured milk, place 2 tsp lemon juice or vinegar in measuring cup; pour in milk to 1 cup level and let stand for 10 minutes, then stir.

Although sorbets are best prepared just before eating so they do not crystallize, they can be prepared up to 2 days in advance.

NUTRIENTS PER SERVING

Calories	99
Carbohydrate	23 g
Fiber	1 g
Protein	2 g
Fat, total	1 g
Fat, saturated	0 g
Cholesterol	2 mg
Sodium	66 mg

EXCHANGES PER SERVING

1½ Other Carbohydrates

1	cup buttermilk or soured milk
½	cup puréed strawberries
¼	cup water
¼	cup liquid honey
½	tsp grated orange zest
1	tbsp freshly squeezed orange juice

1. In a bowl, mix together buttermilk, strawberries, water, honey, orange zest and juice.

2. Freeze in ice cream machine according to manufacturer's directions. (Or pour into cake pan and freeze until nearly solid. Chop into chunks and beat with electric mixer or process in food processor until smooth. Freeze again until solid.)

Makes 4 servings

TULIP COOKIES WITH FRUIT SORBET

Preheat oven to 350°F
Baking sheet, sprayed with baking spray

¾	cup buttermilk
1	egg
6	tbsp granulated sugar
⅓	cup whole wheat flour
⅓	cup all-purpose flour
⅛	tsp ground cinnamon
⅛	tsp salt
	Raspberry or mango sorbet
	Fresh raspberries or sliced ripe mango

1. In a bowl, stir together buttermilk, egg, sugar, whole wheat flour, flour, cinnamon and salt until smooth. Let batter rest for 20 minutes.

2. Place 1 tbsp batter at one end of prepared baking sheet. With the back of a spoon, spread to form a circle 5 inches in diameter. Repeat with another 1 tbsp batter on other half of baking sheet. Bake for 9 to 11 minutes or until golden. With a spatula, remove hot cookies from baking sheet and place each over bottom of a glass, pressing gently to create fluted effect. Cool completely on glass.

3. Repeat with remaining batter, re-spraying baking sheet between batches.

4. Serve each tulip cup with a small scoop of sorbet, garnished with fresh fruit.

Makes 20 cookies (1 cookie per serving)

DIETITIAN'S NOTE *The Nutrients per Serving and Exchanges do not include the sorbet or fruit. Count ¼ cup of Raspberry Ice (page 266) or commercial sherbet as an additional ½ Fruit Exchange.*

TIPS To save time, make the tulip cups assembly-line fashion. Use 2 baking sheets; while one tray bakes, spread the batter on the next tray, then put it in the oven just as you remove the last batch.

The cookies must be shaped while they are warm, so work quickly. If cookie cools and is too firm to shape, return to oven for 30 seconds or until softened.

NUTRIENTS PER SERVING

Calories	36
Carbohydrate	7 g
Fiber	0 g
Protein	1 g
Fat, total	0 g
Fat, saturated	0 g
Cholesterol	10 mg
Sodium	27 mg

EXCHANGES PER SERVING

½ Other Carbohydrate

RASPBERRY ICE WITH FRESH STRAWBERRIES

NUTRIENTS PER SERVING

Calories	51
Carbohydrate	12 g
Fiber	5 g
Protein	1 g
Fat, total	1 g
Fat, saturated	0 g
Cholesterol	0 mg
Sodium	0 mg

EXCHANGES PER SERVING

1 Fruit

4½ cups fresh raspberries
Honey to taste
6 tbsp low-fat yogurt (optional)
6 large fresh strawberries
Fresh mint leaves

1. In a blender or food processor, purée raspberries. Strain to remove seeds. Stir in honey to taste. In an ice cream maker, freeze according to manufacturer's directions.

2. Divide among 6 individual dessert dishes. Spoon 1 tbsp yogurt on top of each serving, if desired. Garnish each serving with a strawberry and mint leaves.

Makes 6 servings

DIETITIAN'S NOTES *If you add honey to this recipe, remember that 1 tbsp will contribute 17 grams of carbohydrate, equivalent to 1 Free Food or Extra per serving. A single tablespoon of low-fat yogurt per serving supplies negligible carbohydrate and fat.*

For help in planning your meals, ask your doctor to refer you to a diabetes education center or a dietitian. Local hospitals may also have referral services. On the Internet, look for the "Find a Nutrition Professional" feature at www.eatright.org.

FROZEN LEMON PIE

9-inch pie plate

1   can (6 oz) frozen lemonade concentrate
3   cups vanilla-flavored frozen yogurt
1   cup lower-fat sour cream
1   cup frozen lower-fat non-dairy whipped topping, divided
    Fresh lemon slices, for garnish

Graham Wafer Crust
¾   cup graham wafer crumbs
3   tbsp melted soft margarine
¼   tsp ground cinnamon
¼   tsp ground nutmeg

1. Thaw the lemonade concentrate slightly. Put semi-frozen concentrate in a large bowl and beat for 30 seconds. Gradually stir in frozen yogurt. Fold in sour cream and ½ cup of the whipped topping and stir until blended and smooth. Freeze until the mixture will mound on a spoon, about 30 minutes.

2. *Graham Wafer Crust:* In a small bowl, combine graham wafer crumbs, margarine, cinnamon and nutmeg. Press into pie plate.

3. Spoon lemonade mixture into prepared piecrust and freeze for at least 4 hours, until firm, or overnight.

4. Cut pie into 8 servings, and garnish each with 1 tbsp whipped topping and lemon slices.

Makes 8 servings

NUTRIENTS PER SERVING

Calories	265
Carbohydrate	38 g
Fiber	0 g
Protein	5 g
Fat, total	11 g
Fat, saturated	4 g
Cholesterol	10 mg
Sodium	152 mg

EXCHANGES PER SERVING

½	Starch
2	Other Carbohydrates
1	Medium-Fat Meat
1½	Fat

FROZEN VANILLA YOGURT

TIPS Add 1 tsp each lemon extract and grated lemon zest to make lemon yogurt.

This dessert can be prepared up to 2 days in advance, but it is best if served right after freezing.

NUTRIENTS PER SERVING

Calories	114
Carbohydrate	17 g
Fiber	0 g
Protein	5 g
Fat, total	3 g
Fat, saturated	2 g
Sodium	60 mg
Cholesterol	43 mg

EXCHANGES PER SERVING

½ Low-Fat Milk
⅔ Other Carbohydrate

1	egg
⅓	cup brown sugar
½	cup 2% milk
1½	cups 2% yogurt
1½	tsp vanilla

1. In bowl, beat egg with sugar until combined; set aside. In saucepan, heat milk just until bubbles appear around side of pan. Stir a little into egg mixture, then pour back into saucepan. Cook over low heat, stirring, just until thickened, 2 to 4 minutes. (Do not let boil or egg will curdle.) Remove from heat and let cool completely.

2. Beat yogurt and vanilla into cooled mixture. Freeze in ice cream machine according to manufacturer's directions. (Or pour into cake pan and freeze until nearly solid. Chop into chunks and beat with electric mixer or process in food processor until smooth. Freeze again until solid.)

Serves 4 to 6

QUICK CHOCOLATE MOUSSE

1   package (1½ oz) fat-free instant chocolate pudding mix, sweetened with aspartame

1½   cups cold 1% milk

2   cups lower-fat non-dairy whipped topping

In a medium bowl, add chocolate pudding mix to milk. Beat for 1 minute, then fold in whipped topping. Let stand for 5 minutes to set; serve immediately or cover with waxed paper and refrigerate overnight.

Makes 6 servings

NUTRIENTS PER SERVING

Calories	84
Carbohydrate	14 g
Fiber	0 g
Protein	3 g
Fat, total	2 g
Fat, saturated	1 g
Cholesterol	9 mg
Sodium	124 mg

EXCHANGES PER SERVING

1½ Low-Fat Milk

½ Other Carbohydrate

FROZEN JAMOCA MOUSSE

TIPS Buy extra-smooth ricotta for the smoothest mousse.

If you don't have an ice cream maker, pour into a baking dish and freeze until solid. Break into small pieces; in a food processor, pulse on and off until smooth. Store in freezer until ready to serve.

1	cup 5% ricotta cheese
2	cups low-fat yogurt
½	cup fructose
4	tsp unsweetened cocoa powder
2	tsp instant coffee granules
1	tsp vanilla

1. In a food processor or blender, purée ricotta, yogurt, fructose, cocoa, coffee granules and vanilla until smooth.

2. In an ice cream maker, freeze according to manufacturer's directions.

Makes 10 servings

NUTRIENTS PER SERVING

Calories	98
Carbohydrate	14 g
Fiber	0 g
Protein	6 g
Fat, total	2 g
Fat, saturated	1 g
Cholesterol	7 mg
Sodium	66 mg

EXCHANGES PER SERVING

1 Other Carbohydrates
½ Lean Meat

DIETITIAN'S NOTE *Fructose is a sugar that occurs naturally in small amounts in many foods. It can also be refined into a pure form. Gram for gram, it is sweeter than ordinary sugar (sucrose), but it does not raise blood sugar as much. It is not, however, a sugar substitute or Free Food/Extra. As with ordinary sugar, 1 tbsp counts as an Other Carbohydrate Exchange. Look for it in specialty grocery stores and some health food stores.*

ROCKY ROAD MOUSSE

1	package (1½ oz) fat-free instant chocolate pudding mix, sweetened with aspartame
1½	cups cold 1% milk
1	cup lower-fat non-dairy whipped topping
½	cup plain yogurt
6	lower-fat graham wafers
1	cup miniature marshmallows
½	cup Chocolate Sauce (see recipe, page 293)

1. In a medium bowl, add chocolate pudding mix to milk. Beat for 1 minute, then fold in whipped topping and yogurt. Divide among 6 dessert dishes or parfait glasses. Let stand for 5 minutes until set, or cover and refrigerate for up to 4 hours.

2. Just before serving, break graham wafers into small pieces and sprinkle one wafer on each mousse. Top with mini marshmallows and drizzle with chocolate sauce.

Makes 6 servings

NUTRIENTS PER SERVING

Calories	130
Carbohydrate	24 g
Fiber	0 g
Protein	4 g
Fat, total	2 g
Fat, saturated	1 g
Cholesterol	6 mg
Sodium	176 mg

EXCHANGES PER SERVING

½ Starch
1 Other Carbohydrates
½ Medium-Fat Meat

SUNSHINE LEMON MOUSSE

TIP This recipe contains raw eggs. If the food safety of raw eggs is a concern for you, use pasteurized eggs. Many grocery stores now carry pasteurized eggs in their shells.

Stand mixer

1	envelope (¼ oz) unflavored gelatin
¼	cup cold water
3	egg yolks
¾	cup granulated sugar, divided
2	tsp grated lemon zest
⅓	cup freshly squeezed lemon juice
1	cup cold whipping (35%) cream
3	egg whites, at room temperature

Topping

½	cup cold whipping (35%) cream
1	tsp confectioner's sugar, sifted
1	lemon, cut lengthwise into halves and thinly sliced (optional)

1. In a small microwave-safe bowl, sprinkle gelatin over water and let soften for 5 minutes. Microwave on High for 10 seconds. Stir, then heat for 5 seconds. The gelatin should be melted. If it isn't, heat for 5 seconds more. Stir again and set aside.

2. Place egg yolks and ½ cup of the sugar in the mixer bowl. Attach the whip and mixer bowl to the mixer. Set to Speed 6 and beat until thick and pale yellow. Reduce speed to Stir and mix in dissolved gelatin and lemon zest and juice until incorporated. Transfer to a large bowl. Clean the mixer bowl and whip.

3. Place whipping cream in the mixer bowl. Attach the whip and mixer bowl to the mixer. Set to Speed 8 and beat until firm. Using a large rubber spatula, gently fold into the yolk mixture. Clean the mixer bowl and whip.

4. Place egg whites in the mixer bowl. Attach the whip and mixer bowl to the mixer. Set to Speed 4 and beat until foamy. Increase to Speed 8 and beat until soft peaks form. Beat in the remaining ¼ cup sugar, in 2 additions, and beat until stiff, glossy peaks form. Using a large rubber spatula, gently fold into yolk mixture until no trace of white remains.

5. Spoon mousse into 10 dessert dishes. Cover tightly and refrigerate for at least 3 hours or overnight.

6. *Topping:* Place whipping cream in a clean mixer bowl. Attach the whip and mixer bowl to the mixer. Set to Speed 8 and beat until it starts to thicken, then sprinkle with confectioner's sugar and beat until firm. Top each serving with a dollop of cream and a lemon slice, if using.

Makes 10 servings

DIETITIAN'S NOTES *If you don't have a microwave, in Step 1 pour ¼ cup boiling (not cold) water into a measuring cup. Sprinkle gelatin on top and stir. If the gelatin is not completely dissolved after 2 minutes, set the measuring cup in a saucepan of warm water over low heat until the remaining gelatin particles dissolve.*

By skipping the topping, you can reduce the Fat Exchanges from 3 to 2. This dessert may then fit more easily into your meal plan.

As you prepare the recipes in this book, you will become familiar with the appropriate portion sizes for different types of desserts and the approximate Exchanges assigned to them. Use this knowledge to help you choose wisely when you're eating away from home.

NUTRIENTS PER SERVING

Calories	203
Carbohydrate	17 g
Fiber	0 g
Protein	3 g
Fat, total	14 g
Fat, saturated	8 g
Cholesterol	103 mg
Sodium	33 mg

EXCHANGES PER SERVING

1 Other Carbohydrates
3 Fat

BANANA STRAWBERRY MOUSSE

TIP For attractive orange segments, peel a whole orange with a sharp knife, removing zest, pith and membrane; cut on both sides of dividing membranes to release segments.

NUTRIENTS PER SERVING

Calories	60
Carbohydrate	14 g
Fiber	1 g
Protein	2 g
Fat, total	0 g
Fat, saturated	0 g
Cholesterol	0 mg
Sodium	3 mg

EXCHANGES PER SERVING

1 Fruit

3	small ripe bananas
1	cup orange juice
1	cup strawberries
6	tbsp lemon juice
½	cup cold water
1	package (1 tbsp) gelatin
	Orange segments or sliced strawberries

1. In a blender, combine bananas, orange juice, strawberries and lemon juice; purée until smooth. Put water in a small saucepan; sprinkle with gelatin. Let stand for 1 minute. Heat gently, stirring until gelatin dissolves. With motor running, pour hot gelatin through blender feed tube; purée until smooth. Divide among 8 individual dessert dishes or champagne coupes.

2. Chill for 2 hours. Serve garnished with orange segments or sliced strawberries.

Makes 8 servings

DIETITIAN'S NOTE *Many garnishes are a feast for the eyes without adding significant carbohydrate. Count 2 orange segments or 4 strawberries as a Free Food or Extra. For most fruits, ¼ cup sliced also counts as a Free Food or Extra.*

MANGO RASPBERRY FOOL

Stand mixer

4	mangos, peeled and chopped
⅔	cup granulated sugar
¼	cup freshly squeezed lime juice
1	tsp unflavored gelatin
1	tbsp cold water
1½	cups cold whipping (35%) cream
¼	cup light rum (optional)
1½	cups fresh raspberries
	Additional fresh raspberries

1. Attach the fruit/vegetable strainer to the mixer. Set to Speed 4 and run mangoes through the strainer into a large bowl, with another bowl to catch the solids. Discard solids. You should have about 2 cups purée. Stir in sugar and lime juice.

2. In a small microwave-safe bowl, sprinkle gelatin over water and let soften for 5 minutes. Microwave on High for 10 seconds. Stir, then heat for 5 seconds. The gelatin should be melted. If it isn't, heat for 5 seconds more. Stir again and add to mango purée.

3. Place whipping cream in the mixer bowl. Attach the whip and mixer bowl to the mixer. Set to Speed 8 and beat until firm. Reduce speed to Stir and mix in rum, if using. Using a large rubber spatula, thoroughly fold in mango purée. Fold in raspberries and spoon into 10 serving dishes. Cover and refrigerate for at least 3 hours or overnight. Serve cold, garnished with raspberries.

Makes 10 servings

DIETITIAN'S NOTES *If your mixer doesn't have a fruit/vegetable strainer attachment, process the chopped mango in a blender or food processor until smooth and then strain, reserving juice and discarding solids.*

One-quarter cup rum spikes the flavor but, divided among 10 servings, adds negligible alcohol.

TIP Store, wrapped in plastic wrap, in the refrigerator for up to 2 days.

NUTRIENTS PER SERVING

Calories	218
Carbohydrate	27 g
Fiber	2 g
Protein	1 g
Fat, total	13 g
Fat, saturated	8 g
Cholesterol	46 mg
Sodium	15 mg

EXCHANGES PER SERVING

1	Fruit
1	Other Carbohydrates
2½	Fat

CHOCOLATE BAVARIAN PIE

TIP You can use a store-bought pie shell for this recipe, or you can make your own: In a small bowl, combine 1½ cups chocolate cookie crumbs with 2 tbsp confectioner's sugar, sifted, and 6 tbsp melted unsalted butter or margarine. Stir until completely mixed. Distribute evenly in a 9-inch pie plate, pressing firmly against the sides and bottom. Bake at 350°F for 10 minutes, until firm. Let cool before filling.

Double boiler

1½	cups 1% milk, divided
1	envelope (¼ oz) unflavored gelatin
⅔	cup granulated sugar
¼	cup unsweetened cocoa powder, sifted
½	tsp vanilla
½	cup plain yogurt
	Chocolate cookie crumb pie shell (see Tip)

Strawberry Whipped Topping

½	cup sliced strawberries, fresh or frozen
1	cup lower-fat non-dairy whipped topping

1. Pour 1 cup milk into the top of a double boiler and sprinkle with gelatin; let stand for 2 minutes.

2. In a small bowl, combine granulated sugar and cocoa; whisk into the milk and gelatin mixture. Cook over lightly boiling water, whisking constantly, until thick and smooth, about 10 minutes. Continue to cook, stirring, for 1 minute longer. Remove from heat and stir in the remaining ½ cup milk and vanilla. Let cool to room temperature.

3. Stir in yogurt, cover and refrigerate until mixture begins to set, about 30 minutes.

4. Spoon into chocolate cookie crumb pie shell; chill for at least 4 hours, until set, or overnight.

5. *Strawberry Whipped Topping:* If frozen, thaw and drain the berries well; if fresh, wash and pat them dry. In a food processor, purée the berries. Fold into whipped topping. Dollop onto the chilled pie.

Makes 8 servings

NUTRIENTS PER SERVING

Calories	260
Carbohydrate	40 g
Fiber	1 g
Protein	5 g
Fat, total	10 g
Fat, saturated	3 g
Cholesterol	5 mg
Sodium	219 mg

EXCHANGES PER SERVING

1	Starch
1½	Other Carbohydrates
2	Fat

277

RASPBERRY BROWNIE PARFAIT

NUTRIENTS PER SERVING

Calories	320
Carbohydrate	47 g
Fiber	2 g
Protein	8 g
Fat, total	13 g
Fat, saturated	5 g
Cholesterol	53 mg
Sodium	208 mg

EXCHANGES PER SERVING

½	Starch
2½	Other Carbohydrates
1	Medium-Fat Meat
1½	Fat

6	Chocolate Brownies (see recipe, page 151)
2	cups raspberry-flavored frozen yogurt
½	cup fresh raspberries
¼	cup lower-fat non-dairy whipped topping

1. Cut each brownie into small pieces.

2. In each of 4 dessert dishes or parfait glasses, layer ¼ cup frozen yogurt, ⅛ of the brownie pieces and 1 tbsp fresh raspberries. Repeat layers.

3. Top each parfait with 1 tbsp whipped topping and a "pretty" raspberry.

Makes 4 servings

Recipe photo in color insert.

DIETITIAN'S NOTE *To lower the carbohydrate/sugar and fat content, you can choose a lower-fat frozen yogurt sweetened with artificial sweetener.*

PUMPKIN CUSTARD

Preheat oven to 325°F
4 large or 6 small custard cups

1	cup 2% evaporated milk
1	cup pumpkin purée (not pie filling, if using canned)
2	tbsp granulated sugar
1	egg
¼	tsp ground nutmeg
¼	tsp ground ginger

In a blender or food processor, combine milk, pumpkin, sugar, egg and spices. Process until well blended; pour into 4 large or 6 small custard cups. Bake in preheated oven for about 30 minutes or until knife inserted in center comes out clean. Serve warm or cold.

Serves 6

TIPS Most baked custards have 2 or more eggs. This custard uses 2% evaporated milk and 1 egg to create a slightly softer version.

This is a superb way to use up all the pumpkin you scooped out when making the jack-o'-lantern for Halloween. The custard is rich in vitamin A and calcium and makes a good finish for a lighter meal.

This recipe courtesy of Cynthia Chace, Dietitian.

NUTRIENTS PER SERVING

Calories	82
Carbohydrate	12 g
Fiber	1 g
Protein	5 g
Fat, total	2 g
Fat, saturated	1 g
Sodium	56 mg
Cholesterol	39 mg

EXCHANGES PER SERVING

⅓ Fruit
½ Low-Fat Milk

MAPLE CUSTARD WITH FRESH FRUIT

TIP Any kind of fresh, frozen or drained canned fruit can be used. Try sliced strawberries, raspberries, blueberries, peaches or plums, or a combination of several seasonal fresh fruits.

NUTRIENTS PER SERVING

Calories	165
Carbohydrate	30 g
Fiber	1 g
Protein	4 g
Fat, total	3 g
Fat, saturated	1 g
Sodium	45 mg
Cholesterol	98 mg

EXCHANGES PER SERVING

½ Fruit
1½ Other Carbohydrates
1 Fat

2	egg yolks
1⅓	cups milk
⅓	cup pure maple syrup
2	tbsp cornstarch
2	peaches, pears or bananas, peeled and sliced

1. In a small saucepan, whisk together egg yolks, milk, maple syrup and cornstarch until smooth. Cook over medium-low heat, whisking constantly, for 2 to 4 minutes or until boiling and thickened.

2. Arrange fruit in 4 individual serving dishes; pour hot custard over. Cover and refrigerate for 1 hour or until cool.

Serves 4

ORANGE CAPPUCCINO PUDDING CAKE

Preheat oven to 350°F
8-inch square baking dish, sprayed with vegetable spray

1	cup all-purpose flour
1	cup packed brown sugar
2	tsp baking powder
2	tsp grated orange zest
½	cup orange juice
2	tbsp vegetable oil
1	egg
2	tsp vanilla
¼	cup semisweet chocolate chips
⅓	cup granulated sugar
¼	cup instant coffee mix powder or hot chocolate mix
¼	cup unsweetened cocoa powder

1. In a bowl, stir together flour, brown sugar and baking powder. In a separate bowl, whisk together orange zest, orange juice, oil, egg and vanilla. Add the wet ingredients to the dry, blending just until mixed. Batter will be thick. Pour into prepared pan. Sprinkle chocolate chips over top.

2. In a bowl, whisk together 1¼ cups hot water, sugar, coffee mix and cocoa. Pour carefully over cake batter. Bake 35 minutes or until cake springs back when touched lightly in center. Serve warm; spoon cake and underlying sauce into individual dessert dishes.

Makes 10 servings

TIPS Use a flavored coffee mix powder, like Irish cream or vanilla, or a cappuccino mix.

Pudding cakes are fantastic because they give you the added bonus of a low-fat sauce.

Best served right out of the oven, but can be reheated in microwave for similar texture.

FROZEN, CHILLED & OTHER DESSERTS

NUTRIENTS PER SERVING

Calories	241
Carbohydrate	47 g
Fiber	1 g
Protein	3 g
Fat, total	6 g
Fat, saturated	1 g
Cholesterol	19 mg
Sodium	101 mg

EXCHANGES PER SERVING

½	Starch
2½	Other Carbohydrates
1	Fat

INDIAN-STYLE RICE PUDDING

TIPS For 1 cup cooked brown rice, cook ⅓ cup rice with ⅔ cup water.

Freshly grated nutmeg has more aroma and flavor than ground. If you only have ground, it is fine to use it, but try grinding fresh sometime—you will really taste and smell the difference.

NUTRIENTS PER SERVING

Calories	148
Carbohydrate	22 g
Fiber	1 g
Protein	5 g
Fat, total	6 g
Fat, saturated	4 g
Cholesterol	3 mg
Sodium	45 mg

EXCHANGES PER SERVING

½ Starch
½ Other Carbohydrate
½ Reduced-Fat Milk
½ Fat

Preheat oven to 350°F
Glass baking dish with cover
Baking sheet

1	cup cooked brown rice
1	can (14 oz) light coconut milk
3	cups milk
½	cup raisins
¼	cup finely chopped almonds
¼	cup unsweetened shredded coconut
¼	cup granulated sugar
½	tsp ground cardamom
1	cinnamon stick
½	tsp grated nutmeg (see Tips)

1. Place rice in baking dish. Add coconut milk, milk, raisins, almonds, coconut, sugar, cardamom and cinnamon stick. Cover, place dish on baking sheet and bake in preheated oven for 1 hour or until sauce has thickened.

2. Serve warm or chilled, sprinkled with nutmeg.

Makes 10 servings

DIETITIAN'S NOTE *Coconut milk contains coconut oil, which is high in saturated fat. Always use the light version, and only as much as you really need.*

APPLE OATMEAL PUDDING

Small (3½ quart) slow cooker
Greased slow cooker stoneware

2	tbsp melted butter or extra virgin olive oil
1	cup rolled oats (not quick-cooking)
⅓	cup demerara sugar
½	cup all-purpose flour
1	tsp baking soda
2	eggs, beaten
1	cup rice milk
6	apples, peeled, cored and thinly sliced
1	tbsp freshly squeezed lemon juice
1	tsp ground cinnamon
1	tbsp packed brown sugar

1. In a bowl, mix together butter, oats and sugar. Stir in flour and baking soda. Gradually add eggs and rice milk, mixing until blended. Spoon into prepared slow cooker stoneware.

2. In a separate bowl, combine apples, lemon juice, cinnamon and brown sugar. Spread evenly over oatmeal mixture. Cover and cook on High for 3½ to 4 hours, until apples are tender.

Makes 10 servings

TIP Oats, in the form of oatmeal, are the most popular whole grain in North America, largely because, unlike other whole grains, they do not need to be refined to enjoy a relatively long shelf life. Oats contain a natural chemical that acts as a preservative, which means that normal processing consists of hulling and roasting, which leaves the bran and germ intact.

NUTRIENTS PER SERVING

Calories	177
Carbohydrate	32 g
Fiber	3 g
Protein	3 g
Fat, total	4 g
Fat, saturated	2 g
Cholesterol	43 mg
Sodium	102 mg

EXCHANGES PER SERVING

2	Starch
1	Fruit
½	Fat

CORNMEAL PUDDING

TIP The nutrient analysis for this recipe was done using 2% milk. If you are concerned about your fat intake, use skim milk instead.

NUTRIENTS PER SERVING

Calories	181
Carbohydrate	27 g
Fiber	1 g
Protein	6 g
Fat, total	6 g
Fat, saturated	2 g
Cholesterol	56 mg
Sodium	227 mg

EXCHANGES PER SERVING

1 Starch

1 Other Carbohydrates

1 Fat

Small (3½ quart) slow cooker
Greased slow cooker stoneware

4	cups 2% milk (see Tip)
½	cup yellow cornmeal, preferably stone-ground
2	eggs, beaten
1	tbsp extra virgin olive oil
½	cup fancy molasses
½	tsp ground ginger
½	tsp ground cinnamon
½	tsp freshly grated nutmeg
½	tsp salt
	Fresh berries, optional
	Vanilla ice cream, optional
	Whipped cream, optional

1. In a saucepan, heat milk over medium-high heat, stirring often to prevent scorching, until boiling. Gradually whisk in cornmeal in a steady stream. Cook, stirring, until mixture begins to thicken and bubbles like lava, about 5 minutes. Remove from heat.

2. In a small bowl, combine beaten eggs with about ½ cup of the hot cornmeal, beating until combined. Gradually return to pot, mixing well. Stir in olive oil, molasses, ginger, cinnamon, nutmeg and salt. Transfer to prepared slow cooker stoneware.

3. Cover and cook on High for 3 hours, until set. Spoon into individual serving bowls and top with fresh berries, vanilla ice cream or a dollop of whipped cream, if using.

Makes 8 servings

LEMON BLUEBERRY PANNA COTTA

Ten ¾-cup custard cups or ramekins, sprayed with vegetable spray

1	cup milk
1½	tbsp unflavored gelatin
¾	cup granulated sugar
3	cups evaporated milk
1	tsp grated lemon zest
2	cups fresh blueberries, divided

1. Pour milk into a small saucepan and sprinkle with gelatin; let stand for 10 minutes. Cook over medium-low heat, stirring constantly with a whisk, until gelatin dissolves, about 2 minutes. Increase heat to medium and add sugar. Continue whisking until sugar dissolves, about 2 minutes. Remove from heat. Stir in evaporated milk and lemon zest, stirring well to combine.

2. Divide mixture evenly among prepared custard cups and add 2 tbsp blueberries to each cup. Cover and refrigerate for at least 4 hours or overnight.

3. To serve, slide a knife around the edge of each cup to loosen the panna cotta. Invert onto a dessert plate and spoon 2 tbsp blueberries onto the side of each plate.

Makes 10 servings

VARIATION Vary the berries and the flavoring for a different taste: raspberries with grated orange zest; sliced strawberries with a splash of vanilla; diced mango with grated ginger. Ask your family to choose their favorites.

NUTRIENTS PER SERVING

Calories	158
Carbohydrate	29 g
Fiber	1 g
Protein	8 g
Fat, total	2 g
Fat, saturated	1 g
Cholesterol	7 mg
Sodium	100 mg

EXCHANGES PER SERVING

1 Other Carbohydrates
1 Fat-Free/1% Milk

ORANGE SABAYON WITH FRESH BERRIES

FROZEN, CHILLED & OTHER DESSERTS

TIP Use an instant-read thermometer to check the temperature of the egg yolk mixture. Food that contains eggs should be heated to at least 160°F to ensure that any salmonella bacteria present in the eggs are destroyed.

NUTRIENTS PER SERVING

Calories	113
Carbohydrate	19 g
Fiber	4 g
Protein	3 g
Fat, total	4 g
Fat, saturated	1 g
Cholesterol	126 mg
Sodium	6 mg

EXCHANGES PER SERVING

½ Fruit

½ Other Carbohydrate

1 Fat

Stand mixer

4	egg yolks
3	tbsp granulated sugar
	Grated zest of 1 orange
⅓	cup freshly squeezed orange juice
4	cups berries, such as blueberries, strawberries, blackberries or raspberries

1. In the mixer bowl, whisk together egg yolks, sugar, and orange zest and juice. Set over a saucepan of simmering water, making sure the bottom of the bowl doesn't touch the water. Cook, whisking constantly, until mixture reaches 160°F. Continue to cook until thick and doubled in volume, about 5 minutes. Do not overheat or the egg yolks will scramble.

2. Attach the whip and mixer bowl to the mixer. Set to Speed 6 and beat until sabayon reaches room temperature, about 5 minutes. Spoon into 6 serving bowls, garnish with berries and serve.

Makes 6 servings

BANANA CREAM TIRAMISU

9- by 5-inch loaf pan, lined with waxed paper

12	giant ladyfinger biscuits (about 5 oz)
3	tbsp pure maple syrup, divided
1	cup lower-fat non-dairy whipped topping
1	cup prepared fat-free chocolate pudding, made with 1% milk
1	large banana
¼	cup chopped walnuts

1. Arrange 6 ladyfingers in a single layer across the bottom of prepared loaf pan. Drizzle evenly with 2 tbsp of the maple syrup.

2. In a medium bowl, fold whipped topping into chocolate pudding.

3. Slice ⅔ banana and arrange in single layer over the ladyfingers. Spoon ½ of the pudding mixture over the banana slices and spread evenly. Wrap the remaining banana and set aside.

4. Arrange the remaining 6 ladyfingers in single layer over the pudding and drizzle the remaining 1 tbsp maple syrup over the ladyfingers. Dollop (or pipe) the rest of the pudding mixture onto the ladyfingers. Cover and refrigerate for at least 1 hour or for up to 1 day.

5. Just before serving, slice the remaining banana and arrange decoratively down the center of the tiramisu. Sprinkle with chopped walnuts.

Makes 8 servings

VARIATION: MAPLE WALNUT & PEAR TIRAMISU: Substitute vanilla pudding for the chocolate pudding and a 14-oz can of pear halves (packed in pear juice) for the bananas. Add ¼ cup chopped walnuts to the middle layer. Do not put pears in the middle layer, but add ¼ cup pear juice to the pudding mixture. Garnish the top of the tiramisu with the pear halves down the middle.

NUTRIENTS PER SERVING

Calories	150
Carbohydrate	24 g
Fiber	1 g
Protein	4 g
Fat, total	5 g
Fat, saturated	1 g
Cholesterol	64 mg
Sodium	48 mg

EXCHANGES PER SERVING

1	Starch
½	Other Carbohydrate
1	Fat

CHOCOLATE COFFEE TIRAMISU

TIPS Sift some cocoa on top of each just before serving. This tastes so decadent, you'll never believe it hasn't the same calories and fat as one made with mascarpone.

Spongy or harder ladyfingers can be used.

The longer this chills, the better it is. The liqueur-coffee mixture penetrates the cookies.

Prepare up to 2 days ahead. It tastes best after 8 hours of refrigeration.

NUTRIENTS PER SERVING

Calories	150
Carbohydrate	21 g
Fiber	0 g
Protein	6 g
Fat, total	5 g
Fat, saturated	2 g
Sodium	102 mg
Cholesterol	66 mg

EXCHANGES PER SERVING

½ Starch
1 Other Carbohydrates
½ Lean Meat
½ Fat

9-inch square baking dish sprayed with vegetable spray

1½	cups 5% ricotta cheese
½	cup light cream cheese
½	cup granulated sugar
3	tbsp cocoa
1	egg yolk
1	tsp vanilla
3	egg whites
⅓	cup granulated sugar
¾	cup strong, prepared coffee
3	tbsp chocolate or coffee-flavored liqueur
16	ladyfinger cookies

1. In food processor, combine ricotta cheese, cream cheese, sugar, cocoa, egg yolk and vanilla until smooth; transfer to a bowl.

2. In bowl, beat egg whites until soft peaks form. Gradually add sugar and continue to beat until stiff peaks form. Gently fold the egg whites into the ricotta mixture.

3. Combine coffee and liqueur in a small bowl.

4. Put half of ladyfingers in bottom of dish. Sprinkle with half of coffee-liqueur mixture. Spread half of ricotta mixture on top. Repeat layers. Cover and chill for at least 3 hours, or overnight.

Serves 16

Recipe photo in color insert.

BLUEBERRY FLAN

Preheat oven to 425°F
9-inch flan pan with removable bottom

1½	cups all-purpose flour
¼	cup granulated sugar
1½	tsp baking powder
¼	cup soft margarine
2	egg whites
¼	tsp almond extract

Filling

3	cups fresh blueberries
⅓	cup granulated sugar
1	tbsp all-purpose flour
1	tbsp lemon juice
2	tsp ground cinnamon

1. In a bowl, combine flour, sugar and baking powder; stir in margarine, egg whites and almond extract to form dough. Press into 9-inch flan pan with removable bottom. Freeze for 15 minutes.

2. *Filling:* In a bowl, mix together blueberries, sugar, flour, lemon juice and cinnamon; pour over crust. Bake in preheated oven for 15 minutes. Reduce temperature to 350°F ; bake for 20 to 25 minutes longer. Cool on rack. Refrigerate for at least 1 hour before serving.

Serves 8

TIPS Try this recipe using wild or low-bush blueberries when they are in season. They have a delicious and more intense flavor than the cultivated variety.

Blueberries are gaining in popularity because of their antioxidant properties. This delicious flan contains a minimal amount of fat.

This recipe courtesy of dietitians Pamela Good and Carrie Roach.

NUTRIENTS PER SERVING

Calories	234
Carbohydrate	42 g
Fiber	2 g
Protein	4 g
Fat, total	6 g
Fat, saturated	1 g
Sodium	135 mg
Cholesterol	0 mg

EXCHANGES PER SERVING

1½	Starch
⅓	Fruit
1	Other Carbohydrates
1	Fat

MAPLE FLAN WITH WALNUTS

TIP For extra maple flavor, omit the vanilla and use 2 tsp maple extract.

NUTRIENTS PER SERVING

Calories	74
Carbohydrate	9 g
Fiber	0 g
Protein	4 g
Fat, total	2 g
Fat, saturated	1 g
Cholesterol	36 mg
Sodium	60 mg

EXCHANGES PER SERVING

½ Other Carbohydrate
½ Fat

Preheat oven to 325°F
4-cup soufflé or casserole dish

2	egg whites
1	egg
2½	tbsp maple syrup
1	tsp vanilla
1	tsp maple extract
1½	cups 2% milk
	Toasted chopped walnuts (optional)
	Cinnamon Cream (optional) (see recipe, opposite)

1. In a bowl, whisk together egg whites, whole egg, maple syrup, vanilla and maple extract until smooth. Gradually add milk, whisking constantly. Pour into soufflé dish.

2. Set dish in larger pan; pour in enough hot water to come halfway up sides. Bake for 60 minutes or until set. Remove from water bath; cool on wire rack. Chill.

3. Serve with toasted chopped walnuts and/or Cinnamon Cream, if desired.

Makes 6 servings

DIETITIAN'S NOTE *Remember that garnishes are not included in Nutrients per Serving or Exchanges, so be mindful of what they will add.*

A garnish of ¼ cup chopped toasted walnuts will add an extra ½ Fat Exchange per serving.

If you use the Cinnamon Cream topping, count one-sixth of the recipe as a Free Food or Extra, plus ½ Fat Exchange.

PUMPKIN FLAN

Preheat oven to 325°F
4-cup soufflé or casserole dish

¾	cup canned pumpkin
2½	tbsp fructose
2	egg whites
1	egg
½	tsp almond extract
½	tsp vanilla
¼	tsp ground cinnamon
⅛	tsp ground cloves
1	cup 2% milk

Cinnamon Cream

1	cup 5% ricotta cheese
4	tsp maple syrup or liquid honey
¾	tsp ground cinnamon

1. In a bowl, beat pumpkin, fructose, egg whites, whole egg, almond extract, vanilla, cinnamon and cloves until smooth. In a saucepan, heat milk until almost boiling; remove from heat. Whisk hot milk into pumpkin mixture. Pour into dish.

2. Set dish in larger pan; pour in enough hot water to come halfway up sides. Bake for 40 minutes or until set. Remove from water bath; cool on wire rack. Chill.

3. *Cinnamon Cream:* In a food processor, purée ricotta, maple syrup and cinnamon until smooth. Serve with flan.

Makes 6 servings

DIETITIAN'S NOTES *Be sure to use pure canned pumpkin, not pumpkin pie filling, in this recipe.*

You will find fructose in specialty grocery stores and some health food stores.

TIP For individual servings, use six ¾-cup custard cups or ramekins and bake for 20 minutes.

NUTRIENTS PER SERVING

Calories	128
Carbohydrate	14 g
Fiber	1 g
Protein	9 g
Fat, total	4 g
Fat, saturated	2 g
Cholesterol	40 mg
Sodium	103 mg

EXCHANGES PER SERVING

½	Vegetable
½	Other Carbohydrate
1	Lean Meat

CHOCOLATE CRÊPES

TIP You can make the crêpes the day before; wrap them in plastic wrap and refrigerate until ready to use.

NUTRIENTS PER SERVING

Calories	99
Carbohydrate	15 g
Fiber	1 g
Protein	3 g
Fat, total	3 g
Fat, saturated	1 g
Cholesterol	26 mg
Sodium	24 mg

EXCHANGES PER SERVING

½ Starch

½ Other Carbohydrate

½ Fat

Sixteen 6-inch squares of parchment or waxed paper

1½	cups all-purpose flour
½	cup unsweetened cocoa powder
6	tbsp confectioner's sugar
Pinch	salt
2	eggs
2	cups milk
2	tbsp vegetable oil
½	tsp vanilla

1. In a large bowl, sift flour, cocoa powder, sugar and salt.

2. In a medium bowl, whisk eggs, milk, oil and vanilla until blended. Add a little at a time to the flour mixture, whisking to dissolve lumps, until smooth. Cover and refrigerate for 1 hour.

3. Heat a small skillet over medium heat and spray lightly with vegetable spray. When skillet is hot, remove from heat and pour in ¼ cup of the batter. Swirl skillet to spread batter evenly over the bottom. Return to heat and cook for 30 to 40 seconds, until bottom is light golden. Turn crêpe over and cook for about 15 seconds, until bottom is light golden. Remove from skillet.

4. Repeat until all batter is used, stacking crêpes between squares of parchment or waxed paper to prevent them from sticking together.

Makes 16 servings

DIETITIAN'S NOTE *The Nutrients per Serving and Exchanges are for the crêpe only. The taste panel chose strawberries and frozen yogurt as their favorite additions: count 2 tbsp low-fat frozen yogurt with ¼ cup unsweetened sliced strawberries as ½ Other Carbohydrate Exchange.*

CHOCOLATE SAUCE

¼ cup unsweetened cocoa powder, sifted
1 tbsp cornstarch
¾ cup evaporated skim milk
½ cup granulated sugar
1 tsp vanilla

1. In a small saucepan, combine cocoa and cornstarch. Whisk in ¼ cup of water until smooth. Whisk in milk and cook over low heat, stirring constantly, until the mixture comes to a boil, about 5 minutes. Cook for 1 minute longer, stirring constantly, until thickened (it will thicken more as it cools).

2. Remove from heat and stir in sugar and vanilla. Let cool to room temperature. Cover and refrigerate for up to 3 days.

Makes 1 cup or 8 servings (2 tbsp per serving)

NUTRIENTS PER SERVING

Calories	85
Carbohydrate	18 g
Fiber	1 g
Protein	2 g
Fat, total	0 g
Fat, saturated	0 g
Cholesterol	1 mg
Sodium	27 mg

EXCHANGES PER SERVING

1 Other Carbohydrates

293

FROZEN, CHILLED & OTHER DESSERTS

DIETITIAN'S NOTE *This sauce is delicious over vanilla ice cream or fresh strawberries. If the carbohydrate content is higher than you would like, replace the sugar with an amount of artificial sweetener that has the same amount of sweetening power as ½ cup sugar. Using artificial sweetener will reduce the calories to 37 and the carbohydrate content to 7 g per serving.*

BEVERAGES

295	Blender Breakfast Blast
296	Peach Melba Smoothie
297	Peanut Butter & Banana Smoothie
298	Peachy Banana Shake
299	Old-Fashioned Chocolate Soda
300	Frosty Chocolate Shake
301	Frosty Strawberry Shake
302	A Perfect Cup of Cocoa
303	Hot Mulled Cider
304	Spiced Iced Tea
305	Lemon Iced Tea

BLENDER BREAKFAST BLAST

Blender or food processor

1	banana, fresh or frozen, sliced
1	cup frozen sliced strawberries
1	cup 1% milk
½	cup plain yogurt
¼	cup wheat germ
2	tsp liquid honey (optional)

In blender, combine banana, strawberries, milk, yogurt and wheat germ. Blend for 1 to 2 minutes, or until smooth. Sweeten with honey, if desired.

Makes 2 servings

TIP When your bananas become too ripe, freeze them to make smoothies. They don't even have to be peeled! Just toss them in the freezer whole, and thaw slightly to remove the peel easily just before using. Don't thaw them too much, though—use them frozen for a good milk shake consistency.

NUTRIENTS PER SERVING

Calories	238
Carbohydrate	44 g
Fiber	5 g
Protein	12 g
Fat, total	3 g
Fat, saturated	1 g
Cholesterol	6 mg
Sodium	108 mg

EXCHANGES PER SERVING

1	Fruit
1	Reduced-Fat Milk
½	Other Carbohydrate
½	Medium-Fat Meat

DIETITIAN'S NOTE *When you don't feel like eating breakfast, have a blast! A Blender Breakfast Blast, that is. With milk, yogurt, fruit and wheat germ, it's full of nutrients: protein, calcium, vitamins A, B, C and E, carbohydrate and fiber. It's an awesome way to start the day!*

PEACH MELBA SMOOTHIE

VARIATION Use regular 1% milk instead of soy milk or, for a dairy-free smoothie, substitute frozen soy beverage for the frozen yogurt.

NUTRIENTS PER SERVING

Calories	165
Carbohydrate	24 g
Fiber	5 g
Protein	7 g
Fat, total	6 g
Fat, saturated	2 g
Cholesterol	1 mg
Sodium	53 mg

EXCHANGES PER SERVING

½ Starch
½ Other Carbohydrate
1 Medium-Fat Meat

Blender or food processor

1	peach, pitted and chopped
1½	cups soy milk
1	cup frozen raspberries
½	cup vanilla-flavored frozen yogurt

In blender, combine peach, soy milk, raspberries and frozen yogurt. Blend for 1 to 2 minutes, or until smooth. Serve immediately.

Makes 2 servings

DIETITIAN'S NOTE *When choosing soy milk, check the label for the amount of carbohydrate per serving. Depending on the brand and flavor chosen, the carbohydrate can vary a lot. For example, one brand of vanilla-flavored soy milk has 9.4 g carbohydrate per 1-cup serving; another has 26 g. This can make quite a difference in the blood glucose response. Also, most flavored soy milks (Chocolate, Mocha, Strawberry, Soyaccino) have a higher sugar content than the original (plain) flavor. Check to make sure the soy milk you choose is "fortified." This means nutrients are added, such as calcium and vitamins D, B_{12} and B_2, and other vitamins and minerals that are normally present in or added to cow's milk.*

PEANUT BUTTER & BANANA SMOOTHIE

Blender or food processor

1	frozen banana, sliced
1½	cups soy milk
1	cup frozen sliced strawberries
2	tbsp peanut butter

In blender, combine banana, soy milk, strawberries and peanut butter. Blend for 1 to 2 minutes, or until smooth. Serve immediately.

Makes 2 servings

TIP To make a smoothie for one, halve the ingredients and use an "electric wand" (immersion/hand-held blender) instead of a regular blender for easy cleanup.

VARIATION Substitute chocolate milk or chocolate-flavored soy milk for the soy milk in this smoothie.

NUTRIENTS PER SERVING

Calories	292
Carbohydrate	38 g
Fiber	5 g
Protein	12 g
Fat, total	13 g
Fat, saturated	2 g
Cholesterol	0 mg
Sodium	107 mg

EXCHANGES PER SERVING

1	Fruit
½	Reduced-Fat Milk
½	Other Carbohydrate
1	High-Fat Meat
1	Fat

DIETITIAN'S NOTE *Soy milk makes a healthy addition to your diet because it's an additional source of phytochemicals. It's a good idea to use soy milk in smoothies because mixing it with other ingredients masks the slightly unusual taste. You can substitute 1% milk for soy milk in any of these smoothies.*

PEACHY BANANA SHAKE

TIP You can make this recipe with all fresh fruit, but using some frozen results in a thicker "milk shake" consistency.

VARIATION Substitute your favorite seasonal fruit or berries for the peach and banana.

NUTRIENTS PER SERVING

Calories	320
Carbohydrate	57 g
Fiber	4 g
Protein	5 g
Fat, total	10 g
Fat, saturated	6 g
Cholesterol	39 mg
Sodium	72 mg

EXCHANGES PER SERVING

2	Fruit
1½	Other Carbohydrates
½	High-Fat Meat
1	Fat

Blender or food processor

1	ripe peach, pitted, peeled and sliced
1	frozen banana, sliced
⅔	cup vanilla ice cream

In blender, combine peach, banana and ice cream. Blend for 1 to 2 minutes, or until smooth. Serve immediately.

Makes 2 servings

DIETITIAN'S NOTE *Fruit shakes are a great way to increase your fruit and fiber intake for the day and can be a fun surprise to tempt a reluctant breakfast eater.*

OLD-FASHIONED CHOCOLATE SODA

2 tsp unsweetened cocoa powder, sifted
2 tsp granulated sugar
2 tbsp 1% milk
½ cup vanilla ice cream
1 can (13 oz) sugar-free lemon-lime soda

1. In a tall glass, combine cocoa and sugar. Add milk and stir until completely blended. Spoon in ice cream and slowly pour in soda. Wait until bubbles disappear, then keep adding soda slowly.

2. Serve immediately with a spoon and a straw.

Makes 1 serving

**NUTRIENTS
PER SERVING**

Calories	186
Carbohydrate	28 g
Fiber	1 g
Protein	4 g
Fat, total	8 g
Fat, saturated	5 g
Cholesterol	30 mg
Sodium	90 mg

**EXCHANGES
PER SERVING**

1½ Other Carbohydrates
1 High-Fat Meat
1 Fat

FROSTY CHOCOLATE SHAKE

NUTRIENTS PER SERVING

Calories	179
Carbohydrate	23 g
Fiber	0 g
Protein	5 g
Fat, total	8 g
Fat, saturated	5 g
Cholesterol	32 mg
Sodium	90 mg

EXCHANGES PER SERVING

1½ Other Carbohydrates
1 High-Fat Meat
1 Fat

Blender or food processor

2	cups vanilla ice cream	
1	cup 1% milk	
¼	cup Chocolate Sauce (see recipe, page 293)	

In blender, combine ice cream, milk and Chocolate Sauce. Blend for 30 seconds, until smooth. Serve immediately.

Makes 4 servings

FROSTY STRAWBERRY SHAKE

Blender or food processor

- ½   cup boiling water
- 1   package (⅓ oz) no-sugar-added strawberry-flavored gelatin
- 2   cups vanilla ice cream
- 1   cup 1% milk
- ½   cup ice cubes, crushed

1. Pour boiling water into the blender. Add gelatin powder and blend for 1 minute. Keep the blender running and add ice cream by large spoonfuls through hole in lid.

2. Turn off the blender; add milk and ice. Blend for another 30 seconds, or until smooth and thick. Serve immediately.

Makes 4 servings

NUTRIENTS PER SERVING

Calories	167
Carbohydrate	19 g
Fiber	0 g
Protein	6 g
Fat, total	8 g
Fat, saturated	5 g
Cholesterol	31 mg
Sodium	143 mg

EXCHANGES PER SERVING

- 1 Other Carbohydrates
- 1 Medium-Fat Meat
- ½ Fat

A PERFECT CUP OF COCOA

TIPS For a Christmas treat, use a candy cane or cinnamon stick for a stir stick.

Mexicans make their hot chocolate with chocolate tablets. You can duplicate the flavor more closely by using squares of semisweet chocolate, but be aware that this will change the nutrient analysis.

NUTRIENTS PER SERVING

Calories	166
Carbohydrate	26 g
Fiber	1 g
Protein	9 g
Fat, total	3 g
Fat, saturated	2 g
Cholesterol	10 mg
Sodium	711 mg

EXCHANGES PER SERVING

1½ Carbohydrates

1	cup 1% milk
2	tsp unsweetened cocoa powder, sifted
2	tsp granulated sugar
½	tsp ground cinnamon
¼	tsp salt
½	tsp vanilla
¼	tsp almond extract
5	mini marshmallows

1. In a small saucepan, heat milk over medium-high heat for about 5 minutes, until hot but not boiling. (Or, in a microwave-safe measuring cup, microwave on High for 1½ to 2 minutes, depending on your microwave. Do not overheat, or it will form a "skin.")

2. In a large mug, combine cocoa, sugar, cinnamon and salt. Add 2 tbsp water and stir to form a smooth paste. Add hot milk, vanilla and almond extract.

3. Top with marshmallows and serve immediately.

Makes 1 serving

DIETITIAN'S NOTE *With cinnamon, vanilla and almond extract, this is indeed the perfect cup of cocoa—and miniature marshmallows add fun. If you wish, replace sugar with an amount of artificial sweetener that has the same amount of sweetening power as 2 tsp sugar. Using artificial sweetener will reduce the calories to 130 and the carbohydrate content to 17 g per serving.*

HOT MULLED CIDER

4	cups unsweetened apple juice
2	tbsp packed brown sugar
1	tsp ground cinnamon
½	tsp ground nutmeg
½	tsp ground allspice
10	whole cloves
2 to 3	cinnamon sticks
1	orange, sliced
1	lemon, sliced

1. In a large saucepan, over medium heat, heat apple juice, brown sugar, cinnamon, nutmeg and allspice for about 10 minutes, until simmering but not boiling.

2. Reduce heat to medium-low. Add cloves, cinnamon sticks, orange slices and lemon slices and simmer for 30 minutes or more to allow flavors to blend. Use a slotted spoon to remove the flavorings before serving.

Makes 6 servings

NUTRIENTS PER SERVING

Calories	97
Carbohydrate	24 g
Fiber	0 g
Protein	0 g
Fat, total	0 g
Fat, saturated	0 g
Cholesterol	0 mg
Sodium	7 mg

EXCHANGES PER SERVING

1½ Fruit

DIETITIAN'S NOTE *A hot beverage such as this is a welcome treat after a winter activity such as skiing or ice skating. To reduce the carbohydrates, replace sugar with an amount of artificial sweetener that has the same amount of sweetening power as 2 tbsp brown sugar. Using artificial sweetener will reduce the calories to 80 and the carbohydrate content to 20 g per serving.*

SPICED ICED TEA

NUTRIENTS PER SERVING

Calories	42
Carbohydrate	11 g
Fiber	1 g
Protein	0 g
Fat, total	0 g
Fat, saturated	0 g
Cholesterol	0 mg
Sodium	3 mg

EXCHANGES PER SERVING

½ Other Carbohydrate

16-cup non-metal beverage container

8	orange pekoe tea bags (regular or decaffeinated)
1	tsp whole cloves
4	cups boiling water
½	cup granulated sugar
10	cups cold water
2	cups orange juice
2	lemons, sliced

1. Place tea bags and cloves in the beverage container. Pour in boiling water, cover and let steep for 10 minutes. Remove tea bags and cloves with a slotted spoon and stir in sugar. Let cool to room temperature, then stir in cold water and orange juice.

2. Serve over ice, garnished with lemon slices.

Makes 16 servings

DIETITIAN'S NOTE *To reduce the calories and carbohydrate count, replace sugar with an amount of artificial sweetener that has the same sweetening power as ½ cup sugar. Using artificial sweetener will reduce the calories to 21 and the carbohydrate content to 6 g per serving.*

LEMON ICED TEA

16-cup non-metal beverage container

12   orange pekoe tea bags (regular or decaffeinated)
6   lemon-flavored tea bags
6   cups boiling water
½   cup granulated sugar
9   cups cold water
2   lemons, sliced

1. Place orange pekoe and lemon tea bags in the beverage container. Pour in boiling water, cover and let steep for 10 minutes. Remove tea bags and stir in sugar. Let cool to room temperature, then stir in cold water.

2. Serve over ice, garnished with lemon slices.

Makes 15 servings

NUTRIENTS PER SERVING

Calories	30
Carbohydrate	9 g
Fiber	0 g
Protein	0 g
Fat, total	0 g
Fat, saturated	0 g
Cholesterol	0 mg
Sodium	3 mg

EXCHANGES PER SERVING

½ Other Carbohydrate

DIETITIAN'S NOTE *To make sugar-free iced tea, replace sugar with an amount of artificial sweetener that has the same sweetening power as ½ cup sugar. Using artificial sweetener will reduce the calories to 7 and the carbohydrate content to 3 g per serving.*

APPENDIX A

HOW MUCH SUGAR IS OKAY?

It is now accepted that, even when a person has diabetes, added sugar is not a bad thing when eaten in measured amounts. As a matter of fact, up to 10% of the total calories eaten in a day can come from added sugar. This means that if a person eats 1,800 calories a day, 180 of them can be derived from added sugar, which works out to 45 grams of sugar. This translates in real food to 1 chewy trail-mix granola bar (13 g sugar), 1 lower-fat chocolate pudding (19 g sugar), and ¾ cup oatmeal crisp maple nut cereal (13 g sugar). It doesn't take much! Foods containing added sugar can be substituted for fruit or starch in the meal plan or can be used when a person taking insulin is more active than usual and chooses to have more carbohydrate to keep the blood sugar level normal. (Some people may prefer to compensate for activity by decreasing their insulin.)

Sugar can come in the form of granulated sugar, brown sugar, confectioners' sugar, honey, molasses and regular jam, jelly or syrup. The recipes in this cookbook use real sugar, but if you feel that the sugar or caloric content is too high, a sugar substitute can be used instead. If you are using Equal (aspartame) or Splenda (sucralose) in your baking, substitute an amount that's equivalent to the total sugar or to a portion of the sugar. Both of these products are made to have similar sweetness to sugar. Therefore, ½ cup of sugar can be replaced with ½ cup Equal or Splenda, which would reduce the carbohydrates by about 88 grams and the total calories by 337. Read the package directions carefully for instructions on how to use these sugar substitutes. Splenda, for example, is to be mixed in with the dry ingredients rather than blended in with the fat.

Many parents ask about the safety of sugar substitutes, especially aspartame, which is used most commonly in sugar-free beverages and in ready-to-eat, prepared and packaged products. Safety levels are set for various sweeteners based on body weight, and parents must keep in mind that children have smaller bodies and will therefore reach their safety level with a smaller amount of the sugar substitute. Talk to your dietitian about how much is safe for your child.

Another type of sugar substitute is the sugar alcohol used in products such as sugar-free chocolate bars, candies, chewing gum, syrups and fruit spreads. Examples of sugar alcohols are isomalt, lactitol, mannitol, maltitol, sorbitol and xylitol. Note that all except isomalt end with "-itol"—it will help you remember the names. Sweets with sugar alcohols should be limited, as large amounts can cause stomach upset, bloating and diarrhea.

Approximately 50% of total sugar alcohol turns into blood glucose. So, for carbohydrate counting, if a label tells you how much total sugar alcohol is present in the food, count it as half of the total. For example, if an ice cream bar contains 8 grams of sorbitol, only 4 grams would be used toward the carb count. Talk to your dietitian about how to read labels of foods with sugar alcohols.

Polydextrose, a carbohydrate commonly found in sugar-free, low-fat ice creams, is not broken down to sugar, does not affect blood sugar and does not need to be included in carbohydrate counting.

The ingredients in packaged food are listed in order of the amount in the food. If sugar is listed near the beginning of the list, then it is one of the main ingredients in that food. Watch for other words on the ingredient list that mean sugar, such as fructose, glucose-fructose, sucrose, maltose, lactose, honey, liquid sugar, invert sugar, liquid invert sugar, syrup, galactose, dextrose, dextrin, high-fructose corn syrup, corn syrup solids, molasses and raisin syrup.

APPENDIX B

LABEL READING FOR CARBOHYDRATES

The "Nutrition Facts" table on food packaging provides information on 13 nutrients, based on the serving size shown. It is important to keep the serving size in mind, since having a smaller or larger serving changes not only the nutrient content but—especially important in diabetes—the total carbohydrate content. The % Daily Value puts nutrients on a scale from 0% to 100% and tells you if there is a little or a lot of a nutrient in one serving of that packaged food. This value is based on a 2,000-calorie intake.

All packaged food labels include amounts of total carbohydrate, dietary fiber and sugars. The dietary fiber and sugars amounts are indented under total carbohydrate, indicating they are part of the total grams of carbohydrate. To determine the amount of carbohydrate that really counts in raising blood sugar, grams of fiber must be subtracted from total grams of carbohydrate. The remaining amount is referred to as the amount of "available carbohydrate," which will convert into blood glucose.

For examples of food labels and more details on how to read them, see the American Diabetes Association's website (**www.diabetes.org**) or the Food and Drug Administration's Center for Food Safety and Applied Nutrition website (**vm.cfsan.fda.gov/~dms/foodlab.html**).

NUTRITION CLAIMS ON LABELS

Manufacturers may or may not choose to put a nutrition claim on their food label. The food product must meet certain criteria set forth by the Food and Drug Administration to have a nutrition claim displayed on the package. In this way, consumers are assured that claims are credible and are consistent with current scientific and dietary recommendations.

A commonly misunderstood term is "no added sugar." It means there is no sugar *added* to the food. However, there may be sugar in the food to begin with. Don't be fooled by the claim on fruit juice that states "no added sugar": the natural sugar from the fruit is, of course, still there. This fruit juice can be used in regular meal planning or for treating low blood sugar, but it is not considered a sugar-free juice.

"Light" is a claim that is allowed on foods that are "reduced in fat" or "reduced in calories." "Light" can also be used to describe a feature of the food such as "light in color." If the word "light" is used on a food label, it must have a statement that explains what characteristic makes the food "light."

For more information on nutrition labeling, see the Food and Drug Administration's Center for Food Safety and Applied Nutrition website: **vm.cfsan.fda.gov/~dms/fdnewlab.html**.

APPENDIX C

VITAMINS & MINERALS

Vitamins are essential nutrients. This means that your body needs these substances to function properly. Vitamins are needed only in small amounts and have no caloric value, but they help the body transform carbohydrate, protein and fat into energy.

There are two main types of vitamins. Fat-soluble vitamins—vitamins A, D, E and K—are found in and absorbed with the fats in our diet. Water-soluble vitamins include the B vitamins and vitamin C. Enjoy a wide variety of foods to meet your daily requirement of vitamins.

Minerals are naturally occurring inorganic substances required by the body. Calcium, phosphorous, magnesium, sodium, potassium, iodine, iron, zinc, manganese, chromium, copper, selenium and fluoride are all examples of minerals. Minerals are found in a wide variety of foods from each of the different food groups. Just as with vitamins, the most important thing is to remember to choose a wide variety of foods each day.

Children and teens who don't drink enough milk will find it difficult to get their daily requirement for calcium. Bone mineralization takes place primarily during the peak growth years. Therefore, it is essential for children and teens to have an adequate intake of milk or other sources of calcium, along with vitamin D, which the body needs in order to absorb calcium.

VITAMINS & MINERALS ON THE NUTRITION FACTS TABLE

Calcium, iron and vitamins A and C can now be found on all food labels. The amounts of these nutrients are expressed in percentages, so that you can see approximately how much of your daily requirement a serving of this food provides. Remember, though, that the percentages are based on a 2,000-calorie diet, not the requirements for children.

WHAT ARE ANTIOXIDANTS & PHYTOCHEMICALS?

Foods deliver thousands of chemicals and substances other than the handful we call nutrients. As we learn more about the different compounds in foods and the role they may play in helping to prevent cancer and heart disease, the terminology that comes with the research can be confusing. Here are some words you might hear in the news.

Free radicals are unstable molecules that can damage the cells of the body. This damage is called **oxidative stress**. **Antioxidants** and **phytochemicals** are food compounds that help fight free radicals and protect the body. Examples of antioxidants are vitamins A, C and E and phytochemicals, all of which can be found in fruits and vegetables.

The best course of action is to eat a wide variety of fruits and vegetables and not to single out a particular nutrient that you think will be the magical answer. Research shows that it may be the combination and interaction of different chemicals that provides the body with maximum health benefits.

GET MOVING!

All children and youth should be physically active, especially if they have diabetes. Exercise is good for us in many ways. It helps us feel energized, works the heart (which is also a muscle), decreases the risk of chronic disease (such as cardiovascular disease), and prevents the body's metabolism from slowing down. If you're not already active, start with small, simple changes. Meet a friend for a walk or a bicycle ride instead of having another snack; take the stairs instead of the elevator; play a game of pickup basketball with your family; and work your way up from there.

Parents can play an important role by setting a good example: they must show their children that activity can be fun and get them involved in exercise programs. Children who find an activity they enjoy will be set on a path that will guide them for the rest of their lives.

APPENDIX D

ESTIMATING EXCHANGES FOR YOUR FAVORITE RECIPES

The recipe information in this book can help you fit your own recipes into your meal plan. Look for a recipe that has similar quantities of the main ingredients and the same number of servings as your recipe. Because they are similar in these ways, your recipe will have approximately the same number of Exchanges as the similar recipe in the book.

You can also use the worksheet on the following pages to help you get a more precise estimate of the Exchanges for your recipes. Turn to the Exchanges worksheet (pages 314–315) and follow the instructions.

The worksheet is accompanied by an ingredient list that can also be used separately. Here's an example. To find out the number of Carbohydrate Exchanges in 1 cup of granulated sugar, you would look in the "Sugar & Syrups" section on page 317 and see that it contains 13½ Carbohydrate Exchanges.

EXCHANGES RECIPE WORKSHEET

a. In column A, enter names or recipe ingredients that are called for by volume
(i.e., measured in cups, tablespoons or teaspoons)

b. Enter quantities of these ingredients in columns Q1 or Q2.
> Enter Q1 if amount is not in cups; otherwise, enter in Q2.
> Omit salt, baking powder, baking soda, spices and any other ingredients where the quantity is less than 1 tsp.

c. Using the equivalent measures below, convert quantities in column Q1 to cups and enter in Q2.

1 tsp = 0.02 cup	*2 tsp = 0.04 cup*	*3 tsp = 1 tbsp = 0.06 cup*
1 tbsp = 0.06 cup	*2 tbsp = 0.13 cup*	*3 tbsp = 0.19 cup*

d. For each ingredient, find Carbohydrate, Fat and Meat sub Exchanges per cup (see pages 316–319)
and enter in the corresponding columns (C1, F1, M1).

e. Multiply Exchanges per cup in C1 by number of cups in Q2; enter result in C2. Repeat for F1 and M1,
entering results in F2 and M2, respectively.

> **NOTE:** *Calculations on this worksheet yield approximate exchange
> counts. Exchanges calculated here may not agree exactly with those
> based on a complete nutrient calculation of the recipe.*

f. Enter name of ingredient and the number used in the recipe in columns A and Q2.

g. Enter Carbohydrate and Fat Exchanges per unit (see page 320) in columns C1 and F1.

h. Multiply choices in C1 and F1 by value in Q2 and enter results in C2 and F2.

i. Calculate and enter C2, F2 and M2 totals for rows *f* to *h*.

j. Add Section A Subtotal to Section B Subtotal.

k. Enter number of servings that recipe makes.

l. Divide C2, F2 and M2 totals in row *j* by number of servings and enter.

m. Round values in row *l* to nearest 0.5. Exception: Round 0.4 or fewer Meat sub Exchanges to zero.

SECTION A

MEASURED INGREDIENTS (cups, tbsp, etc.) A	MEASURES PER RECIPE convert non-cup amounts to cups		CARBOHYDRATE EXCHANGES PER		FAT EXCHANGES PER		MEAT SUB EXCHANGES PER	
	not cups Q_1	cups Q_2	cup C_1	recipe C_2	cup F_1	recipe F_2	cup M_1	recipe M_2
a. to *e.*	>							
	>							
	>							
	>							
	>							
	>							
	>							
	>							
	>							
	>							
	>							
	>							
	>							
Section A Subtotals								

SECTION B

COUNTED INGREDIENTS (Chocolate, pie crust, eggs, etc.) (See page 319) A		# UNITS PER RECIPE Q_2	CARBOHYDRATE EXCHANGES PER		FAT EXCHANGES PER		MEAT SUB EXCHANGES PER	
			1 unit C_1	Recipe C_2	1 unit F_1	recipe F_2	1 unit M_1	recipe M_2
f. to *h.*								

i.   Section B Subtotals

j.   Total Exchanges per Recipe (Section A + B)

k.   *Recipe Makes* [   ] *Servings*

l.   Total Exchanges per Serving, unrounded

m.   **Exchanges per Serving FINAL**   **Carbohydrate >** [   ]   **Fat >** [   ]   **Meat Sub >** [   ]

EXCHANGES FOR RECIPE INGREDIENTS (USE WITH THE EXCHANGES RECIPE WORKSHEET ON PAGES 314-315.)

INGREDIENT	EXCHANGES		
See corresponding columns on worksheet *Enter measured items in Section A of worksheet*	CARB* C1	FAT F1	MEAT M1
FLOUR *(1 cup)*			
whole wheat flour	6		
rye flour	5½		
all-purpose flour	6½		
rice flour	8½		
cake flour	7		
OTHER DRY GRAIN INGREDIENTS *(1 cup)*			
wheat bran, raw unprocessed	2½		
wheat bran cereal (about 12 g fiber per ½ cup)	3½		
bran flakes (ready-to-eat cereal)	1½		
oat bran, raw unprocessed	4		
rolled oats (not instant)	4		
granola (12 g fat per cup)	5		
cornmeal	8½		
cornstarch	8		
FRUIT & FRUIT JUICE *(1 cup)*			
apple juice	2		
apples, raw, chopped or sliced (about 1 medium)	1		
applesauce, unsweetened	2		
banana, mashed (about 2 medium)	3½		
blueberries, raw or frozen without sugar	1½		
cantaloupe, balls or diced	1		
honeydew melon, balls or diced	1		
kiwifruit, sliced (about 3 medium)	1½		
mango, raw, sliced	2		

For use in dessert Exchange calculator, all carbohydrate is classified as "Other Carbohydrates."

INGREDIENT	EXCHANGES		
See corresponding columns on worksheet	CARB* C1	FAT F1	MEAT M1
FRUIT & FRUIT JUICE *(continued)*			
orange juice, frozen concentrate, not diluted	7		
peaches, raw, sliced (about 2 medium)	1½		
pears, raw, sliced (about 1 large)	1½		
pineapple, raw or canned, diced	1½		
raspberries, raw or frozen (no sugar added)	1		
rhubarb, raw, diced (about 8 oz)	½		
strawberries, whole or sliced	½		
fresh strawberry purée, no sugar added	1		
VEGETABLES *(1 cup)*			
carrot, raw, grated (about 2 medium)	½		
zucchini, raw, grated or shredded (about 1 medium)	½		
pumpkin, canned	1½		
DRIED FRUIT *(1 cup)*			
dates, chopped	8½		
apricots, chopped	8		
prunes	7		
cranberries	6½		
seedless raisins	8½		
golden raisins	7½		
MILK & YOGURT *(1 cup)*			
skim milk	1		
buttermilk	1		
1% milk	1		
2% milk	1		
whole milk	1		
2% evaporated milk, undiluted	2½		
yogurt, plain low-fat (1%–2%)	1½		
SUGAR & SYRUPS *(1 cup)*			
white (granulated) sugar	13½		

(continued)

INGREDIENT	EXCHANGES		
See corresponding columns on worksheet	CARB* C1	FAT F1	MEAT M1
SUGAR & SYRUPS *(continued)*			
brown sugar, packed	14½		
brown sugar, lightly packed	12		
confectioner's sugar (also called icing or powdered sugar)	8		
fructose (powdered form)	13½		
corn syrup	16½		
honey	18½		
maple syrup	14		
molasses	17		
rice syrup	17		
FATS & OILS *(1 cup)*			
vegetable oil (canola, soybean)	43½		
margarine, soft hydrogenated	36½		
butter (2 sticks)	37		
hydrogenated vegetable oil shortening	43½		
SOUR CREAM & CREAM CHEESE *(1 cup)*			
sour cream, light (10%)	4½		
sour cream, regular (20%)	9½		
cream cheese, light (about 20% fat), 8 oz	9		
cream cheese, regular (30% fat), 8 oz	16		
NUTS & SEEDS *(1 cup)*			
almonds, chopped or slivered (3½ oz)	11½		
coconut, dried unsweetened	9½		
coconut, shredded sweetened	6½		
flaxseeds, crushed/ground	9		
hazelnuts/filberts, chopped (3½ oz)	14		
peanut butter	26½		
pecans, chopped (3½ oz)	16		
pistachios, shelled (3½ oz)	11½		
sunflower seed kernels, unsalted	14½		
walnuts, small pieces or chopped (3½ oz)	15		

INGREDIENT	EXCHANGES		
See corresponding columns on worksheet	CARB* C1	FAT F1	MEAT M1
MEAT SUBSTITUTES: EGG (*1 cup*)			
liquid egg product, yolks replaced	3 ½		
liquid egg white	3 ½		
liquid whole egg	4		

For individual eggs, egg yolks and egg whites, see end of list

CHEESE (*1 cup*)			
2% cottage cheese			4 ½
ricotta cheese, light (5%)			4
ricotta cheese, regular (10%)			4

Be sure to copy both Carbohydrate and Fat Exchanges to worksheet for all items below

MISCELLANEOUS INGREDIENTS (*1 cup*)			
cocoa powder, unsweetened	3	2	
semisweet chocolate chips (6 oz)	7	10	
white chocolate chips (6 oz)	6 ½	11	
butterscotch chips (6 oz)	7 ½	10	
chocolate wafer crumbs	5 ½	3	
graham wafer crumbs	4 ½	1 ½	

Enter these "counted" items in Section B of worksheet

PIE SHELLS & CRUSTS, PHYLLO SHEETS & CHOCOLATE (*1 cup*)			
chocolate crumb pie shell, ready-to-use: 8-inch	7 ½	7	
graham wafer pie shell, ready-to-use: 8-inch	7 ½	8	
pie crust, frozen, ready-to-bake: 9-inch	5	10	
phyllo dough sheets (16½- by 12-inch), 1 sheet	½	0	
chocolate, bittersweet/semisweet, 1 square (1 oz)	1 ½	5	

EGGS			
egg, whole			1
egg white			½
egg yolk			½

For measured quantities of eggs, see above

ABOUT THE NUTRIENT ANALYSIS & EXCHANGE

Food Intelligence (Toronto, Ontario) calculated the nutrient values for the recipes in this book and assigned the Exchanges (see pages 316–319).

Calculations were carried out with the assistance of Genesis® R&D SQL software, using current versions of the USDA Nutrient Database for Standard Reference and reviewed data from other sources when required. All nutrient values were rounded to the nearest whole number; the Exchanges were rounded to the nearest half.

The calculations were based on:

• *the first ingredient listed where there is a choice;*

• *the exclusion of "optional" ingredients; and*

• *the exclusion of ingredients with non-specified or "to taste" amounts.*

EXCHANGES			
GROUP/LISTS	CARBOHYDRATE (G)	PROTEIN (G)	FAT (G)
CARBOHYDRATES			
Starches	15	0–3	0–1
Fruit	15	—	—
Milk: Fat-Free, Low-Fat (1%)	12	8	0.3
Reduced-Fat (2%)	12	8	5
Whole	12	8	8
Other Carbohydrates	15	v*	v*
Vegetables	5	2	—
MEAT & MEAT SUBSTITUTES			
Lean	—	7	0–3
Medium-Fat	—	7	4–7
High-Fat	—	7	8
Plant-Based Proteins	v*	7	v*
Fat Group	—	—	5

The Exchanges calculations were based on the American Diabetes Association food Exchange values in the table above.

*v = variable

Adapted from Choose Your Foods—Exchange Lists for Diabetes. American Diabetes Association and American Dietetic Association, 2008.

CONTRIBUTING AUTHORS

We extend our heartfelt appreciation to the following authors for contributing their recipes to this collection:

ESTHER BRODY, *ANOTHER 250 BEST MUFFIN RECIPES*
Wheat Muffins (page 12), Honey Whole Wheat Muffins (page 13), Blueberry Wheat Germ Muffins (page 14)

ESTHER BRODY, *THE 250 BEST COOKIE RECIPES*
Oat Bran Raisin Cookies (page 80), Oatmeal Lace Pennies (page 82), Whole Wheat Spice Cookies (page 110), Sesame Seed Cookies (page 115), Diced Rhubarb Cookies (page 117)

JOHANNA BURKHARD, *300 BEST COMFORT FOOD RECIPES*
Strawberry Rhubarb Cobbler (page 226)

MEREDITH DEEDS & CARLA SNYDER, *THE MIXER BIBLE*
Banana Chocolate Chunk Muffins (page 10), Sunrise Zucchini Muffins (page 22), Crispy Oatmeal Cookies (page 75), Sunshine Lemon Mousse (page 272), Mango Raspberry Fool (page 275), Orange Sabayon with Fresh Berries (page 286)

DIETITIANS OF CANADA, *DIETITIANS OF CANADA COOK GREAT FOOD*
Lemon Sherbet (page 260), Strawberry Sorbet (page 263), Pumpkin Custard (page 279), Blueberry Flan (page 289)

DIETITIANS OF CANADA, *SIMPLY GREAT FOOD*
Orange Cranberry Muffins (page 2), Big-Batch Banana Blueberry Muffins (page 4), Banana Applesauce Muffins (page 5), Chocolate Chip Oatmeal Muffins (page 9), Triple B Health Muffins (page 17), Pumpkin Bran Muffins (page 18), Sweet Potato Muffins (page 24), Oat Bran Banana Bread (page 38), Pumpkin Spice Nut Bread (page 42), Fiber-Power Biscotti (page 52), Holiday Biscotti (page 66), Fruity Oatmeal Cookies (page 81), Soft Apple Cinnamon Cookies (page 88), Best-Ever Chocolate Cookies (page 96), Peanut Butter Flaxseed Cookies (page 105), Ginger Cookies (page 111), Charlie & Emma's Favorite Carrot Cookies (page 118), Apricot Coconut Bars (page 126), Toffee Bars (page 135), Berry Cheesecake Bars (page 136), Almond Butter Cereal Squares (page 142), Carrot Cake (page 177), Chocolate Zucchini Cake (page 181), Cinnamon Streusel Coffee Cake (page 188), Chocolate Chunk Coffee Cake (page 196), Apple, Pear & Cranberry Crisp (page 221), Baked Granola

Apples (page 230), Pears in Tosca Sauce (page 233), Rhubarb Bread Pudding (page 241), Dessert Nachos (page 245), Chocolate Fondue (page 246), Balsamic Strawberry Sauce (page 252), Whipped Cream & Yogurt Topping (page 253), Indian-Style Rice Pudding (page 282), Lemon Blueberry Panna Cotta (page 285), Chocolate Crêpes (page 292)

GEORGE GEARY, *THE COMPLETE BAKING COOKBOOK*
Perfect Bran Muffins (page 15), Oat Berry Muffins (page 20), Pumpkin Raisin Scones (page 44), Pecan Cinnamon Biscuits (page 49), Granola Bars (page 129), Perfect Angel Food Cake (page 155)

JULIE HASSON, *300 BEST CHOCOLATE RECIPES*
Chocolate Cherry Biscotti (page 60), Chocolate Chip Orange Biscotti (page 61), Chocolate Quesadillas (page 244)

LYNN ROBLIN, NUTRITION EDITOR, *300 BEST HEALTHY RECIPES*
Streusel Apple Muffins (page 1), Banana Date Muffins (page 3), Blueberry Lemon Cornmeal Muffins (page 8), Yogurt Bran Muffins (page 16), Pineapple Carrot Date Muffins (page 21), Pumpkin Molasses Raisin Loaf (page 26), Carrot Pineapple Zucchini Loaf (page 27), Lemon Poppy Seed Loaf (page 28), Banana Nut Raisin Loaf (page 29), Banana Walnut Bread (page 40), Apricot Date Biscotti (page 51), Lemon & Lime Poppy Seed Biscotti (page 54), Pecan Biscotti (page 57), Two-Tone Chocolate Orange Biscotti (page 62), Gingerbread Biscotti (page 63), Oatmeal Orange Coconut Cookies (page 76), Oatmeal Raisin Cookies (page 78), Oatmeal Raisin Pecan Cookies (page 79), Oatmeal Date Cookies (page 83), Date Roll-Up Cookies (page 86), Crisp Nut Cookies (page 93), Double Chocolate Raisin Cookies (page 97), Rugelach (Cinnamon Chocolate Twist Cookies) (page 100), Cocoa Kisses (page 102), Peanut Butter Cookies (page 104), Peanut Butter Fudge Cookies (page 106), Vanilla Almond Snaps (page 114), Date Nut Bars (page 128), Peanut Butter-Coconut-Raisin Granola Bars (page 130), Date Oatmeal Squares (page 137), Lemon Poppy Seed Squares (page 139), Triple Chocolate Brownies (page 147), Sour Cream Brownies (page 149), Cream Cheese–Filled Brownies (page 150), Chocolate Angel Food Cake (page 156), Chiffon Cake (page 160), Chocolate Espresso Cake (page 162), Blueberry Honey Cake (page 163), Blueberry Peach Cake (page 164), Sour Cream Orange Apple Cake (page 166), Banana Cake with Lemon Cream Frosting (page 168), Date Cake with Coconut Topping (page 170), Prune Orange Spice Cake (page 172), Banana Spice Cake (page 174), Banana Date Cake (page 176), Applesauce Carrot Cake (page 178), Apple Pecan Streusel Cake (page 184), Apricot Date Streusel Cake (page 186), Orange-Glazed Coffee Cake (page 192), Orange Coffee Cake (page 193), Cinnamon Date Coffee Cake (page 194), Chocolate Marble Coffee Cake (page 198), La Costa Cheesecake with Strawberry Sauce (page 199), Raspberry Cheesecake (page 200), Tangy Banana Cheesecake (page 201), Marble Mocha Cheesecake (page 202), Chocolate Cheesecake (page 204), Chocolate Marble Vanilla Cheesecake (page 206), Sour Cream Apple Pie (page 210),

Sour Cream & Berry Pie (page 212), Lemon Meringue Pie (page 213), Creamy Pumpkin Cheese Pie (page 214), Fresh Fruit Tart (page 218), Tropical Fruit Tart (page 219), Blueberry Strawberry Pear Crisp (page 222), Peach & Blueberry Crisp (page 223), Mango Blueberry Strudel (page 229), Poached Pears in Chocolate Sauce (page 234), Key Lime Dessert (page 236), Fluffy Apricot Soufflé with Raspberry Sauce (page 238), Melon Balls with Ginger Sauce (page 240), Cocoa Roll with Creamy Cheese & Berries (page 242), Honey Vanilla Ice Cream (page 255), Mocha Ice Cream (page 256), Frozen Orange Cream (page 257), Fresh Fruit Sorbet (page 261), Pineapple Lime Sorbet (page 262), Strawberry Orange Buttermilk Sorbet (page 264), Tulip Cookies with Fruit Sorbet (page 264), Raspberry Ice with Fresh Strawberries (page 266), Frozen Jamoca Mousse (page 270), Banana Strawberry Mousse (page 274), Orange Cappuccino Pudding Cake (page 281), Maple Flan with Walnuts (page 290), Pumpkin Flan (page 291)

JILL SNIDER, *BARS & SQUARES: MORE THAN 200 RECIPES*

Oatmeal Shortbread (page 68), Almond Spice Shortbread (page 69), Rice Flour Shortbread (page 71), Cornmeal Shortbread (page 72), Chunky Chocolate Shortbread (page 73), Mixed Fruit Bran Bars (page 121), Apple Cinnamon Bars (page 122), Pick-Me-Up Bars (page 124), Apricot Seed Bars (page 125), Nutty Shortbread Bars (page 131), Chocolate Shortbread Bars (page 132), Hazelnut Shortbread Bars (page 133), Chocolate Hazelnut Bars (page 134), Raisin & Applesauce Squares (page 138), Almond Shortbread Squares (page 140), Coconut Seeds Cereal Squares (page 141), Moist 'n' Chewy Chocolate Brownies (page 145), Chocolate Chunk Banana Brownies (page 146), White Chocolate Brownies (page 148), Orange Cream Cheese Brownies (page 152)

JILL SNIDER, *COOKIES: MORE THAN 200 RECIPES*

Mini Hazelnut Biscotti (page 56), Maple Walnut Biscotti (page 58), Chocolate-Wrapped Ginger Biscotti (page 64), Oatmeal Pecan Shortbread (page 70), Cranberry Pecan Oatmeal Cookies (page 77), Crunchy Apricot Oat Drops (page 85), Lemon Lime Cookies (page 89), Lemon Poppy Seed Balls (page 90), Lemon Cranberry Pistachio Wafers (page 91), Orange Coffee Pecan Slices (page 92), Maple Walnut Slice 'n' Bake Cookies (page 94), Chocolate Chip Refrigerator Cookies (page 98), White Chocolate Cranberry Drops (page 103), Spicy Gingersnaps (page 112)

DONNA WASHBURN AND HEATHER BUTT, *125 BEST QUICK BREAD RECIPES*

Rhubarb Orange Bread (page 31), Poppy Seed Oat Bread (page 32), Blueberry Banana Oat Bread (page 33), Blueberry Buckwheat Bread (page 34), Peach Blueberry Quick Bread (page 35), Low-Fat Applesauce Raisin Bread (page 36), Fruited Barm Brack (page 37), Orange Pumpkin Snacking Cake (page 165)

INDEX

Underscored page references indicate boxed text, Dietitian's Notes, or sidebar tips.

Almond Butter Cereal Squares, 142
Almonds
    Almond Butter Cereal Squares,
      142
    Almond Shortbread Squares,
      140
    Almond Spice Shortbread, 69
    Christmas Brownies, 144
    Cornmeal Shortbread, 72
    Date Nut Bars, 128
    Exchange value, 318
    Fiber-Power Biscotti, 52–53
    Holiday Biscotti, 66–67
    Indian-Style Rice Pudding, 282
    Lemon Almond Biscotti, 55
    Pears in Tosca Sauce, 233
    Vanilla Almond Snaps, 114
Almond Shortbread Squares, 140
Almond Spice Shortbread, 69
American Diabetes Association, xv,
    153, 309
Angel food cake
    Angel Tunnel Cake, 158
    Chocolate Angel Food Cake,
      156
    Fruit-Filled Angel Tunnel Cake,
      159
    Peppermint Angel Cupcakes,
      182
    Perfect Angel Food Cake, 155
    Spiced Angel Food Cake, 157
Angel Tunnel Cake, 158
Antioxidants, 35, 217, 312

Apple, Pear & Cranberry Crisp, 221
Apple Cinnamon Bars, 122–23
Apple juice
    Hot Mulled Cider, 303
Apple Oatmeal Pudding, 283
Apple Pecan Streusel Cake, 184–85
Apples
    Apple, Pear & Cranberry Crisp,
      221
    Apple Cinnamon Bars, 122–23
    Apple Oatmeal Pudding, 283
    Apple Pecan Streusel Cake,
      184–85
    Baked Granola Apples, 230
    best, for baking, 230
    Blueberry Apple Crisp, 220
    Carrot, Apple & Coconut Loaf,
      30
    Creamy Dreamy Fruit Salad, 250
    Exchange value, 316
    Honey Vanilla Ice Cream, 255
    Mixed Fruit Bran Bars, 121
    Peanut Butter Apple Crisp, 224
    Pear, Apple & Raisin Strudel, 228
    Phyllo Apple Pie, 209
    Soft Apple Cinnamon Cookies,
      88
    Sour Cream Apple Pie, 210–11
    Sour Cream Orange Apple
      Cake, 166–67
    Spiced Angel Food Cake, 157
    Streusel Apple Muffins, 1
Applesauce
    Applesauce Carrot Cake, 178–79
    Applesauce Spice Cookies, 109

Banana Applesauce Muffins, 5
Blueberry Peach Cake, 164
Chocolate Brownies, 151
Cinnamon Streusel Coffee Cake, 188–89
Exchange value, 316
Low-Fat Applesauce Raisin Bread, 36
Raisin & Applesauce Squares, 138
replacing oil with, 185
Spicy Apple Cupcakes, 183
Streusel Apple Muffins, 1
Applesauce Carrot Cake, 178–79
Applesauce Spice Cookies, 109
Apricot Coconut Bars, 126–27
Apricot Date Biscotti, 51
Apricot Date Streusel Cake, 186–87
Apricots
Almond Butter Cereal Squares, 142
Apricot Coconut Bars, 126–27
Apricot Date Biscotti, 51
Apricot Date Streusel Cake, 186–87
Apricot Seed Bars, 125
Crunchy Apricot Oat Drops, 85
Exchange value, 317
Fiber-Power Biscotti, 52–53
Fluffy Apricot Soufflé with Raspberry Sauce, 238–39
Fruited Barm Brack, 37
Mixed Fruit Bran Bars, 121
Apricot Seed Bars, 125
Artificial sweeteners, 153, 307–8

Baked Granola Apples, 230
Baking powder and baking soda
leavening properties, 23, 111
sodium in, xiii
Balsamic Strawberry Sauce, 252
Banana Applesauce Muffins, 5

Banana Cake with Lemon Cream Frosting, 168–69
Banana Chocolate Chunk Muffins, 10
Banana Cream Tiramisu, 287
Banana Date Cake, 176
Banana Date Muffins, 3
Banana Nut Raisin Loaf, 29
Bananas
Banana Applesauce Muffins, 5
Banana Cake with Lemon Cream Frosting, 168–69
Banana Chocolate Chunk Muffins, 10
Banana Cream Tiramisu, 287
Banana Date Cake, 176
Banana Date Muffins, 3
Banana Nut Raisin Loaf, 29
Banana Spice Cake, 174–75
Banana Strawberry Mousse, 274
Banana Walnut Bread, 40
Big-Batch Banana Blueberry Muffins, 4
Blender Breakfast Blast, 295
Blueberry Banana Muffins, 6
Blueberry Banana Oat Bread, 33
Chocolate Chunk Banana Brownies, 146
Creamy Dreamy Fruit Salad, 250
Exchange value, 316
Fruity Oatmeal Cookies, 81
Maple Custard with Fresh Fruit, 280
Oat Bran Banana Bread, 38–39
Peachy Banana Shake, 298
Peanut Butter & Banana Smoothie, 297
Raspberry Sauce, 238–39
ripe, freezing, 4
Strawberry Sauce, 199
Tangy Banana Cheesecake, 201
Triple B Health Muffins, 17
Banana Spice Cake, 174–75
Banana Strawberry Mousse, 274
Banana Walnut Bread, 40

Bars
Almond Butter Cereal Squares, 142
Almond Shortbread Squares, 140
Almond Spice Shortbread, 69
Apple Cinnamon Bars, 122–23
Apricot Coconut Bars, 126–27
Apricot Seed Bars, 125
Berry Cheesecake Bars, 136
Chocolate Brownies, 151
Chocolate Chunk Banana Brownies, 146
Chocolate Hazelnut Bars, 134
Chocolate Shortbread Bars, 132
Christmas Brownies, 144
Chunky Chocolate Shortbread, 73
Coconut Seeds Cereal Squares, 141
Cornmeal Shortbread, 72
Cream Cheese–Filled Brownies, 150
Crispy Granola Squares, 143
cutting, after cooling, 68
cutting into correct portion sizes, 127
Date Nut Bars, 128
Date Oatmeal Squares, 137
Granola Bars, 129
Hazelnut Shortbread Bars, 133
Lemon Poppy Seed Squares, 139
Mixed Fruit Bran Bars, 121
Moist 'n' Chewy Chocolate Brownies, 145
Nutty Shortbread Bars, 131
Oatmeal Shortbread, 68
Orange Cream Cheese Brownies, 152–53
Peanut Butter–Coconut-Raisin Granola Bars, 130
Pick-Me-Up Bars, 124
Raisin & Applesauce Squares, 138
Rice Flour Shortbread, 71

Sour Cream Brownies, 149
Toffee Bars, 135
Triple Chocolate Brownies, 147
White Chocolate Brownies, 148
Berries. See also Blueberries; Cranberries; Raspberries; Strawberries
antioxidants and fiber in, 217
Berry Cheesecake Bars, 136
Fresh Fruit Tart, 218
Oat Berry Muffins, 20
Orange Sabayon with Fresh Berries, 286
Sour Cream & Berry Pie, 212
Sweetheart Berry Pie, 217
Berry Cheesecake Bars, 136
Best-Ever Chocolate Cookies, 96
Beta-carotene, 30
Beverages
Blender Breakfast Blast, 295
Frosty Chocolate Shake, 300
Frosty Strawberry Shake, 301
Hot Mulled Cider, 303
Lemon Iced Tea, 305
Old-Fashioned Chocolate Soda, 299
Peach Melba Smoothie, 296
Peachy Banana Shake, 298
Peanut Butter & Banana Smoothie, 297
Perfect Cup of Cocoa, A, 302
Spiced Iced Tea, 304
Big-Batch Banana Blueberry Muffins, 4
Biscotti
Apricot Date Biscotti, 51
Chocolate Cherry Biscotti, 60
Chocolate Chip Orange Biscotti, 61
Chocolate-Wrapped Ginger Biscotti, 64–65
Fiber-Power Biscotti, 52–53
Gingerbread Biscotti, 63
Holiday Biscotti, 66–67
Italian origins of, 65
Lemon Almond Biscotti, 55

Lemon & Lime Poppy Seed
Biscotti, 54
Maple Walnut Biscotti, 58–59
Mini Hazelnut Biscotti, 56
Pecan Biscotti, 57
Two-Tone Chocolate Orange
Biscotti, 62
Biscuits
Lemon Yogurt Biscuits, 48
Pecan Cinnamon Biscuits, 49
Whole Wheat Poppy Biscuits,
47
Blackberries
antioxidants and fiber in, 217
Orange Sabayon with Fresh
Berries, 286
Sweetheart Berry Pie, 217
Blender Breakfast Blast, 295
Blueberries
antioxidants in, 35, 217
Big-Batch Banana Blueberry
Muffins, 4
Blueberry Apple Crisp, 220
Blueberry Banana Muffins, 6
Blueberry Banana Oat Bread, 33
Blueberry Buckwheat Bread, 34
Blueberry Flan, 289
Blueberry Honey Cake, 163
Blueberry Lemon Cornmeal
Muffins, 8
Blueberry Peach Cake, 164
Blueberry Strawberry Pear Crisp,
222
Blueberry Wheat Germ Muffins,
14
Cocoa Roll with Creamy Cheese
& Berries, 242–43
Exchange value, 316
fiber in, 217
Fresh Fruit Parfait, 251
Lemon Blueberry Panna Cotta,
285
Mango Blueberry Strudel, 229
Mennonite Streusel Cake,
190–91

Orange Sabayon with Fresh
Berries, 286
Peach & Blueberry Crisp, 223
Peach Blueberry Quick Bread,
35
storing, 223
Sweetheart Berry Pie, 217
Triple B Health Muffins, 17
washing, 223
Blueberry Apple Crisp, 220
Blueberry Banana Muffins, 6
Blueberry Banana Oat Bread, 33
Blueberry Buckwheat Bread, 34
Blueberry Flan, 289
Blueberry Honey Cake, 163
Blueberry Lemon Cornmeal Muffins, 8
Blueberry Peach Cake, 164
Blueberry Strawberry Pear Crisp, 222
Blueberry Wheat Germ Muffins, 14
Bran. See Bran cereal; Bran flakes
cereal; Oat bran; Wheat bran
Bran cereal
Apricot Date Streusel Cake,
186–87
Banana Date Cake, 176
Best-Ever Chocolate Cookies,
96
Date Oatmeal Squares, 137
Exchange value, 316
Fiber-Power Biscotti, 52–53
note about, 76
Pumpkin Bran Muffins, 18–19
Yogurt Bran Muffins, 16
Bran flakes cereal
Almond Butter Cereal Squares,
142
Banana Date Muffins, 3
Exchange value, 316
Mixed Fruit Bran Bars, 121
note about, 76
Oatmeal Date Cookies, 83
Oatmeal Orange Coconut
Cookies, 76
Peanut Butter–Coconut-Raisin
Granola Bars, 130

Bread pudding
    Rhubarb Bread Pudding, 241
Breads. *See also* Muffins
    Banana Nut Raisin Loaf, 29
    Banana Walnut Bread, 40
    Blueberry Banana Oat Bread, 33
    Blueberry Buckwheat Bread, 34
    Carrot, Apple & Coconut Loaf,
      30
    Carrot Pineapple Zucchini Loaf,
      27
    cutting into correct portion sizes,
      <u>26</u>
    Fruited Barm Brack, 37
    Irish Whole Wheat Soda Bread,
      41
    Lemon Poppy Seed Loaf, 28
    Lemon Yogurt Biscuits, 48
    Low-Fat Applesauce Raisin
      Bread, 36
    Oat Bran Banana Bread, 38–39
    Peach Blueberry Quick Bread, 35
    Pecan Cinnamon Biscuits, 49
    Poppy Seed Oat Bread, 32
    Pumpkin Molasses Raisin Loaf,
      26
    Pumpkin Raisin Scones, 44–45
    Pumpkin Spice Nut Bread,
      42–43
    Rhubarb Orange Bread, 31
    Scottish Oatmeal Scones, 46
    Whole Wheat Poppy Biscuits, 47
Breakfast
    Apple Pecan Streusel Cake,
      184–85
    Apricot Date Streusel Cake,
      186–87
    Banana Applesauce Muffins, 5
    Banana Chocolate Chunk
      Muffins, 10
    Banana Date Muffins, 3
    Big-Batch Banana Blueberry
      Muffins, 4
    Blender Breakfast Blast, 295
    Blueberry Banana Muffins, 6

    Blueberry Lemon Cornmeal
      Muffins, 8
    Blueberry Wheat Germ Muffins,
      14
    Chocolate Chip Oatmeal
      Muffins, 9
    Chocolate Chunk Coffee Cake,
      196–97
    Chocolate Marble Coffee Cake,
      198
    Cinnamon Date Coffee Cake,
      194–95
    Cinnamon Streusel Coffee Cake,
      188–89
    Honey Whole Wheat Muffins, 13
    Kiwi Raspberry Muffins, 7
    Mennonite Streusel Cake,
      190–91
    Oat Berry Muffins, 20
    Orange Coffee Cake, 193
    Orange Cranberry Muffins, 2
    Orange-Glazed Coffee Cake,
      192
    Peach Melba Smoothie, 296
    Peachy Banana Shake, 298
    Peanut Butter & Banana
      Smoothie, 297
    Peanut Butter Surprise Muffins,
      11
    Perfect Bran Muffins, 15
    Pineapple Carrot Date Muffins, 21
    Pumpkin Bran Muffins, 18–19
    Streusel Apple Muffins, 1
    Sunrise Zucchini Muffins, 22–23
    Sweet Potato Muffins, 24–25
    Triple B Health Muffins, 17
    Wheat Muffins, 12
    Yogurt Bran Muffins, 16
Brownies
    Chocolate Brownies, 151
    Christmas Brownies, 144
    Cream Cheese–Filled Brownies,
      150
    Moist 'n' Chewy Chocolate
      Brownies, 145

Orange Cream Cheese Brownies, 152–53
Raspberry Brownie Parfait, 278
Sour Cream Brownies, 149
Triple Chocolate Brownies, 147
White Chocolate Brownies, 148
Brown rice syrup, about, 142
Brown sugar
    Exchange value, 318
    measuring, 53
Buckwheat flour
    Blueberry Buckwheat Bread, 34
Butter
    creaming with sugar, 69
    Exchange value, 318
    replacing, with margarine, 185
    saturated fat in, xii
Buttermilk
    Exchange value, 317
    sour milk substitute for, 18
    Strawberry Orange Buttermilk Sorbet, 264
Butterscotch chips
    Pick-Me-Up Bars, 124

C

Cakes
    Angel Tunnel Cake, 158
    Apple Pecan Streusel Cake, 184–85
    Applesauce Carrot Cake, 178–79
    Apricot Date Streusel Cake, 186–87
    Banana Cake with Lemon Cream Frosting, 168–69
    Banana Date Cake, 176
    Banana Spice Cake, 174–75
    Blueberry Honey Cake, 163
    Blueberry Peach Cake, 164
    Carrot Cake, 177
    Chiffon Cake, 160
    Chocolate Angel Food Cake, 156
    Chocolate Cheesecake, 204–5

Chocolate Chunk Coffee Cake, 196–97
Chocolate Espresso Cake, 162
Chocolate Marble Coffee Cake, 198
Chocolate Marble Vanilla Cheesecake, 206
Chocolate Zucchini Cake, 181
Cinnamon Date Coffee Cake, 194–95
Cinnamon Streusel Coffee Cake, 188–89
Cocoa Roll with Creamy Cheese & Berries, 242–43
cutting into correct portion sizes, 171
Date Cake with Coconut Topping, 170–71
Fruit-Filled Angel Tunnel Cake, 159
Ice Cream Fantasy Cake, 259
Individual Miniature Cheesecakes, 207
La Costa Cheesecake with Strawberry Sauce, 199
Marble Mocha Cheesecake, 202–3
Mennonite Streusel Cake, 190–91
Orange Cappuccino Pudding Cake, 281
Orange Coffee Cake, 193
Orange-Glazed Coffee Cake, 192
Orange Pumpkin Snacking Cake, 165
Peppermint Angel Cupcakes, 182
Perfect Angel Food Cake, 155
Piña Colada Snacking Cake, 180
Prune Orange Spice Cake, 172–73
Raspberry Cheesecake, 200
Sour Cream Orange Apple Cake, 166–67

Cakes (*cont*)
    Spiced Angel Food Cake, 157
    Spicy Apple Cupcakes, 183
    Striped Strawberry Cake, 161
    Tangy Banana Cheesecake, 201
Calcium, 311
Canola oil, xii
Cantaloupe
    Coupe Bircher, 231
    Exchange value, 316
    Melon Balls with Ginger Sauce, 240
Carbohydrates
    daily intake, in diabetes meal plan, x
    listed on food labels, 309
    sources of, x, xii
    types of, in desserts, xii
Carrot, Apple & Coconut Loaf, 30
Carrot Cake, 177
Carrot Pineapple Zucchini Loaf, 27
Carrots
    Applesauce Carrot Cake, 178–79
    beta-carotene and Vitamin A in, 30
    Carrot, Apple & Coconut Loaf, 30
    Carrot Cake, 177
    Carrot Pineapple Zucchini Loaf, 27
    Charlie & Emma's Favorite Carrot Cookies, 118
    Exchange value, 317
    Pineapple Carrot Date Muffins, 21
Charlie & Emma's Favorite Carrot Cookies, 118
Cheese. *See also* Cottage cheese; Cream cheese; Ricotta cheese
    Exchange values, 319
    measuring, note about, 53
Cheesecake
    Berry Cheesecake Bars, 136
    Chocolate Cheesecake, 204–5

Chocolate Marble Vanilla Cheesecake, 206
Individual Miniature Cheese-cakes, 207
La Costa Cheesecake with Strawberry Sauce, 199
Marble Mocha Cheesecake, 202–3
Raspberry Cheesecake, 200
Tangy Banana Cheesecake, 201
Cherries
    Cherry Cobbler, 225
    Chocolate Cherry Biscotti, 60
Cherry Cobbler, 225
Chiffon Cake, 160
Chocolate
    Angel Tunnel Cake, 158
    Banana Chocolate Chunk Muffins, 10
    Banana Cream Tiramisu, 287
    Chocolate Angel Food Cake, 156
    Chocolate Bavarian Pie, 276–77
    Chocolate Brownies, 151
    Chocolate Cheesecake, 204–5
    Chocolate Cherry Biscotti, 60
    Chocolate Chip Oatmeal Muffins, 9
    Chocolate Chip Orange Biscotti, 61
    Chocolate Chip Refrigerator Cookies, 98–99
    chocolate chips, mini, note about, 99
    Chocolate Chunk Banana Brownies, 146
    Chocolate Chunk Coffee Cake, 196–97
    Chocolate Coffee Tiramisu, 288
    chocolate cookie crumb pie shell, 276
    Chocolate Crêpes, 292
    Chocolate Espresso Cake, 162
    Chocolate Fondue, 246
    Chocolate Hazelnut Bars, 134

Chocolate Marble Coffee Cake, 198
Chocolate Marble Vanilla Cheesecake, 206
Chocolate Quesadillas, 244
Chocolate Sauce, 293
Chocolate Shortbread Bars, 132
Chocolate-Wrapped Ginger Biscotti, 64–65
Chocolate Zucchini Cake, 181
Chunky Chocolate Shortbread, 73
Cocoa Kisses, 102
Cocoa Roll with Creamy Cheese & Berries, 242–43
Cream Cheese–Filled Brownies, 150
Crispy Granola Squares, 143
Double Chocolate Raisin Cookies, 97
Exchange value, 319
Flying Saucers, 258
Frosty Chocolate Shake, 300
Frozen Jamoca Mousse, 270
Fruity Oatmeal Cookies, 81
Ice Cream Fantasy Cake, 259
Marble Mocha Cheesecake, 202–3
Mocha Ice Cream, 256
Moist 'n' Chewy Chocolate Brownies, 145
Old-Fashioned Chocolate Soda, 299
Orange Cappuccino Pudding Cake, 281
Orange Cream Cheese Brownies, 152–53
Peanut Butter Chocolate Chip Cookies, 107
Peanut Butter Fudge Cookies, 106
Perfect Cup of Cocoa, A, 302
Poached Pears in Chocolate Sauce, 234
Quick Chocolate Mousse, 269

Raspberry Brownie Parfait, 278
Rocky Road Mousse, 271
Rugelach (Cinnamon Chocolate Twist Cookies), 100–101
Sour Cream Brownies, 149
Strawberry Delights, 247
substituting cocoa powder for, 151
Toffee Bars, 135
Triple Chocolate Brownies, 147
Two-Tone Chocolate Orange Biscotti, 62
Chocolate, white
    Best-Ever Chocolate Cookies, 96
    Christmas Brownies, 144
    Exchange value, 319
    White Chocolate Brownies, 148
    White Chocolate Cranberry Drops, 103
Chocolate Angel Food Cake, 156
Chocolate Bavarian Pie, 276–77
Chocolate Brownies, 151
Chocolate Cheesecake, 204–5
Chocolate Cherry Biscotti, 60
Chocolate Chip Oatmeal Muffins, 9
Chocolate Chip Orange Biscotti, 61
Chocolate Chip Refrigerator Cookies, 98–99
Chocolate Chunk Banana Brownies, 146
Chocolate Chunk Coffee Cake, 196–97
Chocolate Coffee Tiramisu, 288
Chocolate Crêpes, 292
Chocolate Espresso Cake, 162
Chocolate Fondue, 246
Chocolate Hazelnut Bars, 134
Chocolate Marble Coffee Cake, 198
Chocolate Marble Vanilla Cheesecake, 206
Chocolate Quesadillas, 244
Chocolate Sauce, 293
Chocolate Shortbread Bars, 132
Chocolate-Wrapped Ginger Biscotti, 64–65

Chocolate Zucchini Cake, 181
Christmas Brownies, 144
Chunky Chocolate Shortbread, 73
Cider
    Hot Mulled Cider, 303
Cinnamon
    Apple Cinnamon Bars, 122–23
    Cinnamon Cream, 291
    Cinnamon Date Coffee Cake,
        194–95
    Cinnamon Streusel Coffee Cake,
        188–89
    Pecan Cinnamon Biscuits, 49
    Rugelach (Cinnamon Chocolate
        Twist Cookies), 100–101
    Soft Apple Cinnamon Cookies,
        88
Cinnamon Cream, 291
Cinnamon Date Coffee Cake,
    194–95
Cinnamon Streusel Coffee Cake,
    188–89
Cobblers
    Cherry Cobbler, 225
    Strawberry Rhubarb Cobbler,
        226–27
Cocoa Kisses, 102
Cocoa Roll with Creamy Cheese &
    Berries, 242–43
Coconut
    Apricot Coconut Bars, 126–27
    Carrot, Apple & Coconut Loaf,
        30
    Coconut Seeds Cereal Squares,
        141
    Crispy Granola Squares, 143
    Crunchy Apricot Oat Drops, 85
    Date Cake with Coconut
        Topping, 170–71
    Exchange value, 318
    Indian-Style Rice Pudding, 282
    Oatmeal Orange Coconut
        Cookies, 76
    Peanut Butter–Coconut-Raisin
        Granola Bars, 130

Piña Colada Snacking Cake, 180
    Toffee Bars, 135
Coconut milk
    Indian-Style Rice Pudding, 282
    light, buying, 282
    saturated fat in, 282
Coconut Seeds Cereal Squares, 141
Coffee
    Chocolate Coffee Tiramisu, 288
    Chocolate Espresso Cake, 162
    Frozen Jamoca Mousse, 270
    Marble Mocha Cheesecake,
        202–3
    Mocha Ice Cream, 256
    Orange Cappuccino Pudding
        Cake, 281
    Orange Coffee Pecan Slices, 92
Coffee cakes
    Apple Pecan Streusel Cake,
        184–85
    Apricot Date Streusel Cake,
        186–87
    Chocolate Chunk Coffee Cake,
        196–97
    Chocolate Marble Coffee Cake,
        198
    Cinnamon Date Coffee Cake,
        194–95
    Cinnamon Streusel Coffee Cake,
        188–89
    Mennonite Streusel Cake,
        190–91
    Orange Coffee Cake, 193
    Orange-Glazed Coffee Cake,
        192
Cookie calculator, xiii–xv
Cookies. See also Bars; Biscotti
    Applesauce Spice Cookies, 109
    baking, tip for, 85
    Best-Ever Chocolate Cookies, 96
    Charlie & Emma's Favorite
        Carrot Cookies, 118
    Chocolate Chip Refrigerator
        Cookies, 98–99
    Cocoa Kisses, 102

Cranberry Orange Oatmeal
Cookies, 84
Cranberry Pecan Oatmeal
Cookies, 77
Crisp Nut Cookies, 93
Crispy Oatmeal Cookies, 75
Crunchy Apricot Oat Drops, 85
Date Roll-Up Cookies, 86–87
Diced Rhubarb Cookies, 117
Double Chocolate Raisin
Cookies, 97
Fruity Oatmeal Cookies, 81
Ginger Cookies, 111
Lemon Cranberry Pistachio
Wafers, 91
Lemon Lime Cookies, 89
Lemon Poppy Seed Balls, 90
Maple Walnut Slice 'n' Bake
Cookies, 94–95
Meringue Candy Canes, 119
Oat Bran Raisin Cookies, 80
Oatmeal Date Cookies, 83
Oatmeal Lace Pennies, 82
Oatmeal Orange Coconut
Cookies, 76
Oatmeal Pecan Shortbread, 70
Oatmeal Raisin Cookies, 78
Oatmeal Raisin Pecan Cookies,
79
Orange Coffee Pecan Slices, 92
Peanut Butter Chip Cookies, 108
Peanut Butter Chocolate Chip
Cookies, 107
Peanut Butter Cookies, 104
Peanut Butter Flaxseed Cookies,
105
Peanut Butter Fudge Cookies,
106
portion sizes, cookie calculator
for, xiii–xv
rolling out, tip for, 89
Rugelach (Cinnamon Chocolate
Twist Cookies), 100–101
Sesame Seed Cookies, 115
Sesame Snap Wafers, 116

Soft Apple Cinnamon Cookies,
88
Spicy Gingersnaps, 112–13
Tulip Cookies with Fruit Sorbet,
265
Vanilla Almond Snaps, 114
White Chocolate Cranberry
Drops, 103
Whole Wheat Spice Cookies,
110
Corn flakes cereal
Banana Date Muffins, 3
Oatmeal Date Cookies, 83
Oatmeal Orange Coconut
Cookies, 76
Cornmeal
Blueberry Lemon Cornmeal
Muffins, 8
Cornmeal Pudding, 284
Cornmeal Shortbread, 72
Exchange value, 316
Peanut Butter Surprise Muffins,
11
Cornmeal Pudding, 284
Cornmeal Shortbread, 72
Cottage cheese
Chocolate Cheesecake, 204–5
Chocolate Marble Vanilla
Cheesecake, 206
Exchange value, 319
Individual Miniature Cheese-
cakes, 207
La Costa Cheesecake with
Strawberry Sauce, 199
measuring, 53
Raspberry Cheesecake, 200
Tangy Banana Cheesecake, 201
Coupe Bircher, 231
Cranberries
Apple, Pear & Cranberry Crisp,
221
Apricot Seed Bars, 125
Christmas Brownies, 144
Cranberry Orange Oatmeal
Cookies, 84

Cranberries (*cont*)

    Cranberry Pecan Oatmeal Cookies, 77

    Crispy Oatmeal Cookies, 75

    Exchange value, 317

    freezing, before chopping, 84

    Fruited Barm Brack, 37

    Lemon Cranberry Pistachio Wafers, 91

    Mixed Fruit Bran Bars, 121

    Orange Cranberry Muffins, 2

    Spiced Angel Food Cake, 157

    White Chocolate Brownies, 148

    White Chocolate Cranberry Drops, 103

Cranberry Orange Oatmeal Cookies, 84

Cranberry Pecan Oatmeal Cookies, 77

Cream cheese

    Banana Spice Cake, 174–75

    Berry Cheesecake Bars, 136

    Chocolate Coffee Tiramisu, 288

    Cream Cheese–Filled Brownies, 150

    Creamy Pumpkin Cheese Pie, 214–15

    Exchange value, 318

    fat-free, note about, 203

    Fruit on a Cloud, 248–49

    Marble Mocha Cheesecake, 202–3

    Orange Cream Cheese Brownies, 152–53

    reduced-fat, buying, 203

    Strawberry Delights, 247

Cream Cheese–Filled Brownies, 150

Creamy Dreamy Fruit Salad, 250

Creamy Pumpkin Cheese Pie, 214–15

Crêpes

    Chocolate Crêpes, 292

Crisp Nut Cookies, 93

Crisp rice cereal

    B vitamins in, 143

    Crispy Granola Squares, 143

    Crunchy Apricot Oat Drops, 85

Crisps

    Apple, Pear & Cranberry Crisp, 221

    Blueberry Apple Crisp, 220

    Blueberry Strawberry Pear Crisp, 222

    Peach & Blueberry Crisp, 223

    Peanut Butter Apple Crisp, 224

Crispy Granola Squares, 143

Crispy Oatmeal Cookies, 75

Crunchy Apricot Oat Drops, 85

Cupcakes

    Peppermint Angel Cupcakes, 182

    Spicy Apple Cupcakes, 183

Currants

    Applesauce Spice Cookies, 109

    Fruited Barm Brack, 37

Custards and flans

    Blueberry Flan, 289

    Maple Custard with Fresh Fruit, 280

    Maple Flan with Walnuts, 290

    Pumpkin Custard, 279

    Pumpkin Flan, 291

D

Dairy products. *See also* Cheese; Sour cream; Yogurt

    fat-free, note about, 203

    measuring, note about, 53

Date Cake with Coconut Topping, 170–71

Date Nut Bars, 128

Date Oatmeal Squares, 137

Date Roll-Up Cookies, 86–87

Dates

    Apricot Date Biscotti, 51

    Apricot Date Streusel Cake, 186–87

    Banana Date Cake, 176

    Banana Date Muffins, 3

    chopping, tip for, 170

Date Cake with Coconut Topping, 170–71
Date Nut Bars, 128
Date Oatmeal Squares, 137
Date Roll-Up Cookies, 86–87
Exchange value, 317
Granola Bars, 129
Mixed Fruit Bran Bars, 121
Oatmeal Date Cookies, 83
Pineapple Carrot Date Muffins, 21
Dessert Nachos, 245
Diabetes
    eating away from home and, 101, 257
    effective management of, x
    exercise and, 312
    healthy eating recommendations, x–xii
    information and resources, xv, 43
    planning and preparing meals, 205, 257
    referral sources, 43
    three types of, ix
Diced Rhubarb Cookies, 117
Double Chocolate Raisin Cookies, 97

E

Eggs
    Exchange value, 319
    raw, in recipes, note about, 260
    separating, tip for, 119
    size, for recipes, 61
    whites, beating, 119
    whites, warming to room temperature, 119
Exchanges
    cookie calculator and, xii–xv
    estimating, for favorite recipes, 313–15
    for recipe ingredients, 316–19
    ingredient measurements and, xiii

swapping, to make room for dessert, xiii
Exercise, 312

F

Fats, dietary
    daily intake, in diabetes meal plan, xi
    Exchange values, 318
    lowering, in recipes, tips for, 185
    monounsaturated fats, xi, 43
    omega-3 fatty acids, xii, 39
    polyunsaturated fats, xi
    saturated fats, xi, xii, 185, 282
    trans fats, xi, xii, 185
    types of, in desserts, xii
Fiber
    daily intake, in diabetes meal plan, x
    foods high in, xii, 16, 25, 217, 231
Fiber-Power Biscotti, 52–53
Flans
    Blueberry Flan, 289
    Maple Flan with Walnuts, 290
    Pumpkin Flan, 291
Flaxseed
    Almond Butter Cereal Squares, 142
    Apricot Seed Bars, 125
    Big-Batch Banana Blueberry Muffins, 4
    Charlie & Emma's Favorite Carrot Cookies, 118
    Chocolate Chip Oatmeal Muffins, 9
    Coconut Seeds Cereal Squares, 141
    Exchange value, 318
    Fruity Oatmeal Cookies, 81
    ground, buying and storing, 39
    Oat Bran Banana Bread, 38–39
    omega-3 fatty acids in, 39

Flaxseed (*cont*)
Peanut Butter Flaxseed Cookies, 105
Pumpkin Bran Muffins, 18–19
Flour. *See also* Whole wheat flour
Blueberry Buckwheat Bread, 34
Exchange value, 316
gluten in, 243
measuring, 53
Rice Flour Shortbread, 71
self-rising, substitute for, 181
white, about, 23
white, history of, 123
white, replacing with whole wheat flour, 16
Fluffy Apricot Soufflé with Raspberry Sauce, 238–39
Flying Saucers, 258
Fondue
Chocolate Fondue, 246
Food labels
nutrition claims on, 309–10
nutrition facts tables, 308, 311
reading, 308, 309–10
serving sizes on, 309
sugars listed on, 308
Fools
Mango Raspberry Fool, 275
Free radicals, 312
Fresh Fruit Parfait, 251
Fresh Fruit Sorbet, 261
Fresh Fruit Tart, 218
Fried Pineapple, 232
Frostings
Lemon Cream Frosting, 168–69
Frosty Chocolate Shake, 300
Frosty Strawberry Shake, 301
Frozen desserts
Flying Saucers, 258
Fresh Fruit Sorbet, 261
Frozen Jamoca Mousse, 270
Frozen Lemon Pie, 267
Frozen Orange Cream, 257
Frozen Vanilla Yogurt, 268
Honey Vanilla Ice Cream, 255

Ice Cream Fantasy Cake, 259
Lemon Sherbet, 260
Mocha Ice Cream, 256
Pineapple Lime Sorbet, 262
Raspberry Ice with Fresh Strawberries, 266
Strawberry Orange Buttermilk Sorbet, 264
Strawberry Sorbet, 263
Tulip Cookies with Fruit Sorbet, 265
Frozen Jamoca Mousse, 270
Frozen Lemon Pie, 267
Frozen Orange Cream, 257
Frozen Vanilla Yogurt, 268
Fructose
buying, 213
effect on blood sugar, 163
Exchange value, 318
Fruit. *See also* Fruit desserts; *specific fruits*
dried, cutting into small pieces, 25
dried, Exchange values, 317
Exchange values, 316–17
Fresh Fruit Sorbet, 261
Fresh Fruit Tart, 218
frozen unsweetened, buying, 239
Fruited Barm Brack, 37
Fruit-Filled Angel Tunnel Cake, 159
fruit juices, Exchange values, 316–17
Fruity Oatmeal Cookies, 81
grilling and serving, 252
Maple Custard with Fresh Fruit, 280
Mixed Fruit Bran Bars, 121
soluble fiber in, 231
Tropical Fruit Tart, 219
Fruit desserts
Apple, Pear & Cranberry Crisp, 221
Baked Granola Apples, 230
Balsamic Strawberry Sauce, 252
Blueberry Apple Crisp, 220

Blueberry Strawberry Pear Crisp, 222
Cherry Cobbler, 225
Chocolate Fondue, 246
Coupe Bircher, 231
Creamy Dreamy Fruit Salad, 250
Dessert Nachos, 245
Fluffy Apricot Soufflé with Raspberry Sauce, 238–39
Fresh Fruit Parfait, 251
Fried Pineapple, 232
Fruit on a Cloud, 248–49
Key Lime Dessert, 236–37
Mango Blueberry Strudel, 229
Melon Balls with Ginger Sauce, 240
Peach & Blueberry Crisp, 223
Peanut Butter Apple Crisp, 224
Pear, Apple & Raisin Strudel, 228
Pears in Tosca Sauce, 233
Poached Pears in Chocolate Sauce, 234
Rhubarb Bread Pudding, 241
Strawberry Delights, 247
Strawberry Rhubarb Cobbler, 226–27
Tropical Parfait, 251
Wine-Poached Pear Fans, 235
Fruited Barm Brack, 37
Fruit-Filled Angel Tunnel Cake, 159
Fruit on a Cloud, 248–49
Fruity Oatmeal Cookies, 81

Gingerbread Biscotti, 63
Ginger Cookies, 111
Ginger Sauce, 240
Graham Wafer Crust, 267
Graham wafers and crumbs
Chocolate Cheesecake, 204–5
Christmas Brownies, 144
Creamy Pumpkin Cheese Pie, 214–15
Exchange value, 319
Frozen Lemon Pie, 267
Graham Wafer Crust, 267
Pick-Me-Up Bars, 124
Rocky Road Mousse, 271
Sour Cream Apple Pie, 210–11
Strawberry Mousse Pie, 216
Grains. See also Bran; Cornmeal; Oats; Wheat germ; Whole wheat flour
Blueberry Buckwheat Bread, 34
Exchange value, 316
fiber in, xii, 16, 25
Indian-Style Rice Pudding, 282
Granola
Baked Granola Apples, 230
Date Nut Bars, 128
Exchange value, 316
Granola Bars, 129
Granola bars
Crispy Granola Squares, 143
Granola Bars, 129
Peanut Butter–Coconut-Raisin Granola Bars, 130
Grapes
Creamy Dreamy Fruit Salad, 250

Gelatin, working with, 212
Gestational diabetes, ix
Ginger
Chocolate-Wrapped Ginger Biscotti, 64–65
Gingerbread Biscotti, 63
Ginger Cookies, 111
Ginger Sauce, 240
Spicy Gingersnaps, 112–13

Hazelnuts
Chocolate Hazelnut Bars, 134
Exchange value, 318
Hazelnut Shortbread Bars, 133
Mini Hazelnut Biscotti, 56
removing outer skin from, 134
White Chocolate Brownies, 148

Hazelnut Shortbread Bars, 133
Holiday Biscotti, 66–67
Honey, effect on blood sugar, 163
Honeydew
    Exchange value, 316
    Melon Balls with Ginger Sauce,
    240
Honey Vanilla Ice Cream, 255
Honey Whole Wheat Muffins, 13
Hot Mulled Cider, 303

Ice cream
    Frosty Chocolate Shake, 300
    Frosty Strawberry Shake, 301
    Honey Vanilla Ice Cream, 255
    Ice Cream Fantasy Cake, 259
    Mocha Ice Cream, 256
    Old-Fashioned Chocolate Soda,
    299
    Peachy Banana Shake, 298
Ice Cream Fantasy Cake, 259
Indian-Style Rice Pudding, 282
Individual Miniature Cheesecakes, 207
Ingredients. *See also specific
    ingredients*
    Exchange values for, 316–19
    measuring, xiii, 53, 173
Irish Whole Wheat Soda Bread, 41
Italian-style recipes. *See also* Biscotti
    Banana Cream Tiramisu, 287
    Chocolate Coffee Tiramisu, 288
    Lemon Blueberry Panna Cotta,
    285
    Maple, Walnut & Pear Tiramisu,
    287

Key Lime Dessert, 236–37
Kiwifruit
    Exchange value, 316

Fresh Fruit Parfait, 251
Kiwi Raspberry Muffins, 7
Tropical Fruit Tart, 219
Kiwi Raspberry Muffins, 7

La Costa Cheesecake with Strawberry
    Sauce, 199
Ladyfingers
    Banana Cream Tiramisu, 287
    Chocolate Coffee Tiramisu, 288
    Maple, Walnut & Pear Tiramisu,
    287
Lemon Almond Biscotti, 55
Lemon Blueberry Panna Cotta, 285
Lemon Cranberry Pistachio Wafers, 91
Lemon Cream Frosting, 168–69
Lemon Iced Tea, 305
Lemon Lime Cookies, 89
Lemon & Lime Poppy Seed Biscotti,
    54
Lemon Meringue Pie, 213
Lemon Poppy Seed Balls, 90
Lemon Poppy Seed Loaf, 28
Lemon Poppy Seed Squares, 139
Lemons
    Blueberry Lemon Cornmeal
    Muffins, 8
    Frozen Lemon Pie, 267
    Lemon Almond Biscotti, 55
    Lemon Blueberry Panna Cotta,
    285
    Lemon Cranberry Pistachio
    Wafers, 91
    Lemon Cream Frosting, 168–69
    Lemon Iced Tea, 305
    Lemon Lime Cookies, 89
    Lemon & Lime Poppy Seed
    Biscotti, 54
    Lemon Meringue Pie, 213
    Lemon Poppy Seed Balls, 90
    Lemon Poppy Seed Loaf, 28
    Lemon Poppy Seed Squares, 139

Lemon Sherbet, 260
Lemon Yogurt Biscuits, 48
Sunshine Lemon Mousse,
272–73
Lemon Sherbet, 260
Lemon Yogurt Biscuits, 48
Limes
Key Lime Dessert, 236–37
Lemon Lime Cookies, 89
Lemon & Lime Poppy Seed
Biscotti, 54
Pineapple Lime Sorbet, 262
Low-Fat Applesauce Raisin Bread, 36

M

Mango Blueberry Strudel, 229
Mango Raspberry Fool, 275
Mangos
beta-carotene and Vitamin A in, 30
Exchange value, 316
Mango Blueberry Strudel, 229
Mango Raspberry Fool, 275
Tropical Fruit Tart, 219
Tropical Parfait, 251
Tulip Cookies with Fruit Sorbet,
265
Maple, Walnut & Pear Tiramisu, 287
Maple Custard with Fresh Fruit, 280
Maple extract
Maple Walnut Biscotti, 58–59
Maple Walnut Slice 'n' Bake
Cookies, 94–95
note about, 94
Maple Flan with Walnuts, 290
Maple syrup
Banana Cream Tiramisu, 287
Exchange value, 318
Maple, Walnut & Pear Tiramisu,
287
Maple Custard with Fresh Fruit,
280
Maple Flan with Walnuts, 290
Maple Walnut Biscotti, 58–59

Maple Walnut Slice 'n' Bake Cookies,
94–95
Marble Mocha Cheesecake, 202–3
Margarine
Exchange value, 318
light, note about, 85
measuring, 53
replacing butter with, 185
replacing shortening with, 185
soft (non-hydrogenated), buying, xii
solid, avoiding, 185
whipped, note about, 85
Marshmallows
Creamy Dreamy Fruit Salad, 250
Crispy Granola Squares, 143
Fruit on a Cloud, 248–49
Perfect Cup of Cocoa, A, 302
Rocky Road Mousse, 271
Measuring ingredients
dairy products, note about, 53
dry measuring cups, 53, 173
flour and sugar, method for, 53
importance of accurate mea-
surements, xiii, 173
liquid measuring cups, 53, 173
liquids, method for, 53
measuring spoons, 173
Melon
Coupe Bircher, 231
Exchange value, 316
Melon Balls with Ginger Sauce, 240
Melon Balls with Ginger Sauce, 240
Mennonite Streusel Cake, 190–91
Meringue Candy Canes, 119
Meringues
Cocoa Kisses, 102
Meringue Candy Canes, 119
Vanilla Almond Snaps, 114
Milk, Exchange value, 317
Milk, soy
choosing, note about, 296
Peach Melba Smoothie, 296
Peanut Butter & Banana
Smoothie, 297
phytochemicals in, 297

INDEX

Minerals, 311
Mini Hazelnut Biscotti, 56
Mint
    Meringue Candy Canes, 119
    Peppermint Angel Cupcakes,
        182
Mixed Fruit Bran Bars, 121
Mocha
    Frozen Jamoca Mousse, 270
    Marble Mocha Cheesecake,
        202–3
    Mocha Ice Cream, 256
Mocha Ice Cream, 256
Moist 'n' Chewy Chocolate Brownies,
    145
Monounsaturated fats, xi, 43
Mousse
    Banana Strawberry Mousse, 274
    Frozen Jamoca Mousse, 270
    Quick Chocolate Mousse, 269
    Rocky Road Mousse, 271
    Sunshine Lemon Mousse,
        272–73
Muffins
    Banana Applesauce Muffins, 5
    Banana Chocolate Chunk
        Muffins, 10
    Banana Date Muffins, 3
    Big-Batch Banana Blueberry
        Muffins, 4
    Blueberry Banana Muffins, 6
    Blueberry Lemon Cornmeal
        Muffins, 8
    Blueberry Wheat Germ Muffins,
        14
    calculating different portion
        sizes, xiv
    Chocolate Chip Oatmeal
        Muffins, 9
    Honey Whole Wheat Muffins, 13
    Kiwi Raspberry Muffins, 7
    Oat Berry Muffins, 20
    Orange Cranberry Muffins, 2
    Peanut Butter Surprise Muffins, 11
    Perfect Bran Muffins, 15

Pineapple Carrot Date Muffins,
    21
portion sizes, note about, 19
Pumpkin Bran Muffins, 18–19
Streusel Apple Muffins, 1
Sunrise Zucchini Muffins, 22–23
Sweet Potato Muffins, 24–25
Triple B Health Muffins, 17
Wheat Muffins, 12
Yogurt Bran Muffins, 16

N

Nachos
    Dessert Nachos, 245
Nut butters
    Almond Butter Cereal Squares,
        142
    note about, 87
Nutrient analyses, for recipes, 320
Nutrition claims, 309–10
Nutrition facts tables, 308, 311
Nuts. See also Almonds; Hazelnuts;
    Peanut butter; Pecans; Walnuts
    beneficial fats in, 43
    chopping fine, for baked goods,
        169
    Crisp Nut Cookies, 93
    Exchange values, 318
    Holiday Biscotti, 66–67
    Lemon Cranberry Pistachio
        Wafers, 91
    toasting, 43
    Toffee Bars, 135
Nutty Shortbread Bars, 131

O

Oat Berry Muffins, 20
Oat bran
    Apricot Coconut Bars, 126–27
    Exchange value, 316
    Oat Bran Banana Bread, 38–39

Oat Bran Raisin Cookies, 80
Triple B Health Muffins, 17
Oat Bran Banana Bread, 38–39
Oat Bran Raisin Cookies, 80
Oatmeal Date Cookies, 83
Oatmeal Lace Pennies, 82
Oatmeal Orange Coconut Cookies, 76
Oatmeal Pecan Shortbread, 70
Oatmeal Raisin Cookies, 78
Oatmeal Raisin Pecan Cookies, 79
Oatmeal Shortbread, 68
Oats
    Almond Butter Cereal Squares, 142
    Apple, Pear & Cranberry Crisp, 221
    Apple Oatmeal Pudding, 283
    Applesauce Spice Cookies, 109
    Apricot Coconut Bars, 126–27
    Apricot Seed Bars, 125
    Best-Ever Chocolate Cookies, 96
    Blueberry Apple Crisp, 220
    Blueberry Banana Oat Bread, 33
    Blueberry Strawberry Pear Crisp, 222
    Charlie & Emma's Favorite Carrot Cookies, 118
    Chocolate Chip Oatmeal Muffins, 9
    Chocolate Hazelnut Bars, 134
    Coconut Seeds Cereal Squares, 141
    Coupe Bircher, 231
    Cranberry Orange Oatmeal Cookies, 84
    Cranberry Pecan Oatmeal Cookies, 77
    Crispy Granola Squares, 143
    Crispy Oatmeal Cookies, 75
    Crunchy Apricot Oat Drops, 85
    Date Oatmeal Squares, 137
    Exchange value, 316
    Fiber-Power Biscotti, 52–53
    Fruity Oatmeal Cookies, 81

Granola Bars, 129
Oat Berry Muffins, 20
Oat Bran Raisin Cookies, 80
Oatmeal Date Cookies, 83
Oatmeal Lace Pennies, 82
Oatmeal Orange Coconut Cookies, 76
Oatmeal Pecan Shortbread, 70
Oatmeal Raisin Cookies, 78
Oatmeal Raisin Pecan Cookies, 79
Oatmeal Shortbread, 68
Peach & Blueberry Crisp, 223
Peanut Butter Apple Crisp, 224
Peanut Butter Chip Cookies, 108
Peanut Butter–Coconut-Raisin Granola Bars, 130
Pick-Me-Up Bars, 124
Pineapple Carrot Date Muffins, 21
plain, unflavored, for recipes, 21
Poppy Seed Oat Bread, 32
Scottish Oatmeal Scones, 46
shelf life, 283
Soft Apple Cinnamon Cookies, 88
soluble fiber in, 231
Sweet Potato Muffins, 24–25
Toffee Bars, 135
Oils
    Exchange values, 318
    low-fat substitutes for, 185
    types of, in desserts, xii
Old-Fashioned Chocolate Soda, 299
Omega-3 fatty acids, xii, 39
Orange Cappuccino Pudding Cake, 281
Orange Coffee Cake, 193
Orange Coffee Pecan Slices, 92
Orange Cranberry Muffins, 2
Orange Cream Cheese Brownies, 152–53
Orange-Glazed Coffee Cake, 192
Orange Pumpkin Snacking Cake, 165

Oranges
 Banana Strawberry Mousse, 274
 Chocolate Chip Orange Biscotti, 61
 Cranberry Orange Oatmeal Cookies, 84
 Creamy Dreamy Fruit Salad, 250
 Fresh Fruit Parfait, 251
 Frozen Orange Cream, 257
 juiced, yield from, 92
 juicing, tip for, 92
 Oatmeal Orange Coconut Cookies, 76
 Orange Cappuccino Pudding Cake, 281
 Orange Coffee Cake, 193
 Orange Coffee Pecan Slices, 92
 Orange Cranberry Muffins, 2
 Orange Cream Cheese Brownies, 152–53
 Orange-Glazed Coffee Cake, 192
 Orange Pumpkin Snacking Cake, 165
 Orange Sabayon with Fresh Berries, 286
 Prune Orange Spice Cake, 172–73
 Rhubarb Orange Bread, 31
 segmenting, method for, 274
 Sour Cream Orange Apple Cake, 166–67
 Strawberry Orange Buttermilk Sorbet, 264
 Two-Tone Chocolate Orange Biscotti, 62
 zested, yield from, 92
Orange Sabayon with Fresh Berries, 286
Oxidative stress, 312

Panna cotta
 Lemon Blueberry Panna Cotta, 285

Papaya
 Tropical Fruit Tart, 219
 Tropical Parfait, 251
Parchment paper, 45, 59
Parfaits
 Fresh Fruit Parfait, 251
 Raspberry Brownie Parfait, 278
 Tropical Parfait, 251
Pastries
 Mango Blueberry Strudel, 229
 Pear, Apple & Raisin Strudel, 228
Peach & Blueberry Crisp, 223
Peach Blueberry Quick Bread, 35
Peaches
 Blueberry Peach Cake, 164
 Exchange value, 317
 Maple Custard with Fresh Fruit, 280
 Peach & Blueberry Crisp, 223
 Peach Blueberry Quick Bread, 35
 Peach Melba Smoothie, 296
 Peachy Banana Shake, 298
Peach Melba Smoothie, 296
Peachy Banana Shake, 298
Peanut butter
 Exchange value, 318
 Peanut Butter Apple Crisp, 224
 Peanut Butter & Banana Smoothie, 297
 Peanut Butter Chip Cookies, 108
 Peanut Butter Chocolate Chip Cookies, 107
 Peanut Butter–Coconut-Raisin Granola Bars, 130
 Peanut Butter Cookies, 104
 Peanut Butter Flaxseed Cookies, 105
 Peanut Butter Fudge Cookies, 106
 Peanut Butter Surprise Muffins, 11
Peanut Butter Apple Crisp, 224
Peanut Butter & Banana Smoothie, 297
Peanut Butter Chip Cookies, 108

Peanut Butter Chocolate Chip
  Cookies, 107
Peanut Butter–Coconut-Raisin
  Granola Bars, 130
Peanut Butter Cookies, 104
Peanut Butter Flaxseed Cookies, 105
Peanut Butter Fudge Cookies, 106
Peanut Butter Surprise Muffins, 11
Pear, Apple & Raisin Strudel, 228
Pears
    Apple, Pear & Cranberry Crisp,
      221
    Blueberry Strawberry Pear Crisp,
      222
    Exchange value, 317
    Maple, Walnut & Pear Tiramisu,
      287
    Maple Custard with Fresh Fruit,
      280
    Pear, Apple & Raisin Strudel, 228
    Pears in Tosca Sauce, 233
    Poached Pears in Chocolate
      Sauce, 234
    Wine-Poached Pear Fans, 235
Pears in Tosca Sauce, 233
Pecan Biscotti, 57
Pecan Cinnamon Biscuits, 49
Pecans
    Apple Pecan Streusel Cake,
      184–85
    Banana Date Cake, 176
    Banana Nut Raisin Loaf, 29
    Chocolate Chip Refrigerator
      Cookies, 98–99
    Chocolate Quesadillas, 244
    Chunky Chocolate Shortbread,
      73
    Cocoa Kisses, 102
    Cranberry Pecan Oatmeal
      Cookies, 77
    Exchange value, 318
    Granola Bars, 129
    Mixed Fruit Bran Bars, 121
    Nutty Shortbread Bars, 131
    Oatmeal Pecan Shortbread, 70

Oatmeal Raisin Pecan Cookies,
  79
Orange Coffee Pecan Slices, 92
Orange Pumpkin Snacking Cake,
  165
Pecan Biscotti, 57
Pecan Cinnamon Biscuits, 49
Pumpkin Spice Nut Bread, 42–43
Peppermint
    Meringue Candy Canes, 119
    Peppermint Angel Cupcakes,
      182
Peppermint Angel Cupcakes, 182
Perfect Angel Food Cake, 155
Perfect Bran Muffins, 15
Perfect Cup of Cocoa, A, 302
Phyllo Apple Pie, 209
Phyllo pastry
    Exchange value, 319
    Mango Blueberry Strudel, 229
    Pear, Apple & Raisin Strudel,
      228
    Phyllo Apple Pie, 209
    working with, 209
Phytochemicals, 297, 312
Pick-Me-Up Bars, 124
Pies and tarts
    Chocolate Bavarian Pie, 276–77
    Creamy Pumpkin Cheese Pie,
      214–15
    Fresh Fruit Tart, 218
    Frozen Lemon Pie, 267
    Lemon Meringue Pie, 213
    Phyllo Apple Pie, 209
    Sour Cream Apple Pie, 210–11
    Sour Cream & Berry Pie, 212
    Strawberry Mousse Pie, 216
    Sweetheart Berry Pie, 217
    Tropical Fruit Tart, 219
Pie shells and crusts
    chocolate cookie crumb pie
      shell, 276
    Exchange value, 319
    Graham Wafer Crust, 267
Piña Colada Snacking Cake, 180

Pineapple
Carrot Pineapple Zucchini Loaf, 27
Creamy Dreamy Fruit Salad, 250
Exchange value, 317
Fresh Fruit Parfait, 251
Fried Pineapple, 232
Piña Colada Snacking Cake, 180
Pineapple Carrot Date Muffins, 21
Pineapple Lime Sorbet, 262
puréed, preparing, 262
Tropical Parfait, 251
Pineapple Carrot Date Muffins, 21
Pineapple Lime Sorbet, 262
Pistachios
Exchange value, 318
Holiday Biscotti, 66–67
Lemon Cranberry Pistachio Wafers, 91
Poached Pears in Chocolate Sauce, 234
Polyunsaturated fats, xi
Poppy Seed Oat Bread, 32
Poppy seeds
Lemon & Lime Poppy Seed Biscotti, 54
Lemon Poppy Seed Balls, 90
Lemon Poppy Seed Loaf, 28
Lemon Poppy Seed Squares, 139
Poppy Seed Oat Bread, 32
Whole Wheat Poppy Biscuits, 47
Portion sizes, xiv–xv, 19, 26, 127, 171, 205, 309
Pre-diabetes, ix
Protein, in diabetes meal plan, xi–xii
Prune Orange Spice Cake, 172–73
Prunes
Exchange value, 317
Prune Orange Spice Cake, 172–73
Pudding cakes
Orange Cappuccino Pudding Cake, 281

Puddings
Apple Oatmeal Pudding, 283
Cornmeal Pudding, 284
Indian-Style Rice Pudding, 282
Rhubarb Bread Pudding, 241
Pumpkin
beta-carotene and Vitamin A in, 30
canned, buying, 19
Creamy Pumpkin Cheese Pie, 214–15
Exchange value, 317
fresh, baking, 214
Orange Pumpkin Snacking Cake, 165
Pumpkin Bran Muffins, 18–19
Pumpkin Custard, 279
Pumpkin Flan, 291
Pumpkin Molasses Raisin Loaf, 26
Pumpkin Raisin Scones, 44–45
Pumpkin Spice Nut Bread, 42–43
Pumpkin Bran Muffins, 18–19
Pumpkin Custard, 279
Pumpkin Flan, 291
Pumpkin Molasses Raisin Loaf, 26
Pumpkin Raisin Scones, 44–45
Pumpkin Spice Nut Bread, 42–43

Q

Quesadillas
Chocolate Quesadillas, 244
Quick Chocolate Mousse, 269

R

Raisin & Applesauce Squares, 138
Raisins
Apple Pecan Streusel Cake, 184–85
Applesauce Spice Cookies, 109
Banana Nut Raisin Loaf, 29

Carrot, Apple & Coconut Loaf, 30

Carrot Pineapple Zucchini Loaf, 27

Coupe Bircher, 231

Cranberry Orange Oatmeal Cookies, 84

Crispy Granola Squares, 143

Double Chocolate Raisin Cookies, 97

Exchange value, 317

Indian-Style Rice Pudding, 282

Low-Fat Applesauce Raisin Bread, 36

Oat Bran Raisin Cookies, 80

Oatmeal Orange Coconut Cookies, 76

Oatmeal Raisin Cookies, 78

Oatmeal Raisin Pecan Cookies, 79

Peanut Butter Chocolate Chip Cookies, 107

Peanut Butter–Coconut-Raisin Granola Bars, 130

Peanut Butter Fudge Cookies, 106

Pear, Apple & Raisin Strudel, 228

Perfect Bran Muffins, 15

Pumpkin Bran Muffins, 18–19

Pumpkin Molasses Raisin Loaf, 26

Pumpkin Raisin Scones, 44–45

Raisin & Applesauce Squares, 138

Rugelach (Cinnamon Chocolate Twist Cookies), 100–101

Sour Cream Orange Apple Cake, 166–67

Sunrise Zucchini Muffins, 22–23

Yogurt Bran Muffins, 16

Raspberries
antioxidants and fiber in, 217
Exchange value, 317
Kiwi Raspberry Muffins, 7
Mango Raspberry Fool, 275
Orange Sabayon with Fresh Berries, 286
Peach Melba Smoothie, 296
Raspberry Brownie Parfait, 278
Raspberry Cheesecake, 200
Raspberry Ice with Fresh Strawberries, 266
Raspberry Sauce, 238–39
Sweetheart Berry Pie, 217
Tulip Cookies with Fruit Sorbet, 265

Raspberry Brownie Parfait, 278

Raspberry Cheesecake, 200

Raspberry Ice with Fresh Strawberries, 266

Raspberry Sauce, 238–39

Recipes
adding whole wheat flour to, 16
carbohydrates in, xii
Exchange calculations, 320
Exchanges and, xiii
fats and oils in, xii
made with fat-free dairy products, note about, 203
making healthier, tips for, 185
measuring ingredients, 53, 173
nutrient analyses, 320
serving sizes, xiv–xv
sodium in, xiii

Rhubarb
Diced Rhubarb Cookies, 117
Exchange value, 317
Rhubarb Bread Pudding, 241
Rhubarb Orange Bread, 31
Strawberry Rhubarb Cobbler, 226–27

Rhubarb Bread Pudding, 241

Rhubarb Orange Bread, 31

Rice
Indian-Style Rice Pudding, 282

Rice flour
Exchange value, 316
Rice Flour Shortbread, 71

Rice Flour Shortbread, 71

Rice syrup, Exchange value, 318

INDEX

Ricotta cheese
    Chocolate Cheesecake, 204–5
    Chocolate Coffee Tiramisu, 288
    Chocolate Marble Vanilla
        Cheesecake, 206
    Cinnamon Cream, 291
    Cocoa Roll with Creamy Cheese
        & Berries, 242–43
    Creamy Pumpkin Cheese Pie,
        214–15
    Exchange value, 319
    Frozen Jamoca Mousse, 270
    Individual Miniature Cheese-
        cakes, 207
    Lemon Cream Frosting, 168–69
    Marble Mocha Cheesecake,
        202–3
    measuring, 53
    Raspberry Cheesecake, 200
Rocky Road Mousse, 271
Rugelach (Cinnamon Chocolate Twist
    Cookies), 100–101

S

Salads
    Creamy Dreamy Fruit Salad, 250
Salt, sodium in, xiii
Saturated fats, xi, xii, 185, 282
Sauces and toppings
    Chocolate Sauce, 293
    Cinnamon Cream, 291
    Ginger Sauce, 240
    Orange Sabayon with Fresh
        Berries, 286
    Raspberry Sauce, 238–39
    Strawberry Sauce, 199
    Strawberry Whipped Topping,
        276–77
    Whipped Cream & Yogurt
        Topping, 253
Scones
    Pumpkin Raisin Scones, 44–45
    Scottish Oatmeal Scones, 46

Scottish Oatmeal Scones, 46
Seeds. *See also* Flaxseed; Poppy
    seeds; Sesame seeds; Sunflower
    seeds
    Exchange values, 318
    toasting, 169
Serving sizes, xiv–xv, 19, 26, 127, 171,
    205, 309
Sesame Seed Cookies, 115
Sesame seeds
    Almond Butter Cereal Squares,
        142
    Apricot Seed Bars, 125
    Coconut Seeds Cereal Squares,
        141
    Granola Bars, 129
    Peanut Butter Cookies, 104
    Pumpkin Bran Muffins, 18–19
    Sesame Seed Cookies, 115
    Sesame Snap Wafers, 116
Sesame Snap Wafers, 116
Shakes
    Frosty Chocolate Shake, 300
    Frosty Strawberry Shake, 301
    Peachy Banana Shake, 298
Sherbet
    Lemon Sherbet, 260
    note about, 261
Shortbread
    Almond Shortbread Squares,
        140
    Almond Spice Shortbread, 69
    Chocolate Shortbread Bars, 132
    Chunky Chocolate Shortbread,
        73
    Cornmeal Shortbread, 72
    cutting, while still warm, 68
    Hazelnut Shortbread Bars, 133
    Nutty Shortbread Bars, 131
    Oatmeal Pecan Shortbread, 70
    Oatmeal Shortbread, 68
    Rice Flour Shortbread, 71
    Scottish origins of, 68
Shortening
    replacing, with margarine, 185

saturated fat in, xii
substitutes for, 45
Smoothies
Peach Melba Smoothie, 296
Peanut Butter & Banana
Smoothie, 297
Sodium
daily intake, in diabetes meal
plan, xii
types of, in desserts, xiii
Soft Apple Cinnamon Cookies, 88
Sorbet
Fresh Fruit Sorbet, 261
note about, 261
Pineapple Lime Sorbet, 262
Strawberry Orange Buttermilk
Sorbet, 264
Strawberry Sorbet, 263
Tulip Cookies with Fruit Sorbet,
265
Soufflés
Fluffy Apricot Soufflé with
Raspberry Sauce, 238–39
Sour cream
Exchange value, 318
fat-free, note about, 203
measuring, 53
Sour Cream Apple Pie, 210–11
Sour Cream & Berry Pie, 212
Sour Cream Brownies, 149
Sour Cream Orange Apple Cake,
166–67
Southwestern-style recipes
Chocolate Quesadillas, 244
Dessert Nachos, 245
Soy milk
choosing, note about, 296
Peach Melba Smoothie, 296
Peanut Butter & Banana
Smoothie, 297
phytochemicals in, 297
Spiced Angel Food Cake, 157
Spiced Iced Tea, 304
Spicy Apple Cupcakes, 183
Spicy Gingersnaps, 112–13

Squash. See Pumpkin; Zucchini
Strawberries
Balsamic Strawberry Sauce, 252
Banana Strawberry Mousse, 274
Blender Breakfast Blast, 295
Blueberry Strawberry Pear Crisp,
222
Cocoa Roll with Creamy Cheese
& Berries, 242–43
Coupe Bircher, 231
Exchange value, 317
Fresh Fruit Parfait, 251
Frosty Strawberry Shake, 301
Ice Cream Fantasy Cake, 259
Orange Sabayon with Fresh
Berries, 286
Peanut Butter & Banana
Smoothie, 297
Raspberry Ice with Fresh
Strawberries, 266
Strawberry Delights, 247
Strawberry Mousse Pie, 216
Strawberry Orange Buttermilk
Sorbet, 264
Strawberry Rhubarb Cobbler,
226–27
Strawberry Sauce, 199
Strawberry Sorbet, 263
Strawberry Whipped Topping,
276–77
Striped Strawberry Cake, 161
Strawberry Delights, 247
Strawberry Mousse Pie, 216
Strawberry Orange Buttermilk Sorbet,
264
Strawberry Rhubarb Cobbler, 226–27
Strawberry Sauce, 199
Strawberry Sorbet, 263
Strawberry Whipped Topping, 276–77
Streusel Apple Muffins, 1
Striped Strawberry Cake, 161
Strudels
Mango Blueberry Strudel, 229
Pear, Apple & Raisin Strudel,
228

Sugar
    advice about, for diabetics, xi,
        237, 307
    carbohydrates per teaspoon, xii
    confectioners', note about, 167
    creaming butter with, 69
    Exchange values, 317–18
    forms of, xi, 307
    low-calorie sweetener substi-
        tutes, 153, 307–8
    measuring, 53
    superfine, making at home, 73
    turbinado, note about, 113
Sugar alcohols, 307–8
Sugar substitutes, 153, 307–8
Sunflower seeds
    Almond Butter Cereal Squares,
        142
    Apricot Seed Bars, 125
    Coconut Seeds Cereal Squares,
        141
    Cranberry Pecan Oatmeal
        Cookies, 77
    Crunchy Apricot Oat Drops, 85
    Exchange value, 318
    Granola Bars, 129
    Pick-Me-Up Bars, 124
Sunrise Zucchini Muffins, 22–23
Sunshine Lemon Mousse, 272–73
Sweeteners, low-calorie, 153, 307–8
Sweetheart Berry Pie, 217
Sweet potatoes
    Sweet Potato Muffins, 24–25
Sweet Potato Muffins, 24–25

T

Tangy Banana Cheesecake, 201
Tarts
    Fresh Fruit Tart, 218
    Tropical Fruit Tart, 219
Tea
    Lemon Iced Tea, 305
    Spiced Iced Tea, 304

Tiramisu
    Banana Cream Tiramisu, 287
    Chocolate Coffee Tiramisu,
        288
    Maple, Walnut & Pear Tiramisu,
        287
Toffee Bars, 135
Toppings
    Cinnamon Cream, 291
    Strawberry Whipped Topping,
        276–77
    Whipped Cream & Yogurt
        Topping, 253
Tortillas
    Chocolate Quesadillas, 244
    Dessert Nachos, 245
Trans fats, xi, xii, 185
Triple B Health Muffins, 17
Triple Chocolate Brownies, 147
Tropical Fruit Tart, 219
Tropical Parfait, 251
Tulip Cookies with Fruit Sorbet,
    265
Two-Tone Chocolate Orange Biscotti,
    62
Type 1 diabetes, ix
Type 2 diabetes, ix

V

Vanilla Almond Snaps, 114
Vegetables. See also Carrots;
    Pumpkin; Zucchini
        Exchange values, 317
        Sweet Potato Muffins, 24–25
Vitamins
    B vitamins, 25, 143, 311
    fat-soluble, 311
    vitamin A, 30, 311, 312
    vitamin C, 311, 312
    vitamin D, 311
    vitamin E, 25, 311, 312
    vitamin K, 311
    water-soluble, 311

W

Walnuts
- Banana Cream Tiramisu, 287
- Banana Date Cake, 176
- Banana Nut Raisin Loaf, 29
- Banana Walnut Bread, 40
- Chocolate Brownies, 151
- Chocolate Chunk Banana Brownies, 146
- Crispy Oatmeal Cookies, 75
- Date Nut Bars, 128
- Diced Rhubarb Cookies, 117
- Exchange value, 318
- Lemon Cream Frosting, 168–69
- Maple, Walnut & Pear Tiramisu, 287
- Maple Flan with Walnuts, 290
- Maple Walnut Biscotti, 58–59
- Maple Walnut Slice 'n' Bake Cookies, 94–95
- Nutty Shortbread Bars, 131
- Pumpkin Spice Nut Bread, 42–43
- Rhubarb Orange Bread, 31

Wheat bran. *See also* Bran cereal; Bran flakes cereal
- Apricot Coconut Bars, 126–27
- Exchange value, 316
- Granola Bars, 129
- note about, 76
- Perfect Bran Muffins, 15
- Triple B Health Muffins, 17

Wheat germ
- about, 78
- Blender Breakfast Blast, 295
- Blueberry Wheat Germ Muffins, 14
- buying and storing, 78
- B vitamins in, 25
- Crunchy Apricot Oat Drops, 85
- Oatmeal Raisin Cookies, 78
- Oatmeal Raisin Pecan Cookies, 79
- Pumpkin Bran Muffins, 18–19
- Vitamin E in, 25

Wheat Muffins, 12

Whipped Cream & Yogurt Topping, 253

White chocolate
- Best-Ever Chocolate Cookies, 96
- Christmas Brownies, 144
- Exchange value, 319
- White Chocolate Brownies, 148
- White Chocolate Cranberry Drops, 103

White Chocolate Brownies, 148

White Chocolate Cranberry Drops, 103

Whole wheat flour. *See also recipes below*
- buying and storing, 16
- Exchange value, 316
- history of, 123
- replacing all-purpose flour with, 16

Whole wheat flour (in breads)
- Banana Nut Raisin Loaf, 29
- Banana Walnut Bread, 40
- Carrot, Apple & Coconut Loaf, 30
- Carrot Pineapple Zucchini Loaf, 27
- Irish Whole Wheat Soda Bread, 41
- Oat Bran Banana Bread, 38–39
- Poppy Seed Oat Bread, 32
- Pumpkin Molasses Raisin Loaf, 26
- Pumpkin Spice Nut Bread, 42–43
- Scottish Oatmeal Scones, 46
- Whole Wheat Poppy Biscuits, 47

Whole wheat flour (in cakes)
- Apple Pecan Streusel Cake, 184–85
- Applesauce Carrot Cake, 178–79
- Banana Cake with Lemon Cream Frosting, 168–69
- Blueberry Honey Cake, 163
- Blueberry Peach Cake, 164
- Carrot Cake, 177

Whole wheat flour (in cakes) (cont)
  Chocolate Chunk Coffee Cake,
    196–97
  Cinnamon Streusel Coffee Cake,
    188–89
  Orange Coffee Cake, 193
  Orange-Glazed Coffee Cake,
    192
  Orange Pumpkin Snacking Cake,
    165
  Prune Orange Spice Cake,
    172–73
  Tangy Banana Cheesecake,
    201
Whole wheat flour (in cookies and
  bars)
  Apple Cinnamon Bars, 122–23
  Apricot Coconut Bars, 126–27
  Charlie & Emma's Favorite
    Carrot Cookies, 118
  Diced Rhubarb Cookies, 117
  Double Chocolate Raisin
    Cookies, 97
  Fruity Oatmeal Cookies, 81
  Oatmeal Raisin Cookies, 78
  Oatmeal Raisin Pecan Cookies,
    79
  Peanut Butter Chocolate Chip
    Cookies, 107
  Pick-Me-Up Bars, 124
  Raisin & Applesauce Squares,
    138
  Sesame Seed Cookies, 115
  Tulip Cookies with Fruit Sorbet,
    265
  Whole Wheat Spice Cookies,
    110
Whole wheat flour (in fruit desserts)
  Blueberry Apple Crisp, 220
  Tulip Cookies with Fruit Sorbet,
    265
Whole wheat flour (in muffins)
  Banana Applesauce Muffins, 5
  Big-Batch Banana Blueberry
    Muffins, 4

  Chocolate Chip Oatmeal
    Muffins, 9
  Honey Whole Wheat Muffins, 13
  Kiwi Raspberry Muffins, 7
  Pumpkin Bran Muffins, 18–19
  Sunrise Zucchini Muffins, 22–23
  Sweet Potato Muffins, 24–25
  Triple B Health Muffins, 17
  Wheat Muffins, 12
  Yogurt Bran Muffins, 16
Whole Wheat Poppy Biscuits, 47
Whole Wheat Spice Cookies, 110
Wine-Poached Pear Fans, 235

Yogurt
  Creamy Dreamy Fruit Salad, 250
  Dessert Nachos, 245
  Exchange value, 317
  Frozen Jamoca Mousse, 270
  Frozen Lemon Pie, 267
  Frozen Vanilla Yogurt, 268
  Ice Cream Fantasy Cake, 259
  measuring, 53
  Raspberry Brownie Parfait, 278
  replacing oil with, 185
  Tangy Banana Cheesecake, 201
  Whipped Cream & Yogurt
    Topping, 253
Yogurt Bran Muffins, 16

Zucchini
  beta-carotene and Vitamin A in,
    30
  Carrot Pineapple Zucchini Loaf,
    27
  Chocolate Zucchini Cake, 181
  Exchange value, 317
  Sunrise Zucchini Muffins, 22–23